Pediatric Acute Care

Second Edition

Pediatric Acute Care

Second Edition

Editors

Mary W. Lieh-Lai, MD
Director, ICU and Critical Care Medicine Fellowship Program
Associate Professor of Pediatrics
Children's Hospital of Michigan/
Wayne State University School of Medicine

Katherine A. Ling-McGeorge, MD
Vice-Chair for Education
Director, Pediatric Residency Program
Assistant Professor of Pediatrics
Children's Hospital of Michigan/
Wayne State University School of Medicine

Maria C. Asi-Bautista, MD
Associate Director, Pediatric ICU
Chippenham Medical Center
Richmond, Virginia

Pharmacy Editor

Cyndi Reid, PharmD
Department of Pharmaceutical Services
Children's Hospital of Michigan

 LIPPINCOTT WILLIAMS & WILKINS
A **Wolters Kluwer** Company
Philadelphia · Baltimore · New York · London
Buenos Aires · Hong Kong · Sydney · Tokyo

Acquisitions Editor: Timothy Y. Hiscock
Developmental Editor: Michael Standen
Production Editor: Cassie Carey
Manufacturing Manager: Tim Reynolds
Cover Designer: Jeane Norton
Compositor: Lippincott Williams & Wilkins Desktop Division
Printer: RR Donnelley

© 2001 by LIPPINCOTT WILLIAMS & WILKINS
530 Walnut Street
Philadelphia, PA 19106 USA
LWW.com

Printed in the USA

Library of Congress Cataloging-in-Publication Data

Pediatric acute care / editors, Mary W. Lieh-Lai ... [et al.].–2nd ed.
   p. ; cm.
Rev. ed. of: The pediatric acute care handbook. 1st ed. ©1995.
   Includes bibliographical references and index.
   ISBN: 0-7817-2852-5
   1. Pediatric emergencies—Handbooks, manuals, etc. 2. Pediatric intensive care—Handbooks, manuals,
etc. I. Lieh-Lai, Mary. II. Pediatric acute care handbook.
   [DNLM: 1. Acute Disease—Child—Handbooks. 2. Acute Disease—Infant—Handbooks. WS 39 P3701
2001]
RJ370.P38 2001
618.92'0025–dc21   2001029692

10   9   8   7   6   5   4   3   2   1

To our families

Eduardo and Christopher Lai

Francis and Rebecca McGeorge

Lester and Jason Bautista

for their patience and understanding,
without them, this book and our
life's work would not be possible

Contributors

Amin Alousi
Malathi Bathija
Maria C. Asi-Bautista
Cheryl Ackley Bagenstose
Lee Benjamin
Vera Borzova
Thomas Brousseau
Michele Carney
Jeff A. Clark
Russell Clark
Kshama Daphtary
Matthew N. Denenberg
Hrishikesh Dingankar
Michael Fiore
Varsha Gharpure
Susan E. Gunderson
Mustafa H. Kabeer
Sujatha Kannan
Peter Karpawich
U. Olivia Kim
Michael Klein
K. Jane Lee
Mary Lieh-Lai
Katherine Ling-McGeorge
Girija Natarajan
Bulent Ozgonenel
Jyoti Panicker
Athina Pappas
Clarence Parks
Adora Poon
Randy Prescilla
Lawrence S. Quang
Cyndi Reid
Edwin Rodriguez
Renato Roxas, Jr.
Michelle Rubinstein
Shilpa Sangvai
Amit Sarnaik
Ina Shamraj
Christina Shanti
Aditi Sharangpani
Jacqueline Spaulding
Adiaha Spinks
Michael Stargardt
Laila Tutunji
Michael Vish

Contents

Preface - The Critically Ill Child

U. Olivia Kim

> Recognizing, assessing, monitoring and providing appropriate treatment for a critically ill child is the goal of the **Pediatric Acute Care Handbook**. Children with severe disease states may not always have obvious symptoms. The first 60 minutes of presentation is termed the "golden hour". This is a critical period when resuscitation, stabilization and definitive treatment must be initiated in order to ensure optimal survival. Children are not little adults, yet, the same pathophysiologic principles apply to them. A sick patient is a sick patient, whether that patient is a child or an adult. Taking care of children is both a challenge and a joy.

Clinical Manifestations

GEN	poor feeding, inconsolable crying (in nonverbal children)
SKIN	rash, mottling, cyanosis, petechiae, purpura, poor perfusion
HEENT	sunken eyes, signs of traumatic head injury, retinal hemorrhages, epistaxis
CVS	murmurs, tachycardia, bradycardia, arrhythmias, *hypotension is a late sign*,
RESP	dyspnea, tachypnea, apnea, hypoventilation, wheezing, rales, retractions, paradoxical breathing. Children with CNS or neuromuscular disease may not demonstrate respiratory distress while some may appear in respiratory distress, but do not have pulmonary pathology (e.g., Kussmaul breathing)
GI	abdominal pain, vomiting, diarrhea, masses, signs of obstruction or peritonitis
CNS	irritability, lethargy, obtundation, seizures, paralysis, weakness, coma

Diagnostics

Obtain laboratory tests, imaging and other tests according to the suspected problem. Consider inflicted injuries and toxic ingestions.

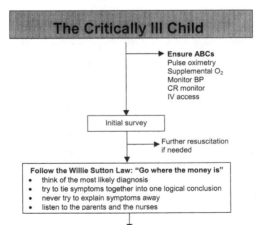

The Critically Ill Child

→ **Ensure ABCs**
Pulse oximetry
Supplemental O$_2$
Monitor BP
CR monitor
IV access

Initial survey

→ Further resuscitation if needed

Follow the Willie Sutton Law: "Go where the money is"
- think of the most likely diagnosis
- try to tie symptoms together into one logical conclusion
- never try to explain symptoms away
- listen to the parents and the nurses

For specifics of disease states and appropriate management, refer to the rest of this book. The Pediatric Acute Care Handbook is based on the Critical Care Resident Educational Series (CCRES), a bi-monthly case-oriented educational series that was started in 1991 by a group of pediatric residents under the guidance of Dr. Mary W. Lieh-Lai at the Children's Hospital of Michigan. Both CCRES and the Handbook are designed to educate and provide a guide for pediatric residents and students in the recognition, stabilization, and management of critically ill children prior to their transfer to, and during their stay in the ICU.
In this second edition, new topics have been added, and old ones revised. The authors and editors hope that this handbook continues to serve the function for which it was written.

Acknowledgments

We wish to extend our sincerest gratitude to the following people who made this project possible

The 1993 graduates of the Pediatric Residency Program who came up with the idea of an educational series (CCRES) upon which this handbook is based: Michael Anderson MD, Brian Engel MD, Maya Heinert MD and Frederick Klingbeil MD

Division of Endocrinology for the Diabetic Protocol

Division of Infectious Diseases for Antibiotic Formulary Agents

Curt Ellis and Dr. Gangadhar Sangvai for the illustrations used in the procedures section

Christopher E. Lai for editorial assistance.

List of Abbreviations

A

ABCs	airway, breathing, circulation
ABG	arterial blood gas
ABO	blood types A, B and O
AC	alternating current
ACh	acetylcholine
AChE	acetylcholinesterase
ACD	acid citrate dextrose
ACTH	adrenocorticotropic hormone
ADH	antidiuretic hormone
ADHD	attention deficit hyperactivity disorder
AED	antiepileptic drug
AFB	acid fast bacilli
A FIB	atrial fibrillation
AIDS	acquired immune deficiency syndrome
ALCAPA	anomalous left coronary arising from the pulmonary artery
ALL	acute lymphocytic leukemia
AL(OH)$_3$	aluminum hydroxide
ALT	alanine transferase
ALTE	apparent life threatening event
AML	acute myelogenous leukemia
ANA	anti-nuclear antibody
ANC	absolute neutrophil count
AP	anterior posterior
ARDS	acute respiratory distress syndrome
ASAP	as soon as possible
ASD	atrial septal defect
ASO	antistreptolysin O
AST	aspartate transferase
ATN	acute tubular necrosis
A fib	atrial fibrillation
AV	arteriovenous, atrioventricular
AVN	AV node
AVP	arginine vasopressin

B

BAL	bronchoalveolar lavage, British anti-Lewisite
BBB	bundle branch block
βhCG	human chorionic gonadotropin
BID	twice a day
BMT	bone marrow transplant
BSA	body surface area
BSAB	body surface area burned
BT	bleeding time
BP	blood pressure
BPD	bronchopulmonary dysplasia
bpm	beats per minute
BUN	blood urea nitrogen

C

C	centigrade
Ca^{++}	calcium
CA	cyclic antidepressant
CaCl$_2$	calcium chloride
CaCO$_3$	calcium carbonate
cap	capsule
CaPO$_4$	calcium phosphate
CBC	complete blood count
CBF	cerebral blood flow
CBG	capillary blood gas
CBZ	carbamazepine
CCB	calcium channel blocker
CF	cystic fibrosis
CHD	congenital heart disease
CK-MB	creatine phosphokinase – myocardial fraction
ChE	cholinesterase
CHF	congestive heart failure
CHO	carbohydrates
CIE	counter immunoelectrophoresis
CLD	chronic lung disease
CMV	cytomegalovirus

CN	cranial nerves, cyanide
CNS	central nervous system
CO	cardiac output, carbon monoxide
coagulation profile	PT, PTT, TT, FSP
COHb	carboxyhemoglobin
CO_2	carbon dioxide
CPB	cardiopulmonary bypass
CPK	creatine phosphokinase
CPR	cardiopulmonary resuscitation
CPS	carbamyl phosphate synthetase
CR monitor	cardiorespiratory monitor
CSF	cerebrospinal fluid
C-spine	cervical spine
CT	computerized axial tomography
CVA	cerebrovascular accident
CVC	central venous catheter
CVP	central venous pressure
CVS	cardiovascular system

D

D	dextrose
D_5W	dextrose with water
DBP	diastolic blood pressure
DDAVP	deamino-D-arginine vasopressin
DFA	direct fluorescent antibody
DFO	deferoxamine
DI	diabetes insipidus
DIC	disseminated intravascular coagulation
div	divided
DKA	diabetic ketoacidosis
dL	deciliter
DO_2	oxygen delivery
DVT	deep vein thrombosis
DPL	diagnostic peritoneal lavage

E

ED	emergency department
ECF	extracellular fluid
ECMO	extracorporeal membrane oxygenation
EDTA	ethylenediaminetetraacetic acid
EEG	electroencephalogram
EKG	electrocardiogram
ELISA	enzyme linked immunosorbent assay
EMG	electromyogram
ENT	otorhinolaryngology
ESR	erythrocyte sedimentation rate
ET	endotracheal
ETT	endotracheal tube
EXT	extremities

F

F	French
Fe^{++}	iron
FE_{Na}	fractional excretion of sodium
FEV_1	forced expiratory volume in 1 second
FFA	free fatty acids
FFP	fresh frozen plasma
FIB	fibrillation
FiO_2	fraction of inspired oxygen
FRC	functional residual capacity
FSP	fibrin split products
FTT	failure to thrive
FVC	forced vital capacity

G

g	gram
GABA	gamma amino butyric acid
GBS	Guillain-Barré syndrome
GCS	Glasgow coma scale
G-CSF	granulocyte colony stimulating factor
GEN	general
GGT	gamma glutamyl transferase
GH	growth hormone
GI	gastrointestinal

GPI	glucose phosphate isomerase
GTC	generalized tonic-clonic
GU	genitourinary
G6PD	glucose-6-phosphate dehydrogenase

H

H^+	hydrogen ion
Hb	hemoglobin
HBO	hyperbaric oxygen
HbSC	hemoglobin SC
HbSS	hemoglobin SS
HCG	human chorionic gonadotropin
HCO_3^-	bicarbonate
Hct	hematocrit
HEENT	head, eyes, ears, nose, throat
HEME	hematology
HeliOx	helium oxygen
HIV	human immunodeficiency virus
h	hours
hpf	high power field
HSV	herpes simplex virus
HTN	hypertension
HR	heart rate
HUS	hemolytic uremic syndrome

I

ICF	intracellular fluid
ICP	intracranial pressure
ICU	intensive care unit
IHSS	idiopathic hypertrophic subaortic stenosis
IM	intramuscular
IA	intraarticular
IABP	intra-aortic balloon pump
IBD	inflammatory bowel disease
ICH	intracranial hemorrhage
IMV	intermittent mandatory ventilation
INH	isoniazid
IO	intraosseous
I's and O's	intake and output
IUGR	intrauterine growth retardation
IV	intravenous
IVB	intravenous bolus
IOP	intraocular pressure
IVH	intraventricular hemorrhage
IVIG	intravenous immunoglobulin

J

J	joules
JRA	juvenile rheumatoid arthritis
JVD	jugular venous distension

K

kg	kilogram
K_2PO_4	potassium phosphate
KCl	potassium chloride

L

L	liter
LAP	left atrial pressure
LD	loading dose
LDH	lactic dehydrogenase
LE	lower extremities
LFT	liver function test
LIP	lymphocyte interstitial pneumonitis
LLQ	left lower quadrant
LMP	last menstrual period
LOC	loss of, level of, consciousness
LP	lumbar puncture
LR	lactated Ringer's solution
LSD	lysergic acid diethylamide
LUQ	left upper quadrant
LV	left ventricle
LVAD	left ventricular assist device
LVOTO	left ventricular outflow tract obstruction

M

mA	milliamps
MAP	mean arterial pressure
MCV	mean corpuscular volume
mEq/kg	milliequivalent per kilogram
mEq/L	milliequivalent per liter
MAX	maximum
Mg^{++}	magnesium
mg	milligram
MH	malignant hyperthermia
MI	myocardial infarction
min	minutes
MIN	minimum
mL	milliliter
mmHg	millimeters of mercury
mos	months
mOsm/L	milliosmoles per liter
MRI	magnetic resonance imaging

N

N	normal, NPH insulin
Na^+	sodium
NaCl	sodium chloride
$NaHCO_3$	sodium bicarbonate
NaOH	sodium hydroxide
NEC	necrotizing enterocolitis
NG	nasogastric
NGT	nasogastric tube
NH_3	ammonia
NICU	neonatal intensive care unit
NO	nitric oxide
NOS	not otherwise specified
NPO	nothing by mouth
NS	normal saline
NSAID	nonsteroidal antiinflammatory drug

O

O_2	oxygen
OCD	obsessive compulsive disorder
OR	operating room
ORT	oral rehydration therapy
Osm	osmolality
OTC	ornithine transcarbamylase
OZ	ounces

P

PD	peritoneal dialysis
P	phosphorus
PA	pulmonary atresia, pulmonary artery
PAC	premature atrial complex
$PaCO_2$	partial pressure of CO_2
PAN	polyarteritis nodosa
PaO_2	partial pressure of O_2
PAT	paroxysmal atrial tachycardia
PB	phenobarbital
PCA	patient controlled analgesia
PCR	polymerase chain reaction
PCC	prothrombin complex concentrate
PCP	pneumocystis carinii pneumonia
PDA	patent ductus arteriosus
PEA	pulseless electrical activity
PEEP	positive end expiratory pressure
PEFR	peak expiratory flow rate
PET	positron emission tomography
PFO	patent foramen ovale
PGE_1	prostaglandin E_1
PGI_2	prostacyclin
PHT	phenytoin
PID	pelvic inflammatory disease
PIH	pregnancy-induced hypertension
PK	pyruvate kinase
PLEDS	paroxysmal lateralizing epileptiform discharges
PMN	polymorphonuclear
PO	by mouth

PPD	purified protein derivative
PPHN	persistent pulmonary hypertension of the newborn
PR	per rectum
prn	as needed
PRBC	packed red blood cells
PROM	prolonged rupture of membranes
PT	prothrombin time
PTH	parathyroid hormone
PTS	pediatric trauma score
PTU	propylthiouracil
PTT	partial thromboplastin time
PVC	premature ventricular complex
PVR	pulmonary vascular resistance
PEEP	positive end expiratory pressure

Q

q	every
QID	four times a day
QTc	corrected QT interval

R

R	regular insulin
RAP	right atrial pressure
RBBB	right bundle branch block
RBC	red blood cells
RDS	respiratory distress syndrome
RESP	respiratory
RDW	red cell distribution width
RLQ	right lower quadrant
RPR	rapid plasma reagent
RSI	rapid sequence intubation
RSV	respiratory syncytial virus
RR	respiratory rate
RTA	renal tubular acidosis
RUQ	right upper quadrant
RV	right ventricle
RVOT	right ventricle outflow tract

S

SBP	systolic blood pressure
SβThal	sickle-beta thalassemia
SC	subcutaneous
SCI	spinal cord injury
SCID	severe combined immunodeficiency
SCIWORA	spinal cord injury without radiographic abnormality
SD	standard deviation
sec	seconds
SGOT	serum glutamic oxalo transferase
SGPT	serum glutamic pyruvate transferase
SI	serum iron
SIADH	syndrome of inappropriate antidiuretic hormone secretion
Sinus tach	sinus tachycardia
SIRS	systemic inflammatory response syndrome
SL	sublingual
SLE	systemic lupus erythematous
SPAG	small particle aerosol generator
Sp. gr.	specific gravity
SpO_2	oxygen saturation
STAT	at once
SV	stroke volume
SVC	superior vena cava
SVR	systemic vascular resistance
SVT	supraventricular tachycardia

T

TAPVR	total anomalous pulmonary venous return
TB	tuberculosis
TBSA	total body surface area
TBW	total body water
^{99}Tc-DMSA	technetium 99m-labeled dimercaptosuccinic acid
TDD	total digitalizing dose
THAM	tris-hydroxy-methyl-amino-methane
Ti	inspiratory time
TIA	transient ischemic attack
TIBC	total iron binding capacity

TID	three times a day
TMP/SMZ	trimethoprim-sulfamethoxazole
TOF	tetralogy of Fallot
TORCH	toxoplasmosis, other (syphilis), rubella, cytomegalovirus, herpes
TPN	total parenteral nutrition
TSH	thyroid stimulating hormone
TT	thrombin time
TTP	thrombotic thrombocytopenic purpura

U

U	unit
u	unit
UA	urinalysis
UAC	umbilical artery catheter
UE	upper extremity
U_{na}	urine sodium
Uosm	urine osmolality
U/P	urine plasma ratio
URI	upper respiratory tract infection
US	ultrasound
UTI	urinary tract infection
UUN	urine urea nitrogen
UVC	umbilical vein catheter

V

VCUG	voiding cystourethrogram
Vd	volume of distribution
V FIB	ventricular fibrillation
VP	ventriculoperitoneal
VPA	valproic acid
VPS	ventriculoperitoneal shunt
V/Q	ventilation/perfusion
VSD	ventricular septal defect
V tach	ventricular tachycardia
VRE	vancomycin resistant enterococcus
vWD	von Willebrand disease
vWF	von Willebrand factor

W

WBC	white blood cell
WIC	women, infant and children's program
WPW	Wolff-Parkinson-White syndrome

Y

y	years

Guidelines for Use

This handbook was developed to help house officers in the initial stabilization and management of acute problems commonly encountered in the care of pediatric patients.

Algorithms begin with presenting signs and symptoms and the minimum workup required at the time of presentation.

 a circled letter in the algorithm refers to annotations on the facing page

☆ denotes a critical point, explained below the algorithm

 is a suggestion that the reader call for assistance or request for a consult

The aim of this book is to help house officers, emergency medicine physicians, family practitioners and other physicians who provide acute care for children, anticipate life-threatening complications, recognize when to call for appropriate services, and transfer patients to a tertiary care facility when those services are not available at their institution.

STAT doses are provided when necessary. The reader is encouraged to refer to standard text for details.

This handbook does not attempt to provide an exhaustive listing of differential diagnosis, and it should not be considered a substitute for recommended textbooks.

Management protocols were patterned after guidelines in use at the Children's Hospital of Michigan. Other modalities are mentioned, but the reader should discuss these options with appropriate subspecialists.

Patients need to be reassessed frequently, and management must be tailored according to the patient's condition.

Section I ♣ ABC's/CPR

- ABC's
- Cardiopulmonary Resuscitation
- Neonatal Resuscitation

ABCs

Shilpa Shangvai

Assessment:
Always assess after each intervention.

(A)
- Listen for air entry
- Check EKG on monitor
- Check pulses (especially after defibrillating)
- Check ETT placement

Measure blood gases/other labs

(B) Access is vital – peripheral venous access should be started immediately. In children < 1 y, consider intraosseous needle placement as first line of vascular access. (See p.270). Never defer these means of securing venous access while waiting for someone to perform a venous cutdown as this may take some time.

(C) Breathing: if the patient is not intubated, use a properly fitting mask to ensure a tight seal. If ventilation is ineffective (no chest rise, no air entry), check mask for seal, reposition head, if not contraindicated (e.g., in spinal cord injury), lift jaw, consider suctioning. Consider the use of laryngeal mask airway (LMA). Remember that not all patients who exhibit spontaneous respirations are able to maintain adequate ventilation/oxygenation. If clinical signs and symptoms suggest overt respiratory failure, begin bag and mask ventilation, while applying cricoid pressure. Patients need ventilatory assistance before they develop apnea. Do not use excessive pressures when ventilating a patient – this may induce pneumothoraces. Use the minimum amount of pressure to achieve chest inflation. If available, attach pressure manometer to bag.

Practical tips:
1. Ensure that the bulb is attached securely to the blade.
2. Endotracheal tube size (internal diameter in mm) estimation:

   Age in years/4 + 4 = ETT size in mm

3. If using a cuffed tube, ascertain cuff integrity by inflating cuff with 3-5 mL of air. Deflate cuff before insertion.
4. After intubating, assess proper placement by auscultation. In addition, use of colorimetric capnography (for CO_2 detection) may provide further confirmation of ETT placement. Tape tube securely at the correct level (See p.305)

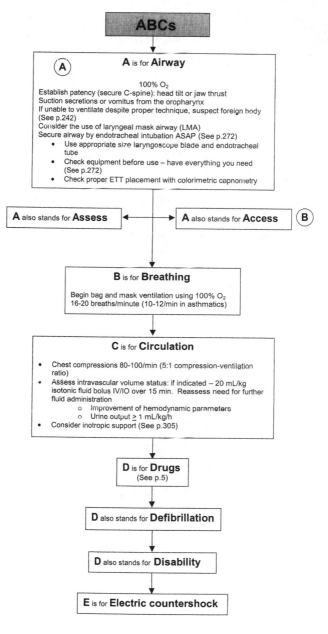

ABCs

A is for **Airway**

(A)

100% O_2
Establish patency (secure C-spine): head tilt or jaw thrust
Suction secretions or vomitus from the oropharynx
If unable to ventilate despite proper technique, suspect foreign body
(See p.242)
Consider the use of laryngeal mask airway (LMA)
Secure airway by endotracheal intubation ASAP (See p.272)
- Use appropriate size laryngoscope blade and endotracheal
  tube
- Check equipment before use – have everything you need
  (See p.272)
- Check proper ETT placement with colorimetric capnometry

A also stands for **Assess**   **A** also stands for **Access**   (B)

B is for **Breathing**

Begin bag and mask ventilation using 100% O_2
16-20 breaths/minute (10-12/min in asthmatics)

C is for **Circulation**

- Chest compressions 80-100/min (5:1 compression-ventilation
  ratio)
- Assess intravascular volume status: if indicated – 20 mL/kg
  isotonic fluid bolus IV/IO over 15 min. Reassess need for further
  fluid administration
    - Improvement of hemodynamic parameters
    - Urine output $\geq$ 1 mL/kg/h
- Consider inotropic support (See p.305)

D is for **Drugs**
(See p.5)

D also stands for **Defibrillation**

D also stands for **Disability**

E is for **Electric countershock**

NOTES

Cardiopulmonary Resuscitation

Cardiopulmonary Arrest → ☎ Call a code

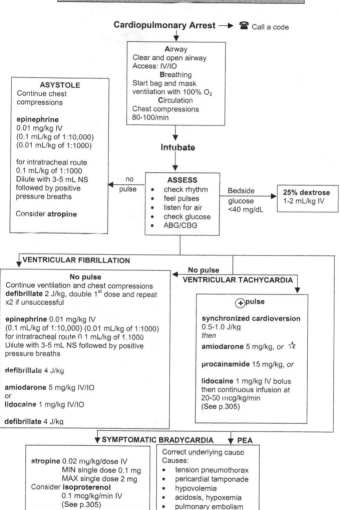

Airway
Clear and open airway
Access: IV/IO
Breathing
Start bag and mask
ventilation with 100% O_2
Circulation
Chest compressions
80-100/min

ASYSTOLE
Continue chest
compressions

epinephrine
0.01 mg/kg IV
(0.1 mL/kg of 1:10,000)
(0.01 mL/kg of 1:1000)

for intratracheal route
0.1 mL/kg of 1:1000
Dilute with 3-5 mL NS
followed by positive
pressure breaths

Consider **atropine**

Intubate

no
pulse

ASSESS
- check rhythm
- feel pulses
- listen for air
- check glucose
- ABG/CBG

Bedside
glucose
<40 mg/dL

25% dextrose
1-2 mL/kg IV

VENTRICULAR FIBRILLATION

No pulse
Continue ventilation and chest compressions
defibrillate 2 J/kg, double 1st dose and repeat
x2 if unsuccessful

epinephrine 0.01 mg/kg IV
(0.1 mL/kg of 1:10,000) (0.01 mL/kg of 1:1000)
for intratracheal route 0.1 mL/kg of 1:1000
Dilute with 3-5 mL NS followed by positive
pressure breaths

defibrillate 4 J/kg

amiodarone 5 mg/kg IV/IO
or
lidocaine 1 mg/kg IV/IO

defibrillate 4 J/kg

No pulse
VENTRICULAR TACHYCARDIA

⊕pulse

synchronized cardioversion
0.5-1.0 J/kg
then
amiodarone 5 mg/kg, *or* ☆

procainamide 15 mg/kg, *or*

lidocaine 1 mg/kg IV bolus
then continuous infusion at
20-50 mcg/kg/min
(See p.305)

SYMPTOMATIC BRADYCARDIA

atropine 0.02 mg/kg/dose IV
MIN single dose 0.1 mg
MAX single dose 2 mg
Consider **isoproterenol**
0.1 mcg/kg/min IV
(See p.305)
external pacemaker (See p.297)

PEA
Correct underlying cause
Causes:
- tension pneumothorax
- pericardial tamponade
- hypovolemia
- acidosis, hypoxemia
- pulmonary embolism

Consider **epinephrine**

Indications for Ca^{++} during CPR
1. Symptomatic hypocalcemia
2. Calcium channel blocker overdose
3. Suspected or documented hyperkalemia
4. Hypermagnesemia

calcium chloride 20 mg/kg IV/IO (0.2 mL/kg of a 10% solution)
Administer over 15 min

☆
Do not routinely
administer
amiodarone and
procainamide
together

Neonatal Resuscitation

Athina Pappas

> Approximately 6% of all full term newborns and 60% of newborns <1500 g require resuscitation. Individuals skilled in newborn resuscitation should be present at every delivery.
> Key elements to successful resuscitation of the newborn include anticipation of potential problems, availability of necessary equipment, and skill of the provider.

Factors which place the infant at risk for cardiorespiratory arrest:

(A)

Maternal factors
- lack of prenatal care
- substance abuse
- age < 16 y or > 35 y
- toxemia of pregnancy
- chronic renal disease
- blood incompatibility
- oligohydramnios
- diabetes
- severe anemia

Intrapartum factors
- use of narcotics within 4 h of delivery
- PROM
- prolonged labor
- precipitous delivery
- excessive maternal bleeding
- prolapsed cord/cord compression
- placenta previa/abruption
- forceps delivery
- abnormal presentation

Fetal factors
- prematurity
- IUGR
- multiple gestation
- thick meconium
- congenital infection
- fetal malformation
- decreased fetal activity
- abnormal heart tones
- postmaturity

(B) Equipment and Supplies:

Suction Equipment	Medications
- bulb syringe - mechanical suction - suction catheters, 5F, 6F, 8F or 10F - 8F feeding tube and 20-mL syringe - meconium aspirator	- **epinephrine** 1:10,000, 1- or 3-mL ampules - **naloxone hydrochloride**, 1-mL of 0.4 mg/mL conc, or 2-mL of 1.0 mg/mL conc - one or more bags: **5% albumin, 0.9 NS**, or **lactated ringers** - **NaHCO₃** 4.2% (5 mEq/10 mL), 10-mL ampule - **10% dextrose**, 250 mL - **sterile water**, 10 mL - **normal saline**, 30 mL

Bag and Mask Equipment	Miscellaneous
- neonatal resuscitation bag with a pressure-release valve or pressure gauge, with a bag capable of delivering 90%-100% O₂ - face masks, newborn and premature sizes (cushioned rim masks preferred) - oral airways, newborn and premature sizes - O₂ with flowmeter and tubing - intubation equipment - laryngoscope with straight blades, #0 (preterm) and #1 (term) - extra bulbs and batteries for laryngoscope - endotracheal tubes, 2.5, 3.0, 3.5, 4.0 mm - stylet - scissors - gloves	- radiant warmer - stethoscope - cardiotachometer with EKG (oscilloscope desirable) - adhesive tape - syringes – 1, 3, 5, 10, 20, 50 mL - needles - 25, 21, 18 gauge - alcohol sponges - umbilical artery catheterization tray - umbilical tape - umbilical catheters – 3.5 or 5F - three-way stopcocks - feeding tube, 5F

Apgar score:

(C) Used to characterize a newborn infant at 1 and 5 minutes following delivery. Should not wait to obtain an Apgar score at 1 minute before beginning resuscitation. If the 5 minute score is < 7, obtain additional scores every 5 minutes for an additional 20 minutes.

Score	0	1	2
heart rate	absent	< 100 bpm	> 100 bpm
respiratory effort	absent, irregular	slow, crying	good cry
muscle tone	limp	some flexion of extremities	good flexion
reflex irritability	no response	grimace	vigorous cry
color	pale	cyanotic	completely pink

✱ Continued on p.8

Algorithm for Resuscitation of the Newly Born Infant

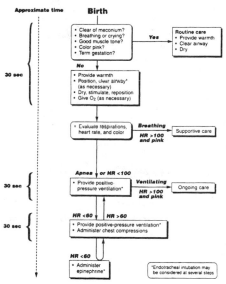

Algorithm for resuscitation of the newly born infant.

From Kattwinkel J, Short J, Niermeyer S, Denson SE, Saichkin J (eds), *Textbook of Neonatal Resuscitation, 4th edition*. 2000, p. 7 of 16. American Heart Association and American Academy of Pediatrics, with permission.

✳ Continued from p.6

(D) Maintain temperature – heat loss with cold stress in a newborn can be very significant if the child is left in wet linen and exposed to room temperature. Dry the infant adequately, remove wet linen and place child under radiant warmer.

Airway – suction mouth and nose with bulb suction or any other appropriate suction device

(E) Assess – perform a 5- to 10-second assessment to determine need for resuscitation, checking heart rate, respiratory effort, color and tone

Initiate breathing – begin bag and mask ventilation if infant is apneic, has gasping respirations or HR <100 bpm. If there is no improvement with correct technique and tight-sealing mask in 15-30 seconds, intubate the trachea.

Endotracheal intubation
- use the appropriate size blade (0 or 1 straight)
- check that handle and blade are in working condition
- select the appropriate size endotracheal tubes
- confirm placement of ETT
- tape ETT securely

Recommended ETT sizes

Weight (g)	ETT size (mm)
< 1000	2.5
1000-2000	3.0
2000-3000	3.5
> 3000	3.5-4.5

(F) Cardiac massage – initiate if heart rate is < 60 bpm after 30 seconds of effective bag and mask ventilation with 100% oxygen.
- Thumb technique (preferred method) – hands encircle infant's chest, using thumbs to compress lower sternum.
- Two-finger technique – tips of middle finger and index or ring finger compress lower third of sternum
- Synchronize ventilation and cardiac massage 1:3

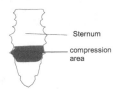

Sternum

compression area

(G) Drug therapy

Administer medications if HR < 60 bpm after 30 seconds of adequate ventilation and cardiac compressions.

Medication	Concentration	Dosage/Route	Volume in mL	Precautions
epinephrine	1:10,000	0.01-0.03 mg/kg IV or ET	0.1-0.3 mL/kg	• give rapidly • may dilute with NS to 1-2 mL if giving via ETT
intravascular volume expansion	whole blood 5% albumin 0.9 NS LR	10 mL/kg IVB		• give over 5-10 min.
NaHCO₃	0.5 mEq/mL (4.2% soln)	2 mEq/kg IV only	4 mL/kg	• give slowly over 1-2 min. • ensure effective ventilation
naloxone	0.4 mg/mL 1.0 mg/mL	0.1 mg/kg IV, SC, ET, IM	0.25 mL/kg of the 0.4 mg/mL conc 0.1 mL/kg of the 1.0 mg/mL conc	• give rapidly • IV, ET preferred; IM, SC acceptable

epinephrine
- β-adrenergic effects - ↑ rate and cardiac contractions
- α-adrenergic effects - ↑ noncerebral peripheral resistance.

NaHCO₃ – may help correct metabolic acidosis

naloxone hydrochloride (Narcan®) – reverses respiratory depression produced by narcotic agents which may have been administered to the mother during labor. It does increase risk of seizures in children born to drug-addicted mothers.

Section II ♣ Critical Conditions

1. Cardiovascular Conditions
- Cardiogenic Shock and Congestive Heart Failure
- Cyanotic Infant
- Cardiac Arrhythmias
- "Tet" Spells of Tetralogy of Fallot (Hypercyanotic Spells)
- Hypovolemic Shock
- Ischemic Heart Disease in Children
- Post-operative Care Following Open-Heart Surgery
- The Infant in Shock
- Ductal Dependent Congenital Heart Lesions

2. Child Abuse

3. Endocrine
- Adrenal Crisis
- Central Diabetes Insipidus
- Diabetic Ketoacidosis (DKA)
- Syndrome of Inappropriate Antidiuretic Hormone Secretion
- Hypoglycemia
- Thyrotoxicosis: Thyroid Storm

4. Gastrointestinal Disorders
- Acute Abdominal Pain
- The Acute Abdomen/Peritonitis
- Lower Gastrointestinal Bleeding
- Upper Gastrointestinal Bleeding
- Gastrointestinal Obstruction

5. Hematological and Oncologic Disorders
- Anemia
- Disseminated Intravascular Coagulation (DIC)
- Hemophilia Emergencies
- Fever in a Neutropenic Patient
- Sickle Cell Disease
- Acute Chest Syndrome in Sickle Cell Disease
- Tumor Lysis Syndrome

6. Immunological Disorders
- Anaphylaxis
- Patient with AIDS and Fever
- Patient with AIDS and Suspected Lung Involvement
- Immunocompromised Host with Fever
- Acute Transfusion Reaction

7. Infectious Diseases
- Encephalitis
- Meningitis
- Tuberculous Meningitis
- Septic Shock

8. Toxicology
- General Poisoning
- Acetaminophen Toxicity
- Alcohol Ingestions: Ethanol, Isopropanol, Methanol, Ethylene Glycol
- Caustic Ingestion/Exposure
- Cyclic Antidepressant Overdose
- Hydrocarbon Exposure
- Iron Poisoning

- Organophosphate/Carbamate Poisoning
- Theophylline Toxicity
- Clonidine Toxicity
- Digoxin Toxicity
- Antiepileptic Drug Overdose: Phenobarbital, Carbamezipine, Phenytoin
- Calcium Channel Blocker Overdose
- Methemoglobinemia
- Envenomations: Spiders, Scorpions
- Snakebites
- Mushroom Poisoning

9. Metabolic Disorders
- Acute Neonatal Hyperammonemia
- Interpretation of Blood Gases
- Inborn Errors of Metabolism
- Malignant Hyperthermia

10. Neurologic Disorders
- Coma
- Guillain-Barré Syndrome
- Increased Intracranial Pressure
- Myasthenia Gravis
- Spinal Cord Injury (SCI)
- Status Epilepticus
- Seizures
- Acute Hemiparesis
- Acute Psychosis
- Suicide

11. Ophthalmologic Emergencies

12. Renal, Fluids and Electrolytes
- Acute Renal Failure
- Hemolytic Uremic Syndrome
- Hypertensive Crisis/Encephalopathy
- Hypernatremic Dehydration
- Hyponatremia
- Hyperkalemia
- Hypermagnesemia
- Hypocalcemia
- Metabolic Acidosis
- Dehydration

13. Respiratory Disorders
- Acute Bronchiolitis
- Acute Respiratory Failure
- Apnea
- Status Asthmaticus
- Dislodged Tracheostomy Tube
- Acute Epiglottitis
- Foreign Body Aspiration
- Wheezing Other than Asthma

14. Smoke Inhalation and Surface Burns
- Burns: Thermal, Chemical, and Electrical
- Smoke Inhalation Injury and Carbon Monoxide (CO) Poisoning

15. Trauma
- Stabilization of the Trauma Patient
- Near Drowning

NOTES

Chapter 1 ⚕ Cardiovascular Conditions

Cardiogenic Shock and Congestive Heart Failure

Lee Benjamin

Congestive heart failure is a syndrome that results from the inability of the heart to provide adequate support for the metabolic requirements of the body. Symptoms are related to the failing heart and venous congestion. These include tachycardia, hepatomegaly, JVD. However, extracardiac symptoms may sometimes be the primary manifestation of CHF, and these include tachypnea, wheezing, poor feeding, and failure to thrive.

oxygen delivery ($\dot{D}O_2$) = cardiac output (CO) x arterial O_2 content (CaO_2)
cardiac output = stroke volume x heart rate
components of stroke volume = preload, cardiac contractility and afterload

In early CHF, ↑ cardiac contractility and other compensatory mechanisms maintain adequate cardiac output. When these compensatory mechanisms are exhausted, cardiogenic shock becomes manifest.

Etiology of CHF and cardiogenic shock

(A)

Age	Myocardial Failure	Volume Overload	Pressure Overload	Others
Birth	asphyxia, sepsis, myocarditis, interrupted aortic arch	systemic AV fistula, valvular regurgitation		anemia, complete heart block, arrhythmias, PPHN, hyperviscosity
< 1 week	ductal dependent CHD (coarctation, hypoplastic left heart syndrome)	TAPVR	aortic stenosis	adrenal insufficiency
1-6 weeks	ALCAPA	PDA, VSD, AV canal	mitral stenosis	
Late infancy	myocarditis, endocardial fibroelastosis, acute rheumatic fever, electrolyte disorders, cardiomyopathy		systemic or pulmonary hypertension	arrhythmias
Childhood/ adolescence	cardiomyopathy, myocarditis, acute rheumatic fever, Kawasaki, toxins/poisons, collagen vascular diseases	endocarditis, valvular regurgitation	IHSS, chronic lung disease, CF, cor pulmonale	arrhythmias, post-operative complications of CHD repair, pericarditis, tamponade

(B) Acute viral myocarditis is most commonly caused by Coxsackie virus. This disorder can affect children at any age. The disease is typically preceded by a few days of URI symptoms. Poor feeding and tachypnea are frequently observed. Physical examination often reveals tachypnea and wheezing and some degree of dehydration (poor oral intake). Children with congestive heart failure develop peribronchial edema and wheezing and are often mistakenly thought to have bronchiolitis or asthma with dehydration. As a result, β-adrenergic agents such as albuterol are administered, along with fluid boluses. **Caution**: β-adrenergic agents may precipitate life-threatening arrhythmias, and repeated fluid boluses may lead to overt heart failure with fluid overload.

(C) Assess EKG for ischemic changes associated with anomalous left coronary artery arising from the pulmonary artery (ALCAPA) and Kawasaki disease (See p.28)

(D) Supraventricular tachycardia (SVT, see p.18), when prolonged, leads to decreased ventricular filling because of shortened diastole, and eventually leads to CHF and cardiogenic shock.

(E) Toddlers may accidentally ingest drugs and toxins, while adolescents may ingest cardiotoxic agents in suicide attempts. Drugs with known cardiotoxicity include cyclic antidepressants, digoxin, calcium channel blockers, β-blockers, and potassium supplements. Children with smoke inhalation or those who have inhaled other noxious fumes may develop cardiotoxicity from carbon monoxide.

✳ Continued on p.14

Clinical Manifestations

(A)
HISTORY	recent infection, possible drug/toxin ingestion, family history
GEN	poor feeding, failure to thrive, increased sweating
SKIN	pale, mottled, cyanosis
HEENT	conjunctival pallor, nasal flaring, periorbital edema
CVS	tachycardia, gallop, decreased or unequal pulses, hypotension
RESP	tachypnea, wheezing, rales, dyspnea (B)
GI	hepatomegaly
CNS	irritability, lethargy

Diagnostics

Blood	ABG/CBG, electrolytes, Ca^{++}, Mg^{++}, BUN, creatinine, CBC, differential, glucose, culture, troponin, CPK, drug screen, AST, ALT, carnitine
Urine	urinalysis, urine output, drug screen
Imaging	chest radiograph, echocardiogram
Other	EKG (C) (D)

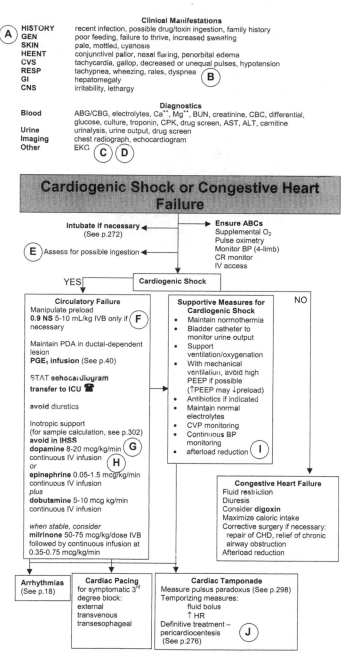

Cardiogenic Shock or Congestive Heart Failure

Intubate if necessary ◀
(See p.272)

▶ **Ensure ABCs**
Supplemental O₂
Pulse oximetry
Monitor BP (4-limb)
CR monitor
IV access

(E) Assess for possible ingestion ◀

YES │

Cardiogenic Shock

Circulatory Failure
Manipulate preload
0.9 NS 5-10 mL/kg IVB only if (F)
necessary

Maintain PDA in ductal-dependent
lesion
PGE₁ infusion (See p.40)

STAT echocardiogram
transfer to ICU ☎

avoid diuretics

Inotropic support
(for sample calculation, see p.302)
avoid in IHSS
dopamine 8-20 mcg/kg/min (G)
continuous IV infusion
or (H)
epinephrine 0.05-1.5 mcg/kg/min
continuous IV infusion
plus
dobutamine 5-10 mcg kg/min
continuous IV infusion

when stable, consider
milrinone 50-75 mcg/kg/dose IVB
followed by continuous infusion at
0.35-0.75 mcg/kg/min

Supportive Measures for Cardiogenic Shock
- Maintain normothermia
- Bladder catheter to monitor urine output
- Support ventilation/oxygenation
- With mechanical ventilation, avoid high PEEP if possible (↑PEEP may ↓preload)
- Antibiotics if indicated
- Maintain normal electrolytes
- CVP monitoring
- Continuous BP monitoring
- afterload reduction (I)

NO

Congestive Heart Failure
Fluid restriction
Diuresis
Consider **digoxin**
Maximize caloric intake
Corrective surgery if necessary:
repair of CHD, relief of chronic
airway obstruction
Afterload reduction

Arrhythmias
(See p.18)

Cardiac Pacing
for symptomatic 3rd
degree block:
external
transvenous
transesophageal

Cardiac Tamponade
Measure pulsus paradoxus (See p.298)
Temporizing measures:
fluid bolus
↑ HR
Definitive treatment –
pericardiocentesis (J)
(See p.276)

✳ Continued from p.12

(F) Optimization of preload: increase preload with judicious intravascular volume expansion. In the presence of significant fluid overload, diuretics may be needed. However, in a patient with cardiogenic shock, diuretics can precipitously decrease preload and lead to further decrease in cardiac output, and should therefore be avoided.

(G) Idiopathic hypertrophic subaortic stenosis (IHSS) is an obstructive valvular disorder that limits stroke volume. Condition may be worsened by inotropic agents. Increase in preload with afterload reduction may be of benefit.

Inotropic Agents

(H)

Drug	Dose	Action	Side Effects
dopamine	2-20 mcg/kg/min	• dopaminergic dose (3-5 mcg/kg/min) - ↑ renal blood flow • β-adrenergic dose (< 10 mcg/kg/min) – inotropic effects • α-adrenergic dose (> 10 mcg/kg/min) - ↑ SVR	• at high doses, hypertension, ↓ splanchnic blood flow, arrhythmias • extravasation leads to tissue necrosis. • not compatible with bicarbonate solution.
dobutamine	2-20 mcg/kg/min	• β-adrenergic • promotes inotropicity and peripheral vasodilation without significant chronotropic effects	• arrhythmias
epinephrine	0.05-1.5 mcg/kg/min	• β and α adrenergic effects • promotes inotropicity • ↑ SVR • ↑ heart rate	• at high doses, hypertension, arrhythmias, tachycardia • extravasation leads to tissue necrosis
milrinone	50-75 mcg/kg IVB over 10-15 min followed by continuous infusion 0.35-0.75 mcg/kg/min	• phosphodiesterase inhibitor • promotes inotropicity • peripheral vasodilatory effects	• hypotension
digoxin	total digitalizing dose 30 mcg/kg slow IV maintenance dose 10 mcg/kg/day PO	• Na$^+$-ATP pump inhibitor • inotropic effects • ↓ HR	• arrhythmias – use with caution or avoid in children with acute myocarditis, hypokalemia or Wenckebach phenomenon
norepinephrine	0.1-2.0 mcg/kg/min	• predominantly α-adrenergic effects, with some β-adrenergic activity • inotropic effect • potent peripheral vasoconstriction	• hypertension • arrhythmias • tissue ischemia
vasopressin	0.018-0.12 units/kg/hour adult dose: 2-6 units/hour	• potent peripheral vasoconstriction	• significant increase in afterload

(I) Afterload reduction: to optimize cardiac output, it may be necessary to reduce afterload to decrease the pressure against which the left ventricle has to work. However, all drugs used for afterload reduction can lead to hypotension because of ↓ SVR and should therefore be avoided during the resuscitation phase of someone with cardiogenic shock.

Nitroprusside, nitroglycerine and captopril may be considered.

(J) Specific interventions
For shock with associated closure of ductus arteriosus in CHD with ductal-dependent lesion (See p.40)
Children with symptomatic 3rd degree heart block require cardiac pacing (See p.297)
Children may occasionally develop cardiac tamponade from infectious or non-infectious pericarditis. Causes include pyogenic, tuberculous, viral, tumors, collagen vascular disease, and chronic renal failure. Pericardiocentesis (See p.276)

NOTES

Cyanotic Infant

Vera Borzova

> Cyanosis is defined as dark blue or purplish discoloration of skin and mucous membranes, classified as central or peripheral.

(A) Consider a respiratory etiology if the patient has symptoms of respiratory distress in addition to tachypnea, which include retractions, grunting, and nasal flaring. The patient who is tachypneic, but is otherwise quiet is more likely to have cyanosis of a cardiac etiology. A single S_2 may be heard in patients with transposition of the great arteries, tetralogy of Fallot, or pulmonary atresia.

(B) *Central cyanosis*: secondary to reduced hemoglobin in excess of 3 g/dL. It is usually associated with low oxygen saturation, is more apparent with polycythemia, less noticeable with anemia and elevated levels of fetal hemoglobin. It is generally more pronounced in mucous membranes, tongue, lips and conjunctivae.

(C) *Peripheral cyanosis*: secondary to (1) decreased cardiac output with subsequent decrease in blood flow and increased peripheral oxygen extraction, and (2) peripheral vasoconstriction. It may be associated with normal arterial oxygen saturation, and is usually observed in the skin of the extremities.

(D)
Hyperoxia Test

- Used to differentiate cardiac versus non cardiac etiology of cyanosis.
- Obtain baseline ABG (PaO_2) with the infant in room air, from the right radial artery (proximal to the patent ductus arteriosus). Then administer 100% oxygen for 5-10 minutes and repeat ABG. The increased level of oxygen may cause closure of the ductus arteriosus; monitor the patient carefully during the procedure.

(E) Abnormal hemoglobins: methemoglobin, carboxyhemoglobin – O_2 administration may not result in clinical improvement of cyanosis.

Respiratory etiology – ventilation/perfusion mismatch:
- intrinsic   hypoventilation, airway obstruction, parenchymal disease
- extrinsic   diaphragmatic hernia, pneumothorax, pneumomediastinum, transient tachypnea of the newborn, RDS

(F) Assess pulmonary vasculature for signs of ↑ vascularity, pulmonary congestion or oligemia
Characteristic chest radiograph findings:
- egg on a string – transposition of the great arteries
- boot-shaped heart – tetralogy of Fallot/pulmonary atresia/VSD
- snowman sign – supracardiac total anomalous pulmonary venous return
- wall to wall heart – Ebstein's anomaly

(G) Characteristic EKG findings:
- superior left axis - tricuspid atresia, endocardial cushion defect, primum ASD
- left axis deviation - pulmonary atresia, +/- tricuspid atresia
- marked right atrial hypertrophy - Ebstein's anomaly

(H) Side effects of **PGE₁** : **apnea**, fever, flushing, tachycardia/bradycardia, **hypotension**. If clinical condition deteriorates, consider total anomalous pulmonary venous return and discontinue infusion.

Clinical Manifestations

HISTORY	known congenital heart disease, exposure to toxins
GEN	failure to thrive, poor feeding
SKIN	cyanosis of skin and mucous membranes
CVS	tachycardia, murmur, unequal pulses, gallop, thrill
RESP	tachypnea, retractions, wheezing, rales
GI	hepatomegaly
CNS	lethargy, irritability

Diagnostics

Blood	ABG, CBC, differential, platelets, electrolytes, glucose, consider carboxyhemoglobin or methemoglobin levels, culture
Urine	culture
Imaging	chest radiograph, echocardiogram
Others	EKG

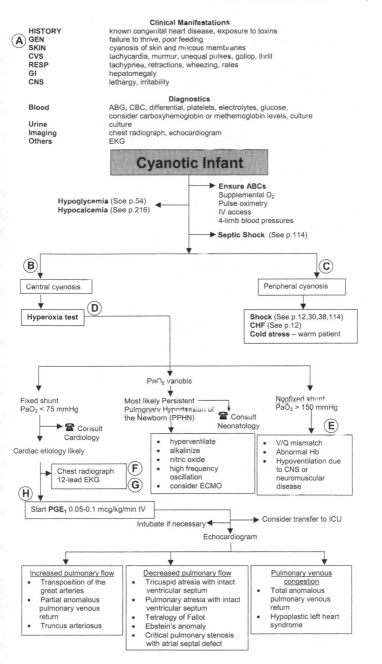

Cyanotic Infant

➤ **Ensure ABCs**
  Supplemental O_2
  Pulse oximetry
  IV access
  4-limb blood pressures

Hypoglycemia (See p.54)
Hypocalcemia (See p.216)

➤ **Septic Shock** (See p.114)

Ⓑ Central cyanosis

Ⓒ Peripheral cyanosis

Hyperoxia test Ⓓ

Shock (See p.12,30,38,114)
CHF (See p.12)
Cold stress – warm patient

PaO_2 variable

Fixed shunt
$PaO_2 < 75$ mmHg

Most likely Persistent Pulmonary Hypertension of the Newborn (PPHN) ☎ Consult Neonatology

Nonfixed shunt
$PaO_2 > 150$ mmHg Ⓔ

➤ ☎ Consult Cardiology

- hyperventilate
- alkalinize
- nitric oxide
- high frequency oscillation
- consider ECMO

- V/Q mismatch
- Abnormal Hb
- Hypoventilation due to CNS or neuromuscular disease

Cardiac etiology likely

Chest radiograph Ⓕ
12-lead EKG Ⓖ

Ⓗ Start **PGE₁** 0.05-0.1 mcg/kg/min IV

Intubate if necessary ◄— ➤ Consider transfer to ICU

Echocardiogram

Increased pulmonary flow	Decreased pulmonary flow	Pulmonary venous congestion
• Transposition of the great arteries • Partial anomalous pulmonary venous return • Truncus arteriosus	• Tricuspid atresia with intact ventricular septum • Pulmonary atresia with intact ventricular septum • Tetralogy of Fallot • Ebstein's anomaly • Critical pulmonary stenosis with atrial septal defect	• Total anomalous pulmonary venous return • Hypoplastic left heart syndrome

Cardiac Arrhythmias

Edwin Rodriguez, Peter Karpawich

Doses for Electrical Countershock

Arrhythmia		Dose	MAX Initial Dose	Subsequent Doses	
				< 50 kg	> 50 kg
V fibrillation		Defibrillate 2→4 J/kg	200J	4 J/kg	200-300J, 360J
Atrial fibrillation*		Synchronized cardioversion 0.5→2 J/kg	100J	2 J/kg	200J, 300J, 360J
Atrial flutter*			50J		100J, 200J, 300J, 360J
SVT/PAT					
(-) pulse	V tach with *regular* form and rate	Defibrillate 2→4 J/kg	100J	4J/kg	200J, 300J, 360J
	V tach with *irregular* form and rate		200J		200-300J, 360J
(+) pulse	V tach with *regular* form and rate	Synchronized cardioversion 0.5→2J/kg	100J	2J/kg	200J, 300J, 360J
	V tach with *irregular* form and rate		200J		200-300J, 360J

*Following surgical correction, children with congenital heart disease (e.g., Fontan procedure) may require 4 J/kg

All values should be corrected for age unless stated otherwise.

(A) Ventricular fibrillation: no discernible P, QRS, or T complexes; may be fine or coarse fibrillation.

(B) PEA: previously referred to as EMD. Investigate underlying cause. Causes: hypoxemia, acidosis, tension pneumothorax, pericardial tamponade, hypovolemia, pulmonary embolism

(C) Sinus tachycardia: normal waveform, with a rate that exceeds the upper limit of normal for age

(D) SVT, PAT: most common arrhythmia in children. Abnormal rate originating proximal to the His bundle bifurcation. Rate usually >230 bpm. P waves may or may not be discernible, and may appear after the QRS, or as a negative deflection (retrograde polarization of the atria). R-R interval usually constant. QRS of normal duration unless conduction is aberrant.

(E) Atrial flutter: atrial rate 250-500 (usually 300) bpm. Saw-tooth pattern may be seen in leads II, III, AVF, and V1. QRS may be normal. Ventricular response may be variable or "fixed", in which case, because of a more regular pattern, diagnosis may be difficult.

(F) Atrial fibrillation: absent P waves (fine fibrillation). R-R interval irregularly irregular (Ashman's phenomenon).

(G) Vagal maneuvers: pharyngeal wall stimulation with nasogastric tube, rectal stimulation, ice pack to nose and mouth for 15 seconds. If able to cooperate, ask patient to perform Valsalva maneuver. Carotid massage may also be attempted. **Do not** press on eyeballs.

(H) PAC without block: premature atrial beat with normal conduction to the ventricles, normal QRS. PAC with aberrant conduction: premature atrial beat with abnormal conduction to the ventricles (during partial refractoriness of the ventricles), creating an abnormal QRS (i.e., RBBB). PAC with block: premature atrial beat with no QRS following the P wave.

(I) PVC: premature beat, wide/aberrant QRS complex with ST segment and T wave in a direction opposite to the QRS (abnormal depolarization leads to abnormal repolarization).

(J) Slow rhythms: treat only in the presence of 3rd degree block or if the patient is symptomatic, i.e., in the presence of CHF or syncope (Stokes-Adams).

✱ Continued on p.20

Patient with Arrhythmia

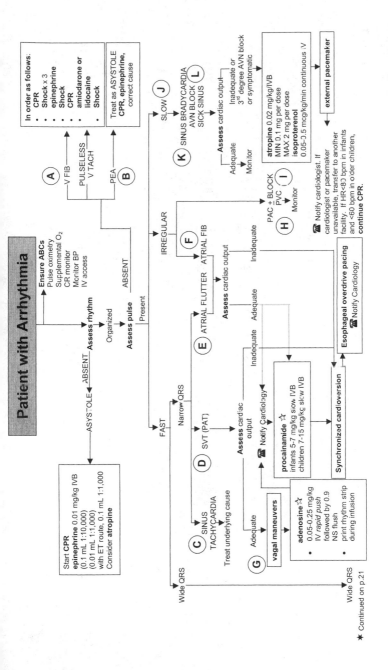

Ensure ABCs
Pulse oximetry
Supplemental O$_2$
CR monitor
Monitor BP
IV access

Assess rhythm

ASYSTOLE ◄— ABSENT

Organized

Assess pulse

Present / ABSENT

(A)
V FIB
PULSELESS
V TACH

(B) PEA

In order as follows:
- CPR
- Shock x 3
- epinephrine
- Shock
- CPR
- amiodarone or lidocaine
- Shock

Treat as ASYSTOLE CPR, epinephrine, correct cause

IRREGULAR

(F) ATRIAL FLUTTER ATRIAL FIB

Assess cardiac output

Inadequate / Adequate

(H) PAC + BLOCK PVC
Monitor **(I)**

☎ Notify cardiologist. If cardiologist or pacemaker unavailable, transfer to another facility. If HR<80 bpm in infants and <60 bpm in older children, **continue CPR.**

SLOW (J)

(K) SINUS BRADYCARDIA AVN BLOCK **(L)**
SICK SINUS

Assess cardiac output

Adequate / Inadequate or 3rd degree AVN block or symptomatic

Monitor

atropine 0.02 mg/kg/IVB
MIN 0.1 mg per dose
MAX 2 mg per dose
isoproterenol
0.05–3.5 mcg/kg/min continuous IV

external pacemaker

Start **CPR**
epinephrine 0.01 mg/kg IVB
(0.1 mL 1:10,000)
(0.01 mL 1:1,000)
with ET route, 0.1 mL 1:1,000
Consider **atropine**

Wide QRS

FAST

Narrow QRS

(C) SINUS TACHYCARDIA
Treat underlying cause

(D) SVT (PAT)

Assess cardiac output

Adequate / Inadequate

(G) vagal maneuvers

adenosine ☆
- 0.05–0.25 mg/kg IV *rapid push* followed by 0.9 NS flush
- print rhythm strip during infusion

☎ Notify Cardiology

procainamide ☆
infants 5–7 mg/kg slow IVB
children 7–15 mg/kg slow IVB

Synchronized cardioversion

Esophageal overdrive pacing
☎ Notify Cardiology

Wide QRS

★ Continued on p.21

✳ Continued from p.18

(K) Sinus bradycardia: normal P wave axis and P-R interval, rate below the lower limit of normal for age. Investigate underlying cause: increased ICP, hypothyroidism, hypothermia, hypoxia, hyperkalemia, gastric distention, drug toxicity.

(L) AVN block:
1st degree: prolonged P-R interval
2nd degree: Mobitz I (Wenckebach) progressive P-R lengthening prior to a non-conducted P wave
                 Mobitz II paroxysmal non-conducted P waves
3rd degree: complete A-V dissociation, independent atrial and ventricular rates.

(M) Ventricular tachycardia: > 3 PVC's in succession. Torsades de pointe is a type of ventricular tachycardia.

(N) SVT with aberrant ventricular conduction (RBBB): uncommon in children (<10%), assume ventricular tachycardia. If there is no improvement following administration of lidocaine, adenosine can be given to slow down rhythm enough to unmask WPW or SVT with block

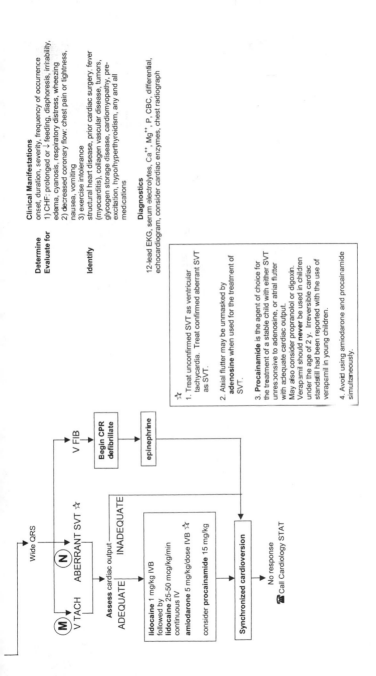

Clinical Manifestations

onset, duration, severity, frequency of occurrence
1) CHF: prolonged or ↓ feeding, diaphoresis, irritability, edema, cyanosis, respiratory distress, wheezing
2) decreased coronary flow: chest pain or tightness, nausea, vomiting
3) exercise intolerance

Determine
Evaluate for

Identify
structural heart disease, prior cardiac surgery, fever (myocarditis), collagen vascular disease, tumors, glycogen storage disease, cardiomyopathy, pre-excitation, hypo/hyperthyroidism, any and all medications

Diagnostics

12-lead EKG, serum electrolytes, Ca⁺⁺, Mg⁺⁺, P, CBC, differential, echocardiogram, consider cardiac enzymes, chest radiograph

☆

1. Treat unconfirmed SVT as ventricular tachycardia. Treat confirmed aberrant SVT as SVT.

2. Atrial flutter may be unmasked by **adenosine** when used for the treatment of SVT.

3. **Procainamide** is the agent of choice for the treatment of a stable child with either SVT unresponsive to adenosine, or atrial flutter with adequate cardiac output.
May also consider propranolol or digoxin. Verapamil should **never** be used in children under the age of 2 y. Irreversible cardiac standstill had been reported with the use of verapamil in young children.

4. Avoid using amiodarone and procainamide simultaneously.

Wide QRS

M V TACH

N ABERRANT SVT ☆

V FIB

Begin CPR
defibrillate

epinephrine

Assess cardiac output

ADEQUATE   INADEQUATE

lidocaine 1 mg/kg IVB followed by
lidocaine 25-50 mcg/kg/min continuous IV

amiodarone 5 mg/kg/dose IVB ☆

consider **procainamide** 15 mg/kg

Synchronized cardioversion

No response
☎ Call Cardiology STAT

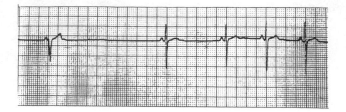

Figure 1.1   **Sinus bradycardia.** Extreme sinus rate variability with P wave rates ranging from 20-75 bpm. The first sinus P wave is followed by a ventricular escape QRS complex.

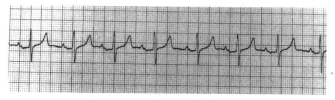

Figure 1.2   **First degree AV block.** Sinus rhythm with all P waves followed by a normal QRS. The P-R interval is prolonged at 0.24 sec. indicating slowed AV conduction. May be seen as a normal response to digoxin or therapy with β-blockers.

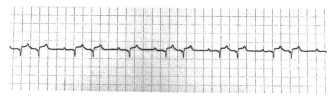
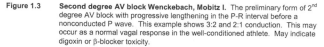

Figure 1.3   **Second degree AV block Wenckebach, Mobitz I.** The preliminary form of 2nd degree AV block with progressive lengthening in the P-R interval before a nonconducted P wave. This example shows 3:2 and 2:1 conduction. This may occur as a normal vagal response in the well-conditioned athlete. May indicate digoxin or β-blocker toxicity.

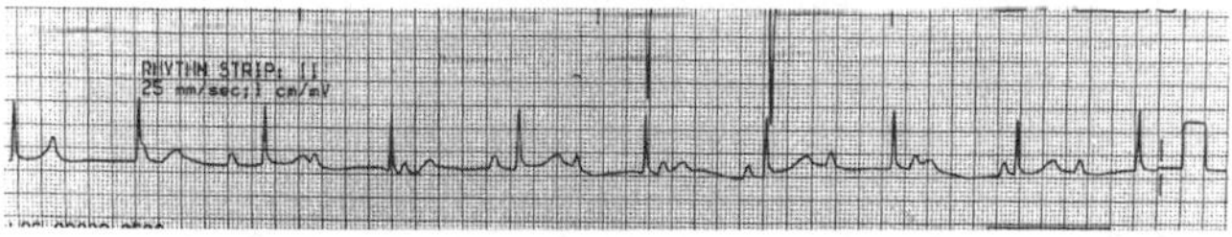

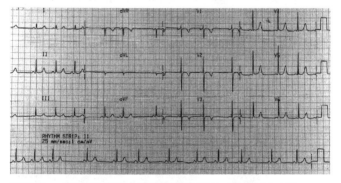

Figure 1.4   **Third degree AV block.** Complete interruption of atrial impulse conduction to the ventricles. The atrial rate is typically faster than the ventricular rate. A normal appearing narrow QRS usually indicates a ventricular escape rhythm high in the conduction system and is usually more stable than a lower origin wide QRS rhythm.

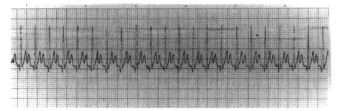

Figure 1.5   **Sinus arrhythmia.** A common finding in infancy and childhood, usually indicating vagal influences on sinus rate. The sinus P wave axis, morphology, and P-R interval are all normal.

Figure 1.6   **Sinus tachycardia.** Accelerated sinus rate for age. P wave axis, morphology, and P-R interval are normal. Typically "speeds up" and "slows down", rather than accelerating or stopping abruptly.

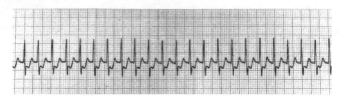

Figure 1.7   **SVT.** Typically a narrow QRS morphology with or without visible P waves at rates >250 bpm. Also referred to as paroxysmal atrial tachycardia (PAT). Often associated with Wolff-Parkinson-White or AV node reentry bypass tracts.

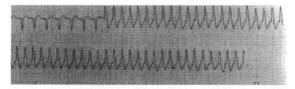

Figure 1.8   **SVT (WPW).** Due to two potential AV connections, the SVT circuit may conduct antegrade to the ventricle via the AV node, giving a narrow QRS (orthodromic conduction). However, a wide QRS resembling ventricular tachycardia may occur if the antegrade conduction utilizes the WPW bypass tract (antidromic conduction). As illustrated, both may occur in the same patient.

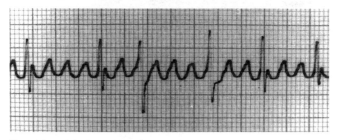

Figure 1.9   **Atrial flutter.** A form of atrial muscle re-entry at a rate approximating 300 bpm. The typical "saw tooth" configuration is often best seen in lead II. This shows variable AV conduction with 4:1, 3:1, and 2:1 conduction.

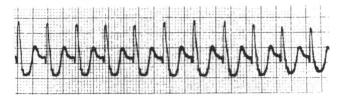

Figure 1.10   **Atrial flutter 2:1.** Due to intrinsic AV node properties, rapid atrial rates of 300 bpm are attenuated, resulting in a common appearance of this tachycardia at 150 bpm. The "saw tooth" pattern is buried in the QRS-T waves.

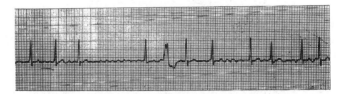

Figure 1.11   **Atrial fibrillation.** A more disorganized atrial muscle tachycardia with nonspecific wavy baseline and variable AV conduction. The commonly associated Ashman phenomenon is illustrated with a wide QRS complex resembling a PVC. This is caused by an atrial impulse conducted to the His-Purkinje system in which the ventricular refractory period has been altered by the preceding long R-R interval.

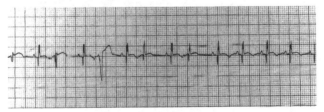

Figure 1.12   **Atrial bigeminy.** A normal sinus P wave followed closely by another, often distorting the preceding T wave, commonly at a fixed "coupled" interval. The resulting QRS may be altered (aberrancy) because of changes in the refractory period and resembles a PVC.

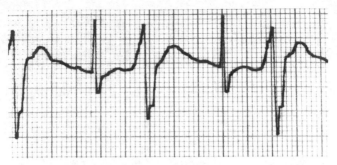

Figure 1.13   Ventricular bigeminy. A normal sinus QRS followed by a premature ventricular complex, often at a fixed coupled interval. Depending on the ventricle of origin, a right or left bundle branch block pattern may result.

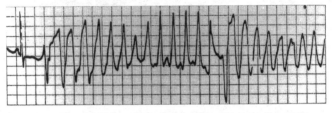

Figure 1.14   Torsade de Pointes. Severe form of ventricular tachycardia with a variable QRS morphology (multiform) giving the impression of "twisting on the baseline".

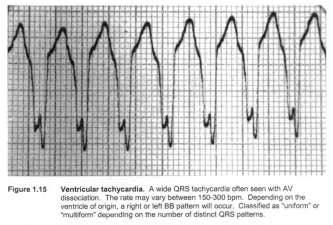

Figure 1.15   **Ventricular tachycardia.** A wide QRS tachycardia often seen with AV
dissociation. The rate may vary between 150-300 bpm. Depending on the
ventricle of origin, a right or left BB pattern will occur. Classified as "uniform" or
"multiform" depending on the number of distinct QRS patterns.

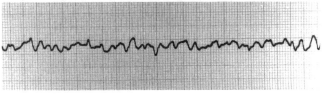

Figure 1.16   **Ventricular fibrillation.** A nonspecific, irregular baseline electrical activity
without organized QRS complexes.

For rhythm strips related to hyperkalemia, see p.212.

Tet Spells of Tetralogy of Fallot (Hypercyanotic Spells)

Michele Carney

Cyanotic episodes generally observed in children with Tetralogy of Fallot who may otherwise be asymptomatic or have only a mild degree of cyanosis. Sudden decrease in pulmonary blood flow may result from increased pulmonary vascular resistance ($\uparrow$PVR) from crying, or a fall in systemic vascular resistance ($\downarrow$SVR) or preload.

With decreased pulmonary blood flow → $\downarrow$ PaO_2, $\downarrow$ pH, $\uparrow$ $PaCO_2$ → hyperventilation → $\uparrow$ systemic venous return → increased blood flow through a fixed obstruction (pulmonary stenosis in TOF) → $\uparrow$ right to left shunt → $\downarrow$ pulmonary blood flow → cycle continues.

(A) Compromised pulmonary blood flow can lead to severe hypoxia, with seizures and death. Patients with unrepaired Tetralogy of Fallot should be instructed to perform maneuvers that will increase systemic vascular resistance and consequently increase blood flow to the lungs. Parents should be instructed to hold an infant into a "balled-up" position, while older children can assume a squatting position. This knee-chest position will trap venous blood in the legs, decreasing venous return, as well as increasing SVR by blocking arterial blood flow through the femoral arteries.

(B) Management principles:
1. Break cycle: try knee-chest position and calming techniques
2. **100% oxygen** to alleviate hypoxemia
3. **Morphine** – sedative effects and increased peripheral venous blood pooling
4. **Fluid bolus** – increases preload
5. **Phenylephrine** – increases systemic vascular resistance
6. **Propranolol** - β-adrenergic blocker, may relax infundibular spasm (controversial)
7. **Esmolol** – same effects as propranolol, but has a much shorter half-life
8. **Sodium bicarbonate** – corrects acidosis and may help in breaking cycle of increased pulmonary vascular resistance.
9. If all the above methods fail, general anesthesia may be attempted.

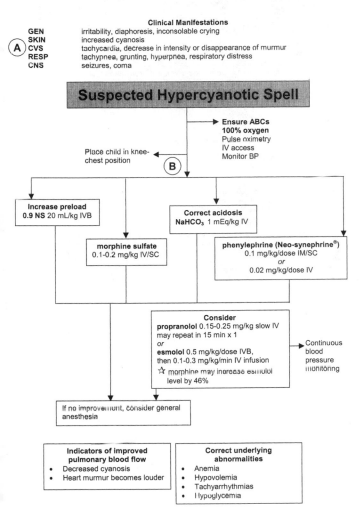

Clinical Manifestations

GEN	irritability, diaphoresis, inconsolable crying
SKIN	increased cyanosis
CVS	tachycardia, decrease in intensity or disappearance of murmur
RESP	tachypnea, grunting, hyperpnea, respiratory distress
CNS	seizures, coma

(A)

Suspected Hypercyanotic Spell

→ **Ensure ABCs**
100% oxygen
Pulse oximetry
IV access
Monitor BP

Place child in knee-
chest position

(B)

Increase preload
0.9 NS 20 mL/kg IVB

Correct acidosis
NaHCO₃ 1 mEq/kg IV

morphine sulfate
0.1-0.2 mg/kg IV/SC

phenylephrine (Neo-synephrine®)
0.1 mg/kg/dose IM/SC
or
0.02 mg/kg/dose IV

Consider
propranolol 0.15-0.25 mg/kg slow IV
may repeat in 15 min x 1
or
esmolol 0.5 mg/kg/dose IVB,
then 0.1-0.3 mg/kg/min IV infusion
☆ morphine may increase esmolol
level by 46%

→ Continuous
blood
pressure
monitoring

If no improvement, consider general
anesthesia

Indicators of improved pulmonary blood flow	**Correct underlying abnormalities**
• Decreased cyanosis	• Anemia
• Heart murmur becomes louder	• Hypovolemia
	• Tachyarrhythmias
	• Hypoglycemia

Hypovolemic Shock

U. Olivia Kim

A state of circulatory decompensation due to a decrease in preload leading to decreased cardiac output and inability to meet the metabolic demands of the body.

Etiology:

(A)

- fluid losses - diarrhea or vomiting
- acute blood loss – trauma, GI bleed
- "third spacing" – hypoalbuminemia, bowel obstruction/peritonitis, burns

Hypovolemia is the most common cause of shock in children.

Stages:

(B)

1. Early, compensated: the loss of fluids or blood activates the sympathetic nervous system and the renin-angiotensin-aldosterone system. This manifests as tachycardia, peripheral vasoconstriction, decreased urine output, and in some cases, even *hypertension*. Mild metabolic acidosis may develop.

2. Late, uncompensated: continued fluid losses result in further decrease in preload and cardiac output. Effects of prolonged vasoconstriction and decreased oxygen delivery to the tissues lead to end-organ damage. Tachycardia may persist, but bradycardia and apnea may be observed. Skin is cool and mottled, patient may develop anuria. Blood gases may show a marked drop in pH from combined respiratory and metabolic acidosis. Disseminated intravascular coagulation may also be seen. Hypotension will manifest during this phase. The metabolic acidosis further aggravates decreased cardiac output because of its myocardial depressant effects.

Clinical Manifestations

History	determine cause, quantitate degree of fluid loss, inquire about risk factors for GI bleeding, history and symptoms of diabetes or diabetes insipidus
GEN	weight loss, poor feeding
HEENT	depressed fontanel, sunken eyes, dry mucous membranes
SKIN	decreased turgor, cold and clammy, mottled, rash
CVS	tachycardia, bradycardia, orthostatic changes, HYPOTENSION is a LATE SIGN
RESP	tachypnea, Kussmaul breathing, grunting, apnea
GI	nausea, vomiting, diarrhea, abdominal pain or tenderness
GU	oliguria, anuria
CNS	lethargy, irritability, seizures

(A)

Diagnostics

Blood	ABG/CBG, electrolytes, BUN, creatinine, CBC, differential, PT, PTT, type and crossmatch if indicated, glucose, Ca^{++}, P, Mg^{++}, lactate, culture
Urine	urinalysis, specific gravity, culture, output (mL/kg/h)
Stool	culture, leucocytes

(B)

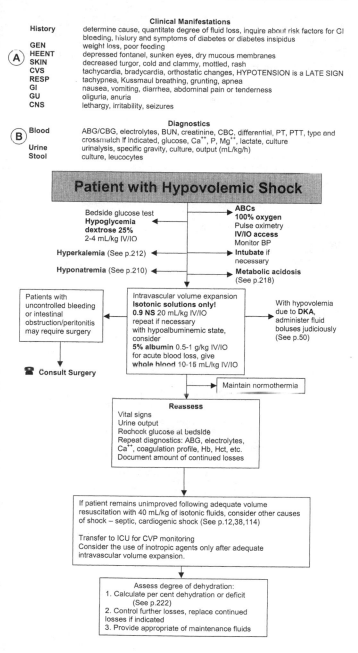

Patient with Hypovolemic Shock

ABCs
100% oxygen
Pulse oximetry
IV/IO access
Monitor BP

Bedside glucose test
Hypoglycemia
dextrose 25%
2-4 mL/kg IV/IO

Intubate if necessary

Hyperkalemia (See p.212)

Hyponatremia (See p.210)

Metabolic acidosis
(See p.218)

Patients with uncontrolled bleeding or intestinal obstruction/peritonitis may require surgery

📞 Consult Surgery

Intravascular volume expansion
Isotonic solutions only!
0.9 NS 20 mL/kg IV/IO
repeat if necessary
with hypoalbuminemic state, consider
5% albumin 0.5-1 g/kg IV/IO
for acute blood loss, give
whole blood 10-15 mL/kg IV/IO

With hypovolemia due to **DKA**, administer fluid boluses judiciously (See p.50)

Maintain normothermia

Reassess
Vital signs
Urine output
Recheck glucose at bedside
Repeat diagnostics: ABG, electrolytes, Ca^{++}, coagulation profile, Hb, Hct, etc.
Document amount of continued losses

If patient remains unimproved following adequate volume resuscitation with 40 mL/kg of isotonic fluids, consider other causes of shock – septic, cardiogenic shock (See p.12,38,114)

Transfer to ICU for CVP monitoring
Consider the use of inotropic agents only after adequate intravascular volume expansion.

Assess degree of dehydration:
1. Calculate per cent dehydration or deficit (See p.222)
2. Control further losses, replace continued losses if indicated
3. Provide appropriate of maintenance fluids

Ischemic Heart Disease in Children

Edwin Rodriguez

> Ischemia – decreased supply of oxygenated blood to an organ.
> Myocardial ischemia – manifests in the EKG as a distortion of the T wave
> Myocardial injury is reflected in the EKG as ST segment changes.
> Myocardial infarction (electrically inert muscle) manifests as Q waves over damaged area

---

(A) Etiology
1. Congenital heart disease
   - Anomalous Left Coronary Arising from the Pulmonary Artery (ALCAPA)
   - Transposition of the Great Arteries
   - Hypertrophic cardiomyopathy

2. Arteritis
   - Kawasaki disease
   - Takayasu's arteritis
   - Vasculitides

3. Post heart transplantation

4. Metabolic/connective tissue diseases:
   - Hyperlipidemia
   - Progeria
   - Diabetes Mellitus
   - Liver disease
   - Chronic renal failure/renal transplant
   - Connective tissue disorders (lupus, polyarteritis nodosa)

5. Embolic
   - Tumors (myxomas)
   - Air emboli (in patients with right to left shunts)

6. Other causes:
   - Following procedures (cardiac catheterization/interventional procedures)
   - Drugs (cocaine)
   - Myocardial bridging of the coronary arteries
   - Following open heart surgery

(B) Indications for thrombolytic therapy **(must be initiated within 1 h of onset of symptoms)**
1. chest pain for > 30 min and < 12 h. In nonverbal children at risk for myocardial ischemia, chest pain may manifest as intermittent crying and irritability with or without diaphoresis.
2. Absence of congestive heart failure or cardiogenic shock
3. EKG evidence of acute ischemia (ST elevation in 2 contiguous leads)

(C) Contraindications for thrombolytic therapy
1. Acute: internal bleeding, systolic and diastolic BP > 2 SD above the 95%ile for age
2. Chronic: AV malformation, CNS tumor
3. Past 6-8 weeks: trauma or surgery in past two weeks, CNS or spinal surgery in past 8 weeks, open-heart surgery in past 8 weeks, recent traumatic brain injury
4. Any time in the past: hemorrhagic stroke, IVH (premature infant), allergy to thrombolytic agent

Clinical Manifestations

GEN	failure to thrive, poor feeding, sudden episodes of crying and irritability may indicate chest pain
SKIN	diaphoresis, pallor
CVS	syncope, chest pain (older children), congestive heart failure
	children with ischemic heart disease following heart transplantation do **not** feel angina or pain because of denervation of the heart
RESP	wheezing, tachypnea, respiratory failure
CNS	irritability, lethargy

Diagnostics

Blood	CK-isoenzymes ($\uparrow$ CK-MB) and index (> 3), $\uparrow$ troponin I and troponin T
Imaging	chest radiograph (cardiomegaly and peribronchial edema)
	if stable, consider dobutamine stress echocardiogram, ultrafast CT, PET scan
Others	exercise stress test, **EKG is the gold standard for the diagnosis of acute myocardial ischemia**

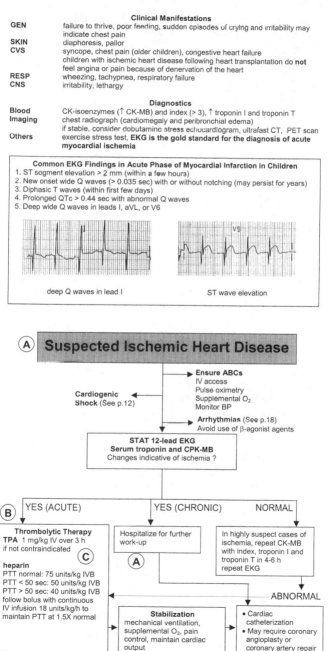

Common EKG Findings in Acute Phase of Myocardial Infarction in Children
1. ST segment elevation > 2 mm (within a few hours)
2. New onset wide Q waves (> 0.035 sec) with or without notching (may persist for years)
3. Diphasic T waves (within first few days)
4. Prolonged QTc > 0.44 sec with abnormal Q waves
5. Deep wide Q waves in leads I, aVL, or V6

deep Q waves in lead I   ST wave elevation

(A) **Suspected Ischemic Heart Disease**

→ **Ensure ABCs**
IV access
Pulse oximetry
Supplemental O₂
Monitor BP

Cardiogenic Shock (See p.12) ←

→ **Arrhythmias** (See p.18)
Avoid use of β-agonist agents

STAT 12-lead EKG
Serum troponin and CPK-MB
Changes indicative of ischemia ?

(B) **YES (ACUTE)**   **YES (CHRONIC)**   **NORMAL**

Thrombolytic Therapy
TPA 1 mg/kg IV over 3 h
if not contraindicated

(C)

heparin
PTT normal: 75 units/kg IVB
PTT < 50 sec: 50 units/kg IVB
PTT > 50 sec: 40 units/kg IVB
follow bolus with continuous
IV infusion 18 units/kg/h to
maintain PTT at 1.5X normal

Hospitalize for further work-up

(A)

In highly suspect cases of ischemia, repeat CK-MB with index, troponin I and troponin T in 4-6 h repeat EKG

——— **ABNORMAL**

Stabilization
mechanical ventilation, supplemental O₂, pain control, maintain cardiac output

• Cardiac catheterization
• May require coronary angioplasty or coronary artery repair

Post-operative Care Following Open-Heart Surgery

Jeff A. Clark

> Cardiac output is dependent on preload, myocardial contractility, and afterload. All three components have to be optimized in order to minimize cardiac work.
> Objectives of care:
> - minimize workload on the heart and lungs
> - prevent secondary injury by maintaining adequate perfusion
> - weaning the patient from artificial support

(A) Complications of open-heart surgery
- Anatomic
  - residual shunts (atrial, ventricular or great vessel)
  - residual obstruction (valvular, subvalvular, supravalvular)
  - residual valvular insufficiency
  - effusions or clots
  - hemorrhage
- Functional
  - ventricular dysfunction
  - end-organ dysfunction (most often involves lungs, kidneys and CNS)

Effects of hypothermic cardiopulmonary bypass and/or circulatory arrest
Determinants
- degree of hypothermia
- duration of bypass
- duration of aortic cross-clamp (if any)

Global effects
- Stress response
  - peaks during rewarming
  - mediated by catecholamines, cortisol, GH, prostaglandins, leukotrienes, other cytokines, insulin, glucose, endorphins and other substances
  - may induce myocardial damage, pulmonary and systemic hypertension, endothelial damage and pulmonary vascular reactivity
- Systemic inflammation and endothelial injury
  - impairs release of vasodilators (nitric oxide, prostacyclin)
  - promotes vasoconstriction (by impaired metabolism of thromboxane and endothelin)
- Non-pulsatile perfusion - may promote capillary sludging and edema

Myocardial effects
- ischemia-reperfusion injury
- decreased contractility
- β-receptor dysfunction - $\downarrow$ cardiac response to adrenergic agonist agents

Pulmonary effects
- reduced static and dynamic compliance
- reduced FRC
- surfactant washout
- atelectasis
- interstitial edema
- endothelial injury
- hemodilution - lower plasma oncotic pressure

Renal effects
- $\uparrow$ renin, angiotensin and catecholamines $\rightarrow$ renal vasoconstriction
- ATN is frequent

CNS effects
- safe duration of DHCA is 30-60 min, after which risk of transient and permanent neurologic sequelae increase significantly
- air and particulate embolism are also causes of post-CPB neurologic dysfunction
- the brain is particularly susceptible to low perfusion during the first 12-24 h after CPB therefore adequate perfusion and substrate delivery must be maintained
- hypothermia is the main protective strategy during CPB

Electrolyte disturbances may be significant
- total body fluid overload
- judicious use of fluids to maintain cardiac output
- rapid K^+ fluxes common
- hypokalemia is relatively better tolerated than hyperkalemia – treatment of hypokalemia should not be overly aggressive

(B) Left ventricular dysfunction
- can occur after any type of cardiac surgery
- may be easier to diagnose and manage than RV dysfunction
- therapy should be directed towards improving cardiac output
- C.O. = stroke volume x HR
  - $\uparrow$ HR will $\uparrow$ cardiac O_2 demands and decrease coronary filling time

✳ Continued on p. 36

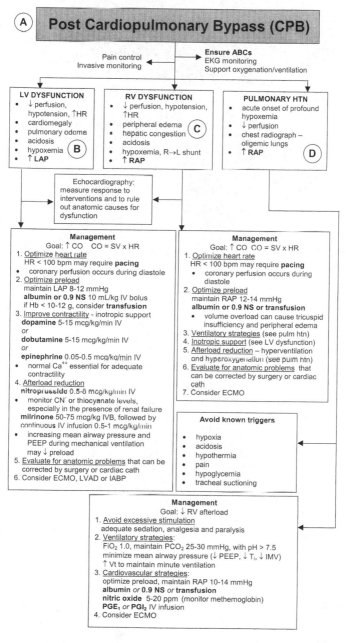

(A) **Post Cardiopulmonary Bypass (CPB)**

Pain control
Invasive monitoring

Ensure ABCs
EKG monitoring
Support oxygenation/ventilation

LV DYSFUNCTION
- ↓ perfusion, hypotension, ↑HR
- cardiomegaly
- pulmonary edema
- acidosis
- hypoxemia (B)
- ↑ LAP

RV DYSFUNCTION
- ↓ perfusion, hypotension, ↑HR
- peripheral edema (C)
- hepatic congestion
- acidosis
- hypoxemia, R→L shunt
- ↑ RAP

PULMONARY HTN
- acute onset of profound hypoxemia
- ↓ perfusion
- chest radiograph – oligemic lungs
- ↑ RAP (D)

Echocardiography: measure response to interventions and to rule out anatomic causes for dysfunction

Management
Goal: ↑ CO   CO = SV x HR
1. Optimize heart rate
   HR < 100 bpm may require **pacing**
   - coronary perfusion occurs during diastole
2. Optimize preload
   maintain LAP 8-12 mmHg
   albumin or 0.9 NS 10 mL/kg IV bolus
   if Hb < 10-12 g, consider **transfusion**
3. Improve contractility - inotropic support
   dopamine 5-15 mcg/kg/min IV
   or
   dobutamine 5-15 mcg/kg/min IV
   or
   epinephrine 0.05-0.5 mcg/kg/min IV
   - normal Ca^{++} essential for adequate contractility
4. Afterload reduction
   nitroprusside 0.5-8 mcg/kg/min IV
   - monitor CN$^-$ or thiocyanate levels, especially in the presence of renal failure
   milrinone 50-75 mcg/kg IVB, followed by continuous IV infusion 0.5-1 mcg/kg/min
   - increasing mean airway pressure and PEEP during mechanical ventilation may ↓ preload
5. Evaluate for anatomic problems that can be corrected by surgery or cardiac cath
6. Consider ECMO, LVAD or IABP

Management
Goal: ↑ CO   CO = SV x HR
1. Optimize heart rate
   HR < 100 bpm may require **pacing**
   - coronary perfusion occurs during diastole
2. Optimize preload
   maintain RAP 12-14 mmHg
   albumin or 0.9 NS or transfusion
   - volume overload can cause tricuspid insufficiency and peripheral edema
3. Ventilatory strategies (see pulm htn)
4. Inotropic support (see LV dysfunction)
5. Afterload reduction – hyperventilation and hyperoxygenation (see pulm htn)
6. Evaluate for anatomic problems that can be corrected by surgery or cardiac cath
7. Consider ECMO

Avoid known triggers
- hypoxia
- acidosis
- hypothermia
- pain
- hypoglycemia
- tracheal suctioning

Management
Goal: ↓ RV afterload
1. Avoid excessive stimulation
   adequate sedation, analgesia and paralysis
2. Ventilatory strategies:
   FiO$_2$ 1.0, maintain PCO$_2$ 25-30 mmHg, with pH > 7.5
   minimize mean airway pressure (↓ PEEP, ↓ T$_i$, ↓ IMV)
   ↑ Vt to maintain minute ventilation
3. Cardiovascular strategies:
   optimize preload, maintain RAP 10-14 mmHg
   albumin or 0.9 NS or transfusion
   nitric oxide 5-20 ppm (monitor methemoglobin)
   PGE$_1$ or PGI$_2$ IV infusion
4. Consider ECMO

✳ Continued from p.34

C Right ventricular dysfunction
- frequently results from anatomic changes after surgery which ↑ workload on RV (e.g., Norwood)
- ↓ SpO_2 related to RV dysfunction are usually due to ↑ RV pressures with R→L shunting through an anatomic communication
- management approach similar to that of LV dysfunction, but RV is usually less responsive to inotropic agents

D Pulmonary hypertension
- more common in newborns because pulmonary vasculature remains hypertrophic and highly responsive to metabolic changes
- usually precipitated by acidosis or hypoxemia
- hallmark: rapid onset of hypoxemia and poor perfusion

NOTES

The Infant in Shock

Athina Pappas

> Shock is a clinical syndrome characterized by inability of cardiac output to meet the metabolic demands of the tissues. It may be due to decreased delivery of substrates, but may also result from excessive needs of tissues that outstrip supply.

(A)

Etiology
- Hypovolemic – due to inadequate intravascular volume or preload, such as acute fluid or blood loss
- Cardiogenic – diminished cardiac output because of pump failure
- Distributive – relative decrease in preload with decreased systemic vascular resistance

(B)

Normal blood pressure in infants and neonates

Age	Systolic pressure (mmHg)	Diastolic pressure (mmHg)
Birth – 12 h of age (<1000 g)	39-59	16-36
Birth – 12 h of age (>3000 g)	50-70	25-45
Neonate up to 96 h of age	60-90	20-60
Infant up to 6 mos of age	87-105	53-66

(C)

There are a number of <u>specific disease states</u> to be considered in the management of an infant with shock:

- Sepsis/septic shock – neonates can present with shock resulting from Group B streptococcus, *E. coli*, listeria, or disseminated herpes. Risk factors for developing such infections include maternal sepsis or infection, poor or no prenatal care, and low birth weight.

- Cardiogenic shock – infants may develop cardiogenic shock from acute viral myocarditis, prolonged/untreated SVT, or ischemic heart disease from ALCAPA. However, in a child who presents with shock within the first week of life, it is important that the physician considers the possibility of ductal-dependent congenital heart disease. These lesions include coarctation of the aorta and hypoplastic left heart syndrome. At birth systemic blood flow is maintained by the patent ductus arteriosus. However, as the ductus closes, circulatory failure results from diminished or no systemic blood flow.
    - Pathophysiology: ductus closes → diminished systemic blood flow → circulatory failure → tissue anoxia and multi-organ failure → anaerobic metabolism and ↑ catecholamine release → tachycardia, hypotension, poor perfusion → ↓ splanchnic blood flow, with renal, hepatic insufficiency and gut ischemia with metabolic and respiratory acidosis → worsened circulatory failure.
    - Goal of therapy is to maintain patency of the ductus arteriosus by **PGE₁** infusion, as well as to provide support for the failing circulation by the correction of metabolic acidosis, judicious volume expansion, ventilatory support with 100% oxygen, and inotropic support.

- Congenital adrenal hyperplasia – is a group of disorders produced by enzyme deficiencies crucial to adrenal steroidogenesis. The most common form is 21-hydroxylase deficiency.
    - The lack of the 21-hydroxylase enzyme results in decreased cortisol synthesis. Two types include the simple virilizing and the salt-losing forms. There is an overproduction of cortisol precursors and sex steroids which do not depend on 21-hydroxylase enzyme for biosynthesis. As a result, the excessive sex hormones can produce a virilizing state. In the salt-losing form, there is diminished or no production of aldosterone. This produces a syndrome of shock, hyponatremia, and hyperkalemia that is often profound. High suspicion for this disease will prompt the physician to look for signs of virilization and/or hyponatremia with hyperkalemia in the infant who is in shock.
    - The goal of therapy is to provide **glucocorticoids** to replace the cortisol and suppress ACTH overproduction. In addition, life-threatening **hyperkalemia** and **hypoglycemia** must be properly managed (See p. 54,212).

- Hypovolemic shock
    - fluid losses from gastroenteritis
    - blood loss from birth trauma, fetofetal transfusion, fetomaternal transfusion, placental tear, severed umbilical cord
    - severe hemolytic anemia

Clinical Manifestations

(A)
| HISTORY | gastrointestinal losses, bleeding, fever or temperature instability, birth history, family history of inherited metabolic disease and/or consanguinity |
| GEN | poor feeding, failure to thrive |
(B)
SKIN	mottled, rash, petechiae, purpura, vesicles, blisters, gray color, pallor or cyanosis
CVS	tachycardia, murmur, gallop, bradycardia, diminished femoral pulses, hypotension
RESP	tachypnea, grunting, retractions, wheezing, rales
CNS	irritability, seizures, obtundation, coma

Diagnostics

Blood	ABG/CBG, electrolytes, glucose, Ca^{++}, P, BUN, creatinine, PT, PTT, platelets, lactic acid, Coomb's test, reticulocyte count, LFTs, type and crossmatch, culture
Urine	output, urinalysis, culture
Imaging	chest radiograph, abdominal films if indicated
Others	EKG, echocardiogram

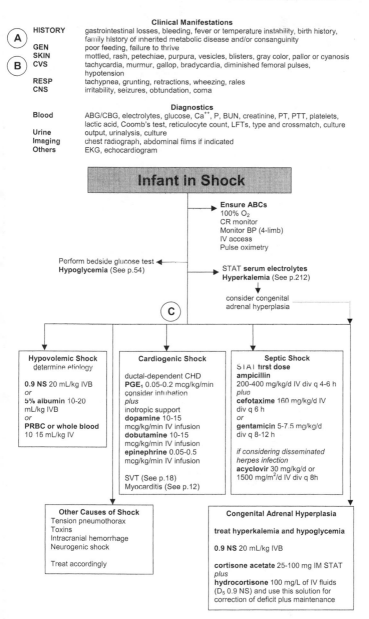

Infant in Shock

Ensure ABCs
100% O_2
CR monitor
Monitor BP (4-limb)
IV access
Pulse oximetry

Perform bedside glucose test ◄———
Hypoglycemia (See p.54)

STAT **serum electrolytes**
Hyperkalemia (See p.212)

consider congenital
adrenal hyperplasia

(C)

Hypovolemic Shock
determine etiology

0.9 NS 20 mL/kg IVB
or
5% albumin 10-20
mL/kg IVB
or
PRBC or whole blood
10-15 mL/kg IV

Cardiogenic Shock

ductal-dependent CHD
PGE₁ 0.05-0.2 mcg/kg/min
consider intubation
plus
inotropic support
dopamine 10-15
mcg/kg/min IV infusion
dobutamine 10-15
mcg/kg/min IV infusion
epinephrine 0.05-0.5
mcg/kg/min IV infusion

SVT (See p.18)
Myocarditis (See p.12)

Septic Shock
STAT first dose
ampicillin
200-400 mg/kg/d IV div q 4-6 h
plus
cefotaxime 160 mg/kg/d IV
div q 6 h
or
gentamicin 5-7.5 mg/kg/d
div q 8-12 h

*if considering disseminated
herpes infection*
acyclovir 30 mg/kg/d or
1500 mg/m²/d IV div q 8h

Other Causes of Shock
Tension pneumothorax
Toxins
Intracranial hemorrhage
Neurogenic shock

Treat accordingly

Congenital Adrenal Hyperplasia

treat hyperkalemia and hypoglycemia

0.9 NS 20 mL/kg IVB

cortisone acetate 25-100 mg IM STAT
plus
hydrocortisone 100 mg/L of IV fluids
(D_5 0.9 NS) and use this solution for
correction of deficit plus maintenance

Ductal Dependent Congenital Heart Lesions

Michele Carney

(A) Congenital heart defects that result in ↓ blood flow to the lungs or ↓ systemic blood flow are dependent on the pulmonary-systemic shunt from the patent ductus arteriosus to maintain pulmonary and systemic blood flow. Closure of the ductus arteriosus causes marked worsening of obstruction to pulmonary blood flow with right to left shunt and cyanosis in right-sided congenital heart lesions and decreased systemic blood flow with shock in left-sided obstructive lesions.

Pattern of blood flow

Obstructive right-sided cardiac lesion

> Right atrium → right ventricle → pulmonary artery (high resistance) → blood shunted from the right atrium through the PFO → left atrium → left ventricle → aorta → through the PDA → lungs → pulmonary veins → left atrium → left ventricle → aorta (and the PDA) → systemic circulation

Obstructive left-sided cardiac lesion

> Right atrium → right ventricle → pulmonary artery → PDA → aorta (low resistance) → systemic circulation
> ↓
> lungs → pulmonary veins
> left atrium → left ventricle
> → aorta (high resistance)

(B) Obstructive right heart lesions
- pulmonary atresia
- pulmonary stenosis
- tricuspid atresia
- tetralogy of Fallot

Obstructive left heart lesions
- aortic stenosis
- severe coarctation of the aorta
- hypoplastic left heart syndrome

Mixed lesion
- D transposition of the great arteries (in the absence of large VSD or ASD)

(C) Side effects of PGE_1
- apnea
- fever
- seizures
- hypotension
- flushing
- decreased platelet aggregation
- diarrhea

PGE_1 should result in improvement in all ductal dependent heart lesions with the exception of TAPVR. If patient's condition worsens on PGE_1 infusion, consider discontinuing infusion.

(D) pH, PaO_2, and $PaCO_2$ levels in CHD

When pulmonary or systemic blood flow is dependent on a patent ductus arteriosus or any pulmonary-systemic shunt, an increase in blood flow in either direction will result in decreased blood flow in the other.

In children with cyanotic heart disease and PDA,

↑ SpO_2 > 80% with or without respiratory alkalosis with $PaCO_2$ < 35 mmHg results in dilation of the pulmonary vasculature → ↑ pulmonary blood flow with flooding of the lungs and CHF + ↓ systemic blood flow

↓ SpO_2 < 70% with or without respiratory or metabolic acidosis → pulmonary vasoconstriction → ↑ pulmonary vascular resistance → ↓ pulmonary blood flow → hypoxemia

Therefore, when providing supplemental oxygen and choosing a ventilatory rate for these patients, PaO_2, $PaCO_2$, HCO_3^- and pH should be maintained at levels which optimize both pulmonary and systemic blood flow, while considering the type of CHD lesion.

Clinical Manifestations

A Infants are generally healthy at birth, then develop symptoms during the next 1-2 weeks of life when the ductus arteriosus closes: poor feeding, tachypnea, cyanosis, irritability, diaphoresis, and overt circulatory collapse.

Diagnostics

If patient is stable, consider hyperoxia test (See p.16)

Blood	ABG, electrolytes, Ca^{++}, Mg^{++}, BUN, creatinine
EKG	In the presence of tricuspid atresia or AV canal with pulmonic stenosis, EKG will show left axis deviation (newborns all have right axis deviation)
B **Chest radiograph**	enlarged heart, altered pulmonary vasculature
Echocardiogram	defines anatomy and patency of ductus arteriosus

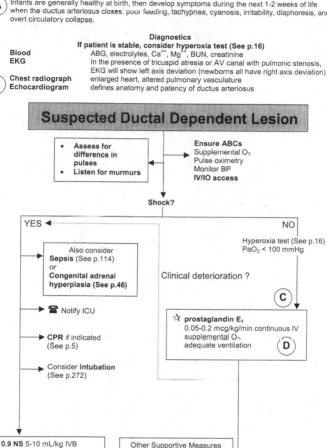

Suspected Ductal Dependent Lesion

- Assess for difference in pulses
- Listen for murmurs

Ensure ABCs
Supplemental O_2
Pulse oximetry
Monitor BP
IV/IO access

Shock?

YES ← ⋯⋯⋯⋯ **NO**

Hyperoxia test (See p.16)
$PaO_2 < 100$ mmHg

Also consider
Sepsis (See p.114)
or
Congenital adrenal hyperplasia (See p.46)

Clinical deterioration ?

C

☎ Notify ICU

☆ **prostaglandin E_1**
0.05-0.2 mcg/kg/min continuous IV
supplemental O_2,
adequate ventilation **D**

CPR if indicated
(See p.5)

Consider **intubation**
(See p.272)

0.9 NS 5-10 mL/kg IVB
☆
prostaglandin E_1 **C**
0.05-0.2 mcg/kg/min
continuous IV infusion

with persistent hypotension,
dopamine
8-10 mcg/kg/min
continuous IV infusion
and/or
dobutamine
5-10 mcg/kg/min
continuous infusion

Other Supportive Measures
STAT bedside glucose
hypoglycemia:
dextrose 25% 1-2 mL/kg IVB

metabolic acidosis:
$NaHCO_3$ 1-2 mEq/kg IVB

correct electrolyte
abnormalities **D**

☎ Notify Cardiology
echocardiogram

☆ During prostaglandin infusion, monitor:
- ABG
- blood pressures
- pulse oximetry
- ventilatory status

Chapter 2 ♣ Child Abuse

Katherine Ling-McGeorge

Essential to the management of children with child abuse is the ability to suspect, recognize, evaluate and treat complications of child abuse. There are characteristic profiles of abused children and their abusive perpetrators, as well as common clinical presentations suspicious for non-accidental trauma, which health care providers should recognize in order to better prevent the 14 million cases of reported abuse and over 2000 deaths annually due to abuse. Health care providers should additionally become familiar with their state and local laws governing child abuse documenting and reporting.

Although child neglect and sexual abuse require urgent medical attention, these issues are not addressed in this handbook in the context of emergent care.

Risk Factors
Any condition that interferes with normal parent-child bonding. 90% of abusive adults are found to be related caretakers. Crosses all socioeconomic and ethnic groups. A child who identifies an adult as the perpetrator is usually truthful. Interview the child and all caretakers and witnesses individually, using non-leading questions.

(A) Suspect the following
- histories that are inconsistent with the injury in severity, distribution, and child's developmental level
- alleged self-inflicted or sibling-inflicted injury
- vague or no explanation given
- varying or changing accounts upon re-interview
- delay in seeking medical care

Profile of abusive caretakers	**Profile of abused children**
unrealistic expectations (e.g., toilet training)	age < 4 yr
young parental age	prematurity
mental illness	multiple birth
history of abusive childhood	congenital defect
previous loss of a child	mental retardation
fear of injury to the child	difficult temperament
domestic violence	
substance abuse	
crisis situation in abuser's life	

(B) Ophthalmologic lesions are similar in both nonaccidental and unintentional trauma. Differential diagnoses include: bleeding disorders, ↑ICP, ↑BP. Normal newborn infants may have hemorrhages that clear within a few weeks. Although the differential diagnosis for retinal hemorrhage is extensive, large blotchy hemorrheages are likely to be caused by shaking. Retinal and preretinal hemorrhages are seen in 80% of children with recognized abusive head trauma. Retinal hemorrhages may persist for > 10d post-injury.

(C) Head injury is the most common cause of death in child abuse. In infants with brain trauma, elicit a history of feeding, sleeping, and behavior patterns 24-48h before presentation. In a study by Helfer, Slovis and Black, of 246 falls from the height of a sofa or bed, only 1.2% demonstrated skull fractures; of those, none were bilateral or diastatic. The most commonly seen abusive brain injury involves violent shaking of infants with or without impact trauma. Children < 2 y are particularly vulnerable to shaking injuries, because of their relatively large cranium and weak neck musculature.

(D) External manifestations of blunt chest trauma are rare due to ↑chest wall compliance in children, and dissipation of energy to internal organs. May result in delay in clinical presentation. Chest injuries include: pulmonary contusion, pneumothorax, pleural effusion, rib fractures, vascular or tracheobronchial injuries.

Abdominal injuries are the second most common cause of death in battered children. Usually associated head and skin injuries. Caution: the abdominal examination may not be reliable in patients with concomitant head injury. Most common abdominal injuries in order of frequency:
- ruptured liver, spleen
- intestinal perforation
- intramural hematoma of the duodenum, proximal jejunum, or retroperitoneal
- ruptured blood vessels
- pancreatic injury
- kidney, bladder injury
- chylous ascites

✳ (Continued on p. 44)

(A) **Clinical Manifestations**

GEN shock, sepsis, toxin exposure (particularly caustic ingestions), failure to thrive, traumatic alopecia

(B) **Fundi** retinal hemorrhages, retinal detachment, dislocated lens, hyphema, corneal abrasion, papilledema

RESP apnea, ALTE, foreign body aspiration

CVS unexplained shock, profound anemia

GI/GU peritonitis, vaginal bleeding from suspected abusive trauma, hematuria

CNS unexplained loss of consciousness, altered mental status, seizures, coma, periorbital ecchymosis, hemotympanum, CSF otorrhea or rhinorrhea, Battle's sign, bruised or scarred/deformed pinna, subgaleal hematoma

SKIN **See below**

Other Factitious Disorder by Proxy: commonly presents with recurrent seizures, bleeding, altered mental status, fever, apnea, diarrhea, vomiting, rash

Diagnostics

History **Document:** date, time, place, address, sequence of events, names, surface of impact, height of fall, length of time in contact with burning agents

Physical **Document:** growth parameters, developmental status, affect, behavior, photographs with scales and labels

Blood CBC, differential, platelets, comprehensive drug and toxicology screens

Urine urinalysis, comprehensive drug and toxicology screens, metabolic screens if indicated

Imaging **See below by system**

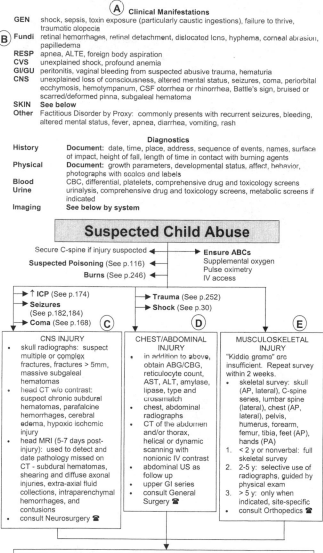

Suspected Child Abuse

Secure C-spine if injury suspected ◄━━━━━► **Ensure ABCs**
Suspected Poisoning (See p.116) ◄━━━━━ Supplemental oxygen
Burns (See p.246) ◄━━━━━ Pulse oximetry
IV access

► ↑ **ICP** (See p.174) ► **Trauma** (See p.252)
► **Seizures** ► **Shock** (See p.30)
(See p.182,184)
► **Coma** (See p.168) (C) (D) (E)

CNS INJURY	CHEST/ABDOMINAL INJURY	MUSCULOSKELETAL INJURY
• skull radiographs: suspect multiple or complex fractures, fractures > 5mm, massive subgaleal hematomas • head CT w/o contrast: suspect chronic subdural hematomas, parafalcine hemorrhages, cerebral edema, hypoxic ischemic injury • head MRI (5-7 days post-injury): used to detect and date pathology missed on CT - subdural hematomas, shearing and diffuse axonal injuries, extra-axial fluid collections, intraparenchymal hemorrhages, and contusions • consult Neurosurgery ☎	• in addition to above, obtain ABG/CBG, reticulocyte count, AST, ALT, amylase, lipase, type and crossmatch • chest, abdominal radiographs • CT of the abdomen and/or thorax, helical or dynamic scanning with nonionic IV contrast • abdominal US as follow up • upper GI series • consult General Surgery ☎	"Kiddie grams" are insufficient. Repeat survey within 2 weeks. • skeletal survey: skull (AP, lateral), C-spine series, lumbar spine (lateral), chest (AP, lateral), pelvis, humerus, forearm, femur, tibia, feet (AP), hands (PA) 1. < 2 y or nonverbal: full skeletal survey 2. 2-5 y: selective use of radiographs, guided by physical exam 3. > 5 y: only when indicated, site-specific • consult Orthopedics ☎

File written report to appropriate department of Social Services
Consult Social Work ☎, consult Child Protection Team if available ☎
Admit for further evaluation if indicated
• visitation restrictions
• review prior medical records
• continue to elicit account of mechanism of injury
• medical examination of all siblings and other minors in the household (others at 20% risk of also being abused)

✱ (Continued on p.45)

✱ (Continued from p.42)

(E) Differential diagnoses of skeletal abnormalities: osteogenesis imperfecta, congenital syphilis, leukemia, primary bone tumors or metastatic lesions, scurvy, rickets, Menkes' kinky hair syndrome (copper deficiency), hyperparathyroidism, birth trauma, Blount's disease, Caffey's disease (infantile cortical hyperostosis).

Suspect the following radiographic abnormalities:
- isolated long-bone fractures, spiral fractures in the pre-ambulatory child
- corner fractures
- acromial fractures (either traction forces jerking upward or direct blow)
- scapular fractures
- sternal fracture (direct blow)
- multiple or posterior rib fractures
- multiple costovertebral or costochondral fractures
- incidental compression fractures of the spine (due to slamming the child down on the buttocks or by hyperflexing and hyperextending the trunk as in shaking injuries)
- multiple fractures in different stages of healing

(F) Differential diagnoses of skin lesions which can be mistaken for abuse: Mongolian spots, allergic shiners, phytophotodermatitis, erythema marginatum, hypersensitivity, eczema, bullous impetigo, Henoch Schönlein purpura, Ehlers-Danlos syndrome, other associated bleeding disorders. Lesions caused by folk medicine practices include cupping, coin rubbing (cao gao), caida de molera, moxibustion.

Although prior studies have suggested that color dating of bruising is possible, current literature shows that bruising cannot be reliably aged on appearance alone.

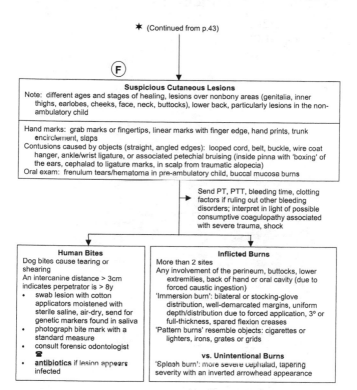

✱ (Continued from p.43)

(F)

Suspicious Cutaneous Lesions

Note: different ages and stages of healing, lesions over nonbony areas (genitalia, inner thighs, earlobes, cheeks, face, neck, buttocks), lower back, particularly lesions in the non-ambulatory child

Hand marks: grab marks or fingertips, linear marks with finger edge, hand prints, trunk encirclement, slaps

Contusions caused by objects (straight, angled edges): looped cord, belt, buckle, wire coat hanger, ankle/wrist ligature, or associated petechial bruising (inside pinna with 'boxing' of the ears, cephalad to ligature marks, in scalp from traumatic alopecia)

Oral exam: frenulum tears/hematoma in pre-ambulatory child, buccal mucosa burns

Send PT, PTT, bleeding time, clotting factors if ruling out other bleeding disorders; interpret in light of possible consumptive coagulopathy associated with severe trauma, shock

Human Bites

Dog bites cause tearing or shearing

An intercanine distance > 3cm indicates perpetrator is > 8y

- swab lesion with cotton applicators moistened with sterile saline, air-dry, send for genetic markers found in saliva
- photograph bite mark with a standard measure
- consult forensic odontologist ☎
- **antibiotics** if lesion appears infected

Inflicted Burns

More than 2 sites

Any involvement of the perineum, buttocks, lower extremities, back of hand or oral cavity (due to forced caustic ingestion)

'Immersion burn': bilateral or stocking-glove distribution, well-demarcated margins, uniform depth/distribution due to forced application, 3° or full-thickness, spared flexion creases

'Pattern burns' resemble objects: cigarettes or lighters, irons, grates or grids

vs. Unintentional Burns

'Splash burn': more severe cephalad, tapering severity with an inverted arrowhead appearance

Chapter 3 ♣ Endocrine

Adrenal Crisis

U. Olivia Kim

(A) Characterized by a rapid, overwhelming and potentially fatal adrenocortical insufficiency that may be either a worsening of a state of chronic adrenal hypofunction, acute damage to previously normal adrenal glands, congenital deficiency, or abrupt withdrawal of chronic steroid administration.

In patients with chronic primary adrenal insufficiency, suspect acute adrenal crisis in the presence of unexplained fever, hypoglycemia, nausea and vomiting, weight loss, dehydration and anorexia, abdominal pain, or cardiovascular collapse. *In previously healthy patients*, suspect adrenal crisis with the above symptoms, especially if associated with sepsis (meningococcemia), following surgery (embolic phenomenon), any hypoxic-ischemic episode, or trauma.
Definitive treatment is based on the patient's exacerbating condition. Majority of adrenal crisis occurs in patients with known chronic adrenal insufficiency.

(B)
Classification of Adrenal Insufficiency
A. Primary adrenal insufficiency
  1. Anatomic destruction of the gland (acute or chronic)
    "Idiopathic atrophy" (autoimmune state) usually polyglandular
    Surgical removal
    Infection (fungal, TB)
    Hemorrhage
    Infiltration (metastatic)
  2. Metabolic failure in hormone production
    Congenital adrenal hyperplasia
    Enzyme inhibitors
    Cytotoxic agents
B. Secondary adrenal insufficiency
  1. Suppression of hypothalamic-pituitary axis
  2. Hypopituitarism secondary to primary pituitary disease
  3. Exogenous or endogenous (neoplastic) corticosteroids

(C) Glucose may be given as **D$_5$ 0.9 NS** or as a separate bolus of **25% dextrose** 2-4 mL/kg (dilute to **12.5% dextrose** for use in infants).

(D) Treat mineralocorticoid deficiency by providing hydrocortisone **and** correcting electrolytes. Load with parenteral hydrocortisone, followed by continuous IV infusion of hydrocortisone to provide adequate protection during acute deterioration. Although mineralocorticoid deficiency exists, replacement is not necessary during acute therapy as high dose glucocorticoids provide mineralocorticoid-like activity.
Use **0.9 NS or D$_5$ 0.9 NS** as rehydrating/maintenance solution until:
  1. Laboratory results become available, adjust accordingly
  2. Patient no longer has significant electrolyte losses
  3. Serum sodium remains stable for 8-12 hours

(E) Ensure that steroid dosage is adjusted in those taking medications that may accelerate hepatic steroid metabolism: phenytoin, barbiturates, rifampin, and mitotane.

Changes in doses of glucocorticoids related to stress
A. Minor illness or stress
  1. Increase glucocorticoid dose 2-3 fold orally for the few days of illness
  2. DO NOT change mineralocorticoid dose
  3. No extra supplementation is needed with uncomplicated dental procedures
  4. If patient is not tolerating oral intake, notify Endocrinology ☎
B. Severe illness, stress of surgery (when patient is unable to take oral fluids)
  1. **Cortisone acetate** 1-5 mg/kg/d IM div q 12-24 h
  2. **Hydrocortisone (Solu-Cortef®)** 100 mg/L of IV fluids (D$_5$ 0.9 NS) at maintenance IV rate
  3. **Fludrocortisone (Florinef®)**, give with sips of water or by NGT

Clinical Manifestations

Life-threatening	Circulatory collapse, hyperkalemia, hypoglycemia with seizures, acidosis
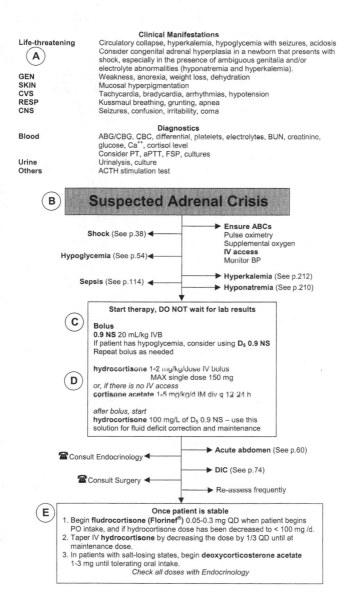 **(A)**	Consider congenital adrenal hyperplasia in a newborn that presents with shock, especially in the presence of ambiguous genitalia and/or electrolyte abnormalities (hyponatremia and hyperkalemia).
GEN	Weakness, anorexia, weight loss, dehydration
SKIN	Mucosal hyperpigmentation
CVS	Tachycardia, bradycardia, arrhythmias, hypotension
RESP	Kussmaul breathing, grunting, apnea
CNS	Seizures, confusion, irritability, coma

Diagnostics

Blood	ABG/CBG, CBC, differential, platelets, electrolytes, BUN, creatinine, glucose, Ca^{++}, cortisol level
	Consider PT, aPTT, FSP, cultures
Urine	Urinalysis, culture
Others	ACTH stimulation test

(B) ## Suspected Adrenal Crisis

Shock (See p.38) ◄─────────── ► **Ensure ABCs**
                                   Pulse oximetry
                                   Supplemental oxygen
Hypoglycemia (See p.54) ◄──────   **IV access**
                                   Monitor BP

Sepsis (See p.114) ◄──────────── ► Hyperkalemia (See p.212)
                                 ► Hyponatremia (See p.210)

Start therapy, DO NOT wait for lab results

(C)

Bolus
0.9 NS 20 mL/kg IVB
If patient has hypoglycemia, consider using **D₅ 0.9 NS**
Repeat bolus as needed

(D)

hydrocortisone 1-2 mg/kg/dose IV bolus
                   MAX single dose 150 mg
or, if there is no IV access
cortisone acetate 1-5 mg/kg/d IM div q 12-24 h

after bolus, start
hydrocortisone 100 mg/L of D₅ 0.9 NS – use this
solution for fluid deficit correction and maintenance

☎ Consult Endocrinology ◄──────── ► **Acute abdomen** (See p.60)

                                 ► **DIC** (See p.74)
☎ Consult Surgery ◄───────────

                                 ► Re-assess frequently

(E)

Once patient is stable
1. Begin **fludrocortisone (Florinef®)** 0.05-0.3 mg QD when patient begins
   PO intake, and if hydrocortisone dose has been decreased to < 100 mg /d.
2. Taper IV **hydrocortisone** by decreasing the dose by 1/3 QD until at
   maintenance dose.
3. In patients with salt-losing states, begin **deoxycorticosterone acetate**
   1-3 mg until tolerating oral intake.
   Check all doses with Endocrinology

Central Diabetes Insipidus

Vera Borzova

> A syndrome that results from the inability of the neurohypophyseal system to produce a sufficient amount of arginine vasopressin (AVP) to maintain normal renal conservation of water.

(A) Typical Findings:
- Large urinary volume (may be > 4 mL/kg/h)
- Urine osmolality < 300 mOsm/kg
- Urine specific gravity < 1.005
- Plasma osmolality > 300 mOsm/kg
- Inappropriately low serum AVP levels (if measured) despite elevated plasma osmolality

(B) Differential diagnosis (partial list):
- Psychogenic polydipsia
- Nephrogenic DI
- Polyuric phase of acute tubular necrosis
- Toxins: lithium, demeclocycline

(C) Etiology:
- Idiopathic
- Familial – autosomal dominant
- Head trauma
- Surgical excision of suprasellar or intrasellar tumors
- Infections – meningitis, encephalitis
- Hypoxic-ischemic CNS injury
- Granulomatous disease

(D) Triple-phase response following neurosurgical destruction of vasopressin-secreting neurons:
1. Initial phase of transient DI lasting a few days (usually due to edema of the area)
2. Second phase of SIADH with decreased urine flow and increased urine osmolality (due to unregulated release of vasopressin by damaged neurons), which can last for $\geq$ 10 days
3. Third phase of permanent polyuria and DI following destruction of $\geq$ 90% of vasopressin-secreting neurons

(E) Management Principles:
1. In the acute treatment phase, continuous intravenous infusion of vasopressin allows titration of dose according to patient response. Intranasal DDAVP or IM pitressin tannate in oil has longer half-lives which do not permit titration.
2. Hyperglycemia is a frequent side effect of treatment.
3. Do not correct elevated serum sodium too rapidly (< 0.5-0.75 mEq/L/h)
4. Hourly laboratory determination may be necessary. Monitor hourly urine output and specific gravity and adjust therapy accordingly.

Clinical Manifestations

History	Post-operative brain tumor excision, history of brain tumor surgery, trauma, ischemia, infections, drug toxicity
GEN	Abrupt onset of polyuria and profound thirst (in awake patients with intact thirst mechanism), eventually leading to hypotension and hypovolemic shock. These symptoms usually follow an inciting event such as hypoxic-ischemic injury, trauma, or surgery
CVS	Hypovolemia may result from significant fluid loss, tachycardia, hypotension
CNS	Irritability, confusion, lethargy, seizures, coma

Diagnostics

Blood	electrolytes, osmolality, BUN, creatinine, glucose, Ca^{++}, Mg^{++}, P
Urine	UUN, electrolytes, osmolality, specific gravity, urine volume
Imaging	Consider CT scan of head
Others	Daily weights, review intake and output

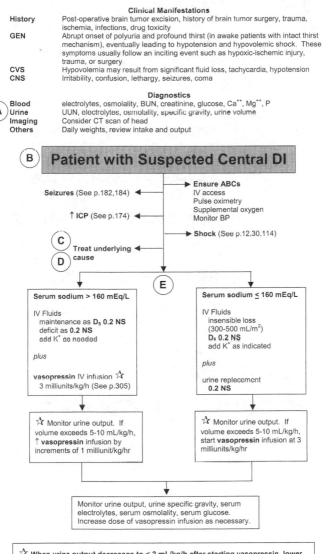

(A)

(B) **Patient with Suspected Central DI**

➤ **Ensure ABCs**
  IV access
  Pulse oximetry
  Supplemental oxygen
  Monitor BP

Seizures (See p.182,184) ◄

↑ **ICP** (See p.174) ◄

➤ **Shock** (See p.12,30,114)

(C)
(D) Treat underlying ◄
    cause

(E)

Serum sodium > 160 mEq/L

IV Fluids
  maintenance as D_5 0.2 NS
  deficit as 0.2 NS
  add K^+ as needed

plus

vasopressin IV infusion ☆
  3 milliunits/kg/h (See p.305)

Serum sodium ≤ 160 mEq/L

IV Fluids
  insensible loss
  (300-500 mL/m^2)
  D_5 0.2 NS
  add K^+ as indicated

plus

urine replacement
  0.2 NS

☆ Monitor urine output. If volume exceeds 5-10 mL/kg/h, ↑ **vasopressin** infusion by increments of 1 milliunit/kg/hr

---

☆ Monitor urine output. If volume exceeds 5-10 mL/kg/h, start **vasopressin** infusion at 3 milliunits/kg/hr

---

Monitor urine output, urine specific gravity, serum electrolytes, serum osmolality, serum glucose.
Increase dose of vasopressin infusion as necessary.

☆ When urine output decreases to < 2 mL/kg/h after starting vasopressin, lower IV fluid rate to prevent water intoxication, e.g., instead of using an IV fluid rate of insensible loss plus urine replacement, switch to maintenance fluid rate or less.

Diabetic Ketoacidosis (DKA)

Maria C. Asi-Bautista

> Suspect DKA in a child who presents with **hyperglycemia** (>300 mg/dl), **ketonemia** (>1:2 dilution) and **acidosis**. 25%-40% of children who develop diabetes present with DKA at the time of diagnosis.

(A) Abdominal pain may sometimes mimic surgical abdomen. The mechanism is unknown. Amylase and transaminases may be elevated.

Infection may be present even if temperature is normal or decreased. Elevated temperature strongly suggests infection.

(B) 15% may have euglycemic DKA (< 350 mg/dl), e.g., alcoholics and pregnant insulin-dependent diabetic teenagers.

Creatinine is spuriously increased due to interference from acetoacetate. Hyponatremia may be present. (See p. 210)

(C) Consider infection/sepsis as a precipitating factor. Perform thorough physical examination to look for possible focus of infection, e.g., non-healing wound/ulcers, abscess, etc.

(D) If a patient is comatose/stuporous and the serum osmolality is < 320 mOsm/L, consider other causes, e.g., toxic ingestion, trauma, etc.

The cause of cerebral edema in DKA is multifactorial, and it has been frequently considered to be a complication of, or aggravated by therapy. However, there has been no consistent biochemical or clinical finding that correlates with neurological decline.

Some of the reported symptoms observed prior to the development of intracranial hypertension include (1) ↓ heart rate, (2) altered sensorium, (3) headache, (4) emesis.

(E) Monitor electrolytes (corrected sodium), osmolality, and neurologic status to detect signs of deterioration. Administer **mannitol** 1 g/kg IV over 15-20 minutes to patients with symptoms of acute neurologic dysfunction. **Ensure availability of mannitol.**

(F) **Insulin is needed to clear ketones.** Continue insulin infusion until ketones are completely clear from plasma.

Insulin concentration for continuous infusion varies at different institutions. Check concentration and dose prior to initiation of infusion. Examples of concentrations: 25 units Regular in 250 mL 0.9 NS (1 mL= 0.1 units), 250 units Regular in 250 mL 0.9 NS (1mL = 1 units)

(G) Serum K^+ will ↓ during treatment because of (1) urinary losses, (2) increase cellular uptake (due to insulin and the correction of metabolic acidosis), (3) dilution from rehydration.

Clinical Manifestations

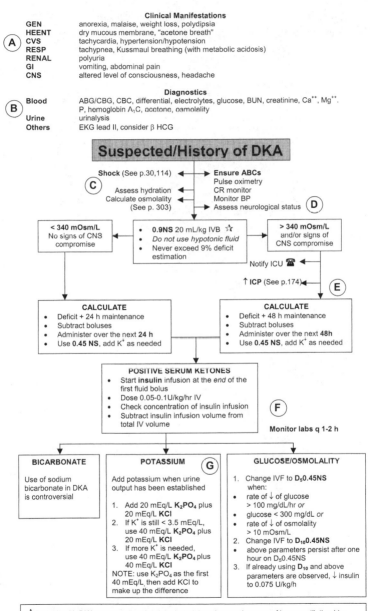

GEN	anorexia, malaise, weight loss, polydipsia
HEENT	dry mucous membrane, "acetone breath"
CVS	tachycardia, hypertension/hypotension
RESP	tachypnea, Kussmaul breathing (with metabolic acidosis)
RENAL	polyuria
GI	vomiting, abdominal pain
CNS	altered level of consciousness, headache

(A)

Diagnostics

Blood	ABG/CBG, CBC, differential, electrolytes, glucose, BUN, creatinine, Ca^{++}, Mg^{++}, P, hemoglobin A_1C, acetone, osmolality
Urine	urinalysis
Others	EKG lead II, consider β HCG

(B)

Suspected/History of DKA

Shock (See p.30,114) ◄──────► **Ensure ABCs**
(C) Pulse oximetry
Assess hydration ◄───── CR monitor
Calculate osmolality ◄───── Monitor BP
(See p. 303) ─────► Assess neurological status (D)

< 340 mOsm/L
No signs of CNS compromise

- **0.9NS** 20 mL/kg IVB ☆
- *Do not use hypotonic fluid*
- Never exceed 9% deficit estimation

> 340 mOsm/L
and/or signs of CNS compromise

Notify ICU ☎ ◄

↑ ICP (See p.174) ◄ (E)

CALCULATE
- Deficit + 24 h maintenance
- Subtract boluses
- Administer over the next **24 h**
- Use **0.45 NS**, add K^+ as needed

CALCULATE
- Deficit + 48 h maintenance
- Subtract boluses
- Administer over the next **48h**
- Use **0.45 NS**, add K^+ as needed

POSITIVE SERUM KETONES
- Start **insulin** infusion at the *end* of the first fluid bolus
- Dose 0.05-0.1U/kg/hr IV
- Check concentration of insulin infusion
- Subtract insulin infusion volume from total IV volume

(F)

Monitor labs q 1-2 h

BICARBONATE

Use of sodium bicarbonate in DKA is controversial

POTASSIUM (G)

Add potassium when urine output has been established

1. Add 20 mEq/L K_2PO_4 plus 20 mEq/L **KCl**
2. If K^+ is still < 3.5 mEq/L, use 40 mEq/L K_2PO_4 plus 20 mEq/L **KCl**
3. If more K^+ is needed, use 40 mEq/L K_2PO_4 plus 40 mEq/L **KCl**

NOTE: use K_2PO_4 as the first 40 mEq/L, then add KCl to make up the difference

GLUCOSE/OSMOLALITY

1. Change IVF to **$D_5$0.45NS** when:
   - rate of ↓ of glucose > 100 mg/dL/hr *or*
   - glucose < 300 mg/dL *or*
   - rate of ↓ of osmolality > 10 mOsm/L
2. Change IVF to **D_{10}0.45NS**
   - above parameters persist after one hour on $D_5$0.45NS
3. If already using D_{10} and above parameters are observed, ↓ insulin to 0.075 U/kg/h

☆Patients with DKA may appear more dehydrated than they are because of hyperventilation (dry lips/mouth) and acidosis (poor myocardial function). In addition, older children have less degree of deficit (3%, 6%, and 9%, respectively for mild, moderate, severe dehydration), as compared to infants.

Syndrome of Inappropriate Antidiuretic Hormone Secretion

Bulent Ozgonenel

Syndrome of inappropriate antidiuretic hormone secretion (SIADH) is characterized by an inappropriate release of ADH in the face of normovolemia or even hypervolemia. The clinical features include hyponatremia and water intoxication. SIADH should be differentiated from cerebral salt wasting syndrome. Hyponatremia and high urine sodium are observed in cerebral salt wasting, but urine volume is appropriate and ADH release is normal in response to hypovolemia. Hyponatremia should be managed with fluid and sodium replacement rather than fluid restriction.

(**A**) SIADH should be suspected in a patient at risk who is well hydrated and suddenly develops oliguria with increased urine specific gravity.

(**B**)

Blood	Urine
• Hyponatremia	• Urine volume ↓
• Low uric acid	• Osmolality inappropriately ↑
• BUN normal or low	• Urine specific gravity >1.020
• Serum osmolality low (<270 mOsm/L)	• $FE_{Na} > 1$
	• $U_{Na} > 30$ mEq/L
	• BUN:UUN > 1:20

Causes of/Risk factors for SIADH (partial list)

(**C**)

Drugs	vincristine, vinblastine, carbamazepine, cyclic antidepressants, NSAIDs, morphine
Neoplasm	brain tumors, Hodgkin's disease, acute leukemia, lung cancer
Surgery	anesthesia, spinal fusion, surgical stress
Neurologic	VP shunt malfunction, head trauma, hypoxic-ischemic encephalopathy, subarachnoid hemorrhage
Infections	pneumonia, bacterial meningitis, tuberculous meningitis

Clinical Manifestations

A	**HISTORY**	causes and risk factors
	GEN	no signs of dehydration
	GI	nausea, vomiting, anorexia
	CNS	confusion, irritability, seizures, coma

Diagnostics

B	**Blood**	electrolytes, osmolality, glucose, BUN, creatinine, uric acid
	Urine	volume, specific gravity, electrolytes, UUN, osmolality
	Others	daily weights, intake and output

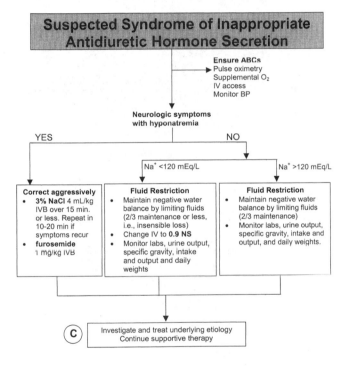

Suspected Syndrome of Inappropriate Antidiuretic Hormone Secretion

Ensure ABCs
→ Pulse oximetry
Supplemental O_2
IV access
Monitor BP

Neurologic symptoms with hyponatremia

YES   NO

Na^+ <120 mEq/L Na^+ >120 mEq/L

Correct aggressively
- **3% NaCl** 4 mL/kg IVB over 15 min. or less. Repeat in 10-20 min if symptoms recur
- **furosemide** 1 mg/kg IVB

Fluid Restriction
- Maintain negative water balance by limiting fluids (2/3 maintenance or less, i.e., insensible loss)
- Change IV to **0.9 NS**
- Monitor labs, urine output, specific gravity, intake and output and daily weights

Fluid Restriction
- Maintain negative water balance by limiting fluids (2/3 maintenance)
- Monitor labs, urine output, specific gravity, intake and output, and daily weights.

C   Investigate and treat underlying etiology
Continue supportive therapy

Hypoglycemia

Amit Sarnaik

(A) Hypoglycemia in infants and children is defined as a blood glucose value of < 40 mg/dl. Hypoglycemia is a sign of an underlying disease process. It generally results from any disorder which interferes with carbohydrate intake, absorption, gluconeogenesis or glycogenolysis. Disorders of gluconeogenesis, ketogenesis and fatty oxidation also increase the risk for developing hypoglycemia. Prompt recognition and treatment is essential to prevent irreversible neurologic injury.

Causes of Hypoglycemia

(B)

Neonates	Infant of diabetic mother, small for gestational age, prematurity, sepsis, infant with respiratory distress, erythroblastosis fetalis, Beckwith-Wiedemann syndrome
Endocrine	Hyperinsulinism (nesidioblastoma, islet cell adenoma, exogenous insulin), hypopituitarism, growth hormone deficiency, hypothyroidism, hypoadrenalism (congenital adrenal hyperplasia)
Inborn errors of metabolism	Carbohydrate metabolism: glycogen storage disease, galactosemia Amino acid metabolism: organic acidemias, ketotic hypoglycemia (most common etiology of hypoglycemia in children) Lipid metabolism: carnitine and acyl CoA dehydrogenase deficiency Disorders affecting gluconeogenesis
Toxic	Oral hypoglycemic agents, salicylates, alcohol, β-blockers, insulin, Jamaican ackee fruit, rat poison, valproic acid, insulin injections (child abuse)
Liver disease	Reye syndrome, hepatitis, cirrhosis
Systemic disorders	Starvation, malnutrition, anorexia nervosa, sepsis, malabsorption, diarrhea

(C) Accuracy of blood glucose determination is essential. Plasma glucose concentration correlates closely with the amount of glucose utilized by the brain. Measurement of glucose in whole blood samples can result in a 10-15% underestimation of glucose since erythrocytes have a relatively lower concentration of glucose. Bedside glucose tests (such as the Accu-Chek®) provide rapid and convenient glucose testing, but are known to have high false positive and negative rates at the lower end of the scale.

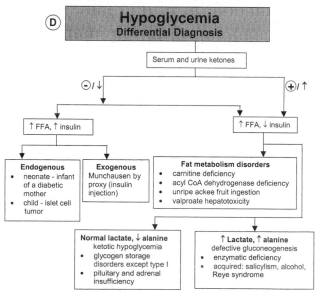

(D) **Hypoglycemia**
Differential Diagnosis

Serum and urine ketones

⊖/↓ ⊕/↑

↑ FFA, ↑ insulin ↑ FFA, ↓ insulin

Endogenous
- neonate - infant of a diabetic mother
- child - islet cell tumor

Exogenous
Munchausen by proxy (insulin injection)

Fat metabolism disorders
- carnitine deficiency
- acyl CoA dehydrogenase deficiency
- unripe ackee fruit ingestion
- valproate hepatotoxicity

Normal lactate, ↓ alanine
ketotic hypoglycemia
- glycogen storage disorders except type I
- pituitary and adrenal insufficiency

↑ Lactate, ↑ alanine
defective gluconeogenesis
- enzymatic deficiency
- acquired: salicylism, alcohol, Reye syndrome

Clinical Manifestations

(A) HISTORY   timing of last meal, toxins (especially alcohols), poor feeding, family history, information which may indicate child abuse
(B) GEN   short stature, failure to thrive, temperature swings
SKIN   abnormal pigmentation, diaphoresis
HEENT   macrosomia
CVS   tachycardia, bradycardia, palpitations
RESP   hyperpnea, bradypnea
GI   hepatomegaly, abdominal pain, nausea, vomiting
CNS   hypotonia, headache, jitteriness, irritability, lethargy, seizures, coma

Diagnostics

(C) Blood   glucose, electrolytes, osmolality, ABG/CBG, comprehensive drug screen, anion gap, BUN, creatinine, acetone, consider LFTs
Urine   drug screen, urinalysis, ketones
Imaging   consider CT or MRI
Others   consider growth hormone, cortisol, ACTH stimulation test, glucose tolerance test

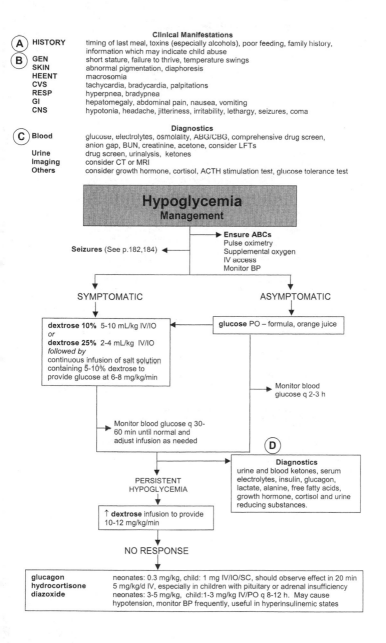

Hypoglycemia
Management

➤ **Ensure ABCs**
Pulse oximetry
Supplemental oxygen
IV access
Monitor BP

Seizures (See p.182,184) ◄

SYMPTOMATIC

ASYMPTOMATIC

dextrose 10% 5-10 mL/kg IV/IO
or
dextrose 25% 2-4 mL/kg IV/IO
followed by
continuous infusion of salt solution containing 5-10% dextrose to provide glucose at 6-8 mg/kg/min

◄ **glucose** PO – formula, orange juice

Monitor blood glucose q 2-3 h

Monitor blood glucose q 30-60 min until normal and adjust infusion as needed

(D) Diagnostics
urine and blood ketones, serum electrolytes, insulin, glucagon, lactate, alanine, free fatty acids, growth hormone, cortisol and urine reducing substances.

PERSISTENT HYPOGLYCEMIA

↑ **dextrose** infusion to provide 10-12 mg/kg/min

NO RESPONSE

glucagon   neonates: 0.3 mg/kg, child: 1 mg IV/IO/SC, should observe effect in 20 min
hydrocortisone   5 mg/kg/d IV, especially in children with pituitary or adrenal insufficiency
diazoxide   neonates: 3-5 mg/kg, child:1-3 mg/kg IV/PO q 8-12 h. May cause hypotension, monitor BP frequently, useful in hyperinsulinemic states

Thyrotoxicosis: Thyroid Storm

Matthew N. Denenberg

> Thyrotoxicosis or thyroid storm is rare in children. It occurs when free thyroid hormones suddenly increase in patients with pre-existing hyperthyroidism. The metabolic and adrenergic effects of thyroid hormones (free T_3) are exaggerated to life-threatening proportions.

(A) Etiology:
- Graves disease
- Thyroiditis
- TSH hypersecretion
- Exogenous thyroid hormone ingestion
- Precipitating factors: infection, DKA

(B) At risk: Observe newborns whose mothers have Graves Disease, especially at two weeks of life, when maternal antithyroid medications taper off.

(C) Blood for thyroid studies should be drawn **before** treatments begin. However, **do not wait** for results to begin treatment. Other routine labs are non-specific, but may be useful in diagnosing the precipitating illness, i.e., sepsis, infection, DKA. Hyperglycemia is common.

(D) Salicylates may increase free T_3 and T_4 via decreasing protein binding. **Supplemental O_2** is needed to support increased O_2 consumption. CHF may be refractory to standard therapy. Avoid atropine and β-adrenergic agents that may further increase heart rate and increase the risk for arrhythmias.

(E) **Propranolol** decreases the adrenergic hyperactivity via β-blockade. In addition, propranolol decreases the conversion of peripheral T_4 to active T_3. Therapeutic effects should be observed within 10 minutes of an IV dose. Repeat IV propranolol until there is a decrease in sympathetic symptoms such as tachcycardia, tremors, diaphoresis, and anxiety. Occasionally, patients may require higher doses of oral propranolol for adequate effect in the first 24 to 48 hours.

(F) **Thiourea medications (PTU and methimazole)** decrease the synthesis of thyroid hormones by inhibiting tyrosine residue organification. In addition, PTU also decreases the peripheral conversion of T_4 to active T_3. Maintenance doses are required for 2 to 6 weeks. No parenteral form is available for either medication.

(G) **Iodide** inhibits the release of stored thyroid hormones. **Administer $\geq$ one hour** after **thiourea** medications, otherwise the iodide will be incorporated in the production of further thyroid hormone.

(H) Although the mechanism is uncertain, glucocorticoids have been shown to increase survival in thyrotoxicosis. **Dexamethasone** decreases peripheral conversion of T_4 to T_3 and may be preferred over hydrocortisone.

(I) Infection, especially pneumonia, is the most common precipitating illness. Other common precipitating factors include sepsis, post-op surgical thyroidectomy, trauma, burns, DKA, hyperosmolar coma, insulin reaction, iodide/iodine-containing medications, thyroid hormone overdose, vascular accidents, pulmonary emboli, toxemia, and emotional stress.

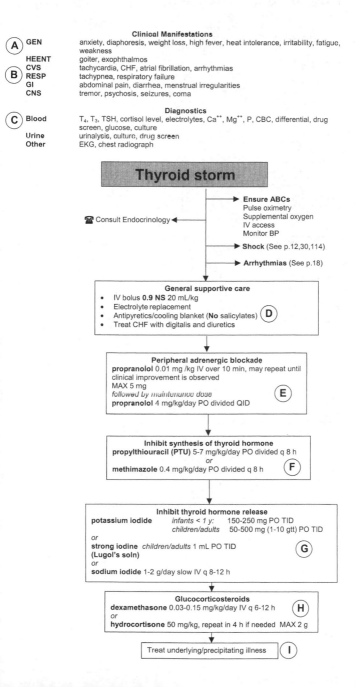

Clinical Manifestations

A GEN   anxiety, diaphoresis, weight loss, high fever, heat intolerance, irritability, fatigue, weakness
    HEENT   goiter, exophthalmos
B CVS   tachycardia, CHF, atrial fibrillation, arrhythmias
    RESP   tachypnea, respiratory failure
    GI   abdominal pain, diarrhea, menstrual irregularities
    CNS   tremor, psychosis, seizures, coma

Diagnostics

C Blood T_4, T_3, TSH, cortisol level, electrolytes, Ca^{++}, Mg^{++}, P, CBC, differential, drug screen, glucose, culture
    Urine   urinalysis, culture, drug screen
    Other   EKG, chest radiograph

Thyroid storm

☎ Consult Endocrinology ◄

► **Ensure ABCs**
Pulse oximetry
Supplemental oxygen
IV access
Monitor BP

► **Shock** (See p.12,30,114)

► **Arrhythmias** (See p.18)

General supportive care
- IV bolus **0.9 NS** 20 mL/kg
- Electrolyte replacement
- Antipyretics/cooling blanket (**No** salicylates) **D**
- Treat CHF with digitalis and diuretics

Peripheral adrenergic blockade
propranolol 0.01 mg/kg IV over 10 min, may repeat until clinical improvement is observed
MAX 5 mg
followed by maintenance dose
propranolol 4 mg/kg/day PO divided QID **E**

Inhibit synthesis of thyroid hormone
propylthiouracil (PTU) 5-7 mg/kg/day PO divided q 8 h
or
methimazole 0.4 mg/kg/day PO divided q 8 h **F**

Inhibit thyroid hormone release
potassium iodide   *infants < 1 y:*   150-250 mg PO TID
    children/adults   50-500 mg (1-10 gtt) PO TID
or
strong iodine   *children/adults* 1 mL PO TID
(Lugol's soln)   **G**
or
sodium iodide 1-2 g/day slow IV q 8-12 h

Glucocorticosteroids
dexamethasone 0.03-0.15 mg/kg/day IV q 6-12 h **H**
or
hydrocortisone 50 mg/kg, repeat in 4 h if needed MAX 2 g

Treat underlying/precipitating illness **I**

Chapter 4 ♣ Gastrointestinal Disorders

Acute Abdominal Pain

Michael Stargardt

Common causes of abdominal pain

Newborns	Infants
Anatomic obstruction: • atresia • stenosis • duplications Functional obstruction: • achalasia • pyloric stenosis • aganglionic megacolon • meconium ileus • necrotizing enterocolitis • malrotation • intussusception Traumatic injury	• GERD • esophagitis • midgut volvulus • intussusception • UTI • hepatitis • ureteropelvic obstruction • tumors • traumatic injury

Location	Child	Adolescent
Epigastric	peptic ulcer disease, hiatal hernia, esophagitis, pancreatitis	
Periumbilical	appendicitis, cholangitis, inflammatory bowel disease, Meckel's diverticulum, pancreatitis	
LUQ	splenic abscess, splenic sequestration, malignancy	splenic abscess, malignancy
RUQ	hepatitis, liver abscess, tumors, cholecystitis, cholangitis	
RLQ/LLQ	appendicitis, inflammatory bowel disease	appendicitis, inflammatory bowel disease, tubo-ovarian abscess, acute ovarian torsion, PID, ectopic pregnancy
Suprapubic	UTI, ureteropelvic obstruction, urolithiasis	UTI, ureteropelvic obstruction, urolithiasis, pregnancy, PID, dysmenorrhea

Abdominal pain resulting from traumatic injury varies in location depending on the site of injury.

Note: referred pain from pneumonia may mimic acute abdomen, therefore a chest radiograph should always be obtained in the work-up of a patient with acute abdominal pain or acute abdomen.

Clinical Manifestations

HISTORY	onset, location, referral of pain, quality, history of trauma
GEN	fever, irritability, weight loss
CV	tachycardia, hypotension
RESP	tachypnea, shallow breathing (splinting), rales (with pneumonia)
GI	acute abdominal pain, localized tenderness, voluntary/involuntary guarding, rebound tenderness, abdominal distention, hypo/hyperactive bowel sounds, history of hematochezia, melena, Murphy's sign, palpable abdominal, inguinal or adnexal mass

Diagnostics

Blood	CBC, differential, electrolytes, Ca^{++}, LFTs, amylase, lipase
Urine	urinalysis, culture, pregnancy test
Imaging	3-views abdominal radiographs, chest radiograph, CT scan, ultrasound, if considering inflicted injuries, obtain skeletal survey
Others	stool guaiac

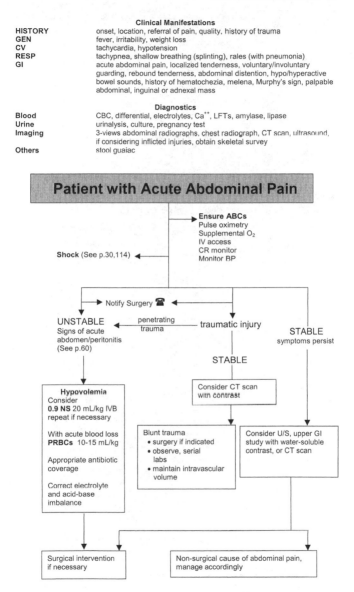

Patient with Acute Abdominal Pain

Ensure ABCs
Pulse oximetry
Supplemental O_2
IV access
CR monitor
Monitor BP

Shock (See p.30,114)

→ Notify Surgery ☎ ←

UNSTABLE
Signs of acute
abdomen/peritonitis
(See p.60)

← penetrating trauma — traumatic injury

STABLE
symptoms persist

STABLE

Hypovolemia
Consider
0.9 NS 20 mL/kg IVB
repeat if necessary

With acute blood loss
PRBCs 10-15 mL/kg

Appropriate antibiotic
coverage

Correct electrolyte
and acid-base
imbalance

Consider CT scan
with contrast

Blunt trauma
• surgery if indicated
• observe, serial labs
• maintain intravascular volume

Consider U/S, upper GI
study with water-soluble
contrast, or CT scan

Surgical intervention
if necessary

Non-surgical cause of abdominal pain,
manage accordingly

The Acute Abdomen/Peritonitis

Christina Shanti, Michael Stargardt, and Michael Klein

(A) A detailed history characterizing the pain is the key to establishing diagnosis:
1. Onset – acute (ischemia in volvulus, intussusception, gonad torsion), insidious or progressive (appendicitis).
2. Location – epigastrium (foregut), umbilicus (midgut), hypogastrium (hindgut), right iliac fossa, left iliac fossa, loin.
3. Pattern – intermittent (intussusception), continuous (appendicitis), colicky (obstruction, nephrolithiasis).
4. Severity and uniqueness
5. Aggravating and alleviating factors
6. Associated symptoms: vomiting (onset, quantity, frequency, projectile, color), change in bowel habit, abnormal micturition, menstruation.
7. Chronology of symptoms
8. Other: travel, family history, extra-abdominal symptoms

(B) *Acute abdomen* is used to describe a group of diseases that can result in life-threatening emergencies, and include intestinal obstruction/perforation, traumatic injury, tumors, ischemic injury and infections with or without peritonitis.

Peritonitis is characterized by the inflammation of the peritoneal lining resulting from infectious, autoimmune, or chemical causes.
Primary peritonitis: the inflammation may result from infection outside of the abdomen which reaches the peritoneal cavity via hematogenous or lymphatic routes.
Secondary peritonitis: inflammation is a result of an intra-abdominal source of infection such as an abscess or following rupture of a visceral structure.

(C) Causes of Acute Abdomen

Immediate Surgical Intervention	Expedited Surgical Intervention	Non-Surgical
• Malrotation • Volvulus • Incarcerated hernia • Nonreducible intussusception • Complete bowel obstruction • Gonad torsion • Perforated NEC/viscus • Ectopic pregnancy • Post-trauma with instability	• Atresia • Appendicitis • Partial bowel obstruction • Abdominal mass (abscess, tumors) • Post-trauma, stable (pancreatic injury, bladder rupture)	• PID • VP shunt/PD catheter infection • NEC without perforation • Pancreatitis • Nephrolithiasis/UTI • Solid organ injury in stable post-trauma patient • Gastroenteritis • Pneumonia (referred pain) • DKA • Mesenteric adenitis • Sickle cell disease • Abdominal pain (See p.58)

(D) Causes of Peritonitis

Acute Primary Peritonitis	Acute Secondary Peritonitis	Special Circumstances
• Ascites due to nephrotic syndrome/hepatic failure • Budd-Chiari syndrome • Lupus • Rheumatoid arthritis • CHF • Systemic infections with *S. pneumoniae*, Group A Streptococcus, Enterococcus, Gram-negative enteric organisms	• Perforated appendicitis • Intussusception • Incarcerated hernias • Perforated NEC • IBD • Perforated peptic ulcer • Traumatic perforation	**Neonatal period** • NEC • meconium ileus • indomethacin-induced perforation **Postpubertal female** • Seeding of peritoneal cavity from GU tract (*N. gonorrhea*, *C. trachomatis*) **Indwelling catheters** • VP shunts, PD catheter

(E) Paracentesis (See p.262)
1. Do not remove a large amount of fluid too rapidly – may cause hypovolemia/hypotension
2. Empty bladder to prevent perforation
3. Do not insert needle through infected skin
4. Analysis: Gram stain, culture, specific gravity, protein, LDH, WBCs, RBCs, glucose, pH

(F) Antibiotics: provide adequate broad-spectrum coverage

Clinical Manifestations (A)

GEN	laying quietly, anxious looking, avoiding deep breaths, crying, with legs drawn up, fever, flushing, pallor, jaundice, signs of hypovolemia
HEENT	sunken eyes, dry mucous membranes
CVS	tachycardia, hypotension (septic shock or hypovolemia)
RESP	Kussmaul breathing, shallow breathing, tachypnea, grunting
GI	distended abdomen, absent or hyperactive bowel sounds, tenderness, local or generalized hyperesthesia, local guarding, board-like rigidity, rebound tenderness, palpable mass, rectal exam may show pelvic mass, bloody or impacted stools, CVA tenderness
GU	vaginal discharge, cervical motion tenderness, adnexal masses/tenderness,
CNS	lethargy, obtundation

Diagnostics

Blood	CBC, differential, electrolytes, ABG/CBG, BUN, creatinine, glucose, cultures Consider LFTs, amylase, lipase, in adolescent females - β-HCG, ESR
Urine	urinalysis, culture
Imaging	3-views abdominal radiograph, chest radiograph (to rule out pneumonia), ultrasound, upper GI series, barium enema, CT scan
Others	stool culture (diarrhea), vaginal culture (PID), fluid cultures (VP, PD), peritoneal fluid for analysis and culture

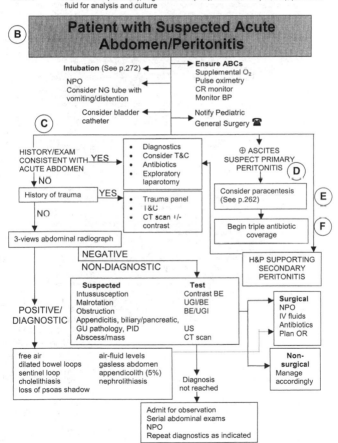

(B) **Patient with Suspected Acute Abdomen/Peritonitis**

Lower Gastrointestinal Bleeding

Kshama Daphtary

(A) Lower gastrointestinal bleeding is defined as bleeding that originates distal to the ligament of Treitz.

Hematochezia is the passage of bright or dark red stools per rectum.
Melena is the passage of black, tarry stools.
Red guaiac-negative stools may be seen with red Jell-O®, fruit punch, licorice, red candy or food coloring, laxatives, rifampin, beets.
Black guaiac-negative stools may be seen with bismuth (Pepto-Bismol®), iron, spinach, activated charcoal.
False positive guaiac stools may be seen after ingestion of red fruits and meats.

Determine the following:
- Is it really blood?
- Is the patient hemodynamically stable?
- Is the bleeding from the upper or lower GI tract? What is the site of the bleeding?
- Is the bleeding acute, chronic, or ongoing?

Causes of Lower Gastrointestinal Bleeding

Newborn	anal fissure, allergic proctocolitis, necrotizing enterocolitis, malrotation with midgut volvulus, Hirschsprung's disease with enterocolitis, vascular malformations
Infant	anal fissure, infectious colitis, allergic proctocolitis, intussusception, Meckel's diverticulum, lymphonodular hyperplasia, intestinal duplication
Toddler	infectious colitis, anal fissure, juvenile polyps, lymphonodular hyperplasia, Meckel's diverticulum, hemolytic uremic syndrome, Henoch-Schönlein purpura
Child/Adolescent	Inflammatory bowel disease, infectious colitis, juvenile polyps

The differential diagnosis of ill-appearing infants with GI bleeding should include *midgut volvulus*, *necrotizing enterocolitis*, and *Hirschsprung's disease*. Necrotizing enterocolitis (NEC) is characterized by nonspecific signs of sepsis (temperature instability, apnea, bradycardia), ileus, abdominal distention, bilious vomiting, GI bleeding, or abdominal wall erythema. Radiologic findings include pneumatosis intestinalis, pneumoperitoneum, or portal venous air.

Children with *inflammatory bowel disease* (IBD) may present with bloody diarrhea, abdominal pain, fever, anemia, and weight loss. Extraintestinal manifestations include arthralgia, skin lesions (erythema nodosum, pyoderma gangrenosum), liver disease (chronic hepatitis, sclerosing cholangitis), uveitis, oral ulceration, and growth retardation. Suspect toxic megacolon in the child with IBD who presents with abdominal distention and fever in 'septic shock'. Perianal ulceration, right lower quadrant abdominal pain associated with a 'mass' may be seen in Crohn's disease.

Inquire about:
- *Nature of bleeding* - hematochezia versus melena, magnitude of bleeding, duration of bleeding, associated GI or systemic symptoms
- *Associated GI symptoms* - vomiting, diarrhea, constipation, cramping, abdominal pain
- *Associated systemic symptoms* - fever, rash, joint pain, shortness of breath, pallor, palpitations, cool extremities, growth retardation, weight loss
- *Medications* - NSAIDs, warfarin, corticosteroids, iron, alcohol, theophylline, antibiotics
- *Past medical history* - GI or liver disorders, bleeding disorders, anesthesia reactions
- *Family history* - of GI disorders (polyps, ulcers, colitis), liver disease, bleeding disorders, anesthesia reactions

(B) Because acidic pH lowers the sensitivity of the guaiac test, use specific cards adjusted for testing for heme in gastric aspirates.

(C) Consider PRBC transfusion to maintain hematocrit > 30% in either the presence of ongoing blood loss or excessive blood loss. Consider transfusing patients with preexisting heart or lung disease early in their presentation.

(D) *Meckel's diverticulum* is the most common source of significant GI bleeding in children. Bleeding is typically painless and may be intermittent or massive. A technetium Tc99 scan may identify heterotopic gastric tissue in the diverticulum.

(A) Clinical Manifestations

SKIN	pallor, jaundice, ecchymosis, spider hemangiomata, prominent vessels over abdomen
HEENT	nasopharyngeal erythema/oozing/clots, tonsillar enlargement or bleeding, mucosal pigmentation
CVS	tachycardia, orthostatic hypotension, hypotension
GI	organomegaly, masses, ascites, tenderness, perianal fissure/fistula/induration, rectal tenderness or gross blood
EXT	soft tissue lesions, bone tumors

Diagnostics

Blood	CBC, differential, PT, PTT, type and cross match, peripheral smear, consider ESR, LFTs, GGT, albumin, total protein
Imaging	abdominal radiograph, consider radionuclide scan (Tc99)
Other	stool culture, fecal leukocytes, consider endoscopy

Lower Gastrointestinal Bleeding

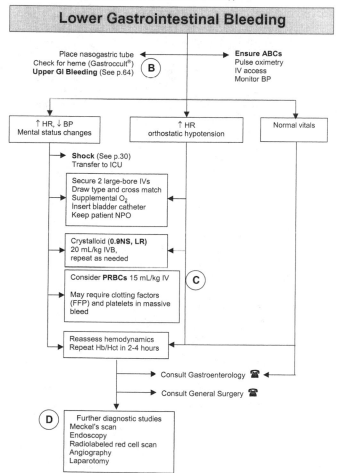

Place nasogastric tube
Check for heme (Gastroccult®)
Upper GI Bleeding (See p.64)

(B)

Ensure ABCs
Pulse oximetry
IV access
Monitor BP

↑ HR, ↓ BP
Mental status changes

↑ HR
orthostatic hypotension

Normal vitals

Shock (See p.30)
Transfer to ICU

Secure 2 large-bore IVs
Draw type and cross match
Supplemental O₂
Insert bladder catheter
Keep patient NPO

Crystalloid (**0.9NS, LR**)
20 mL/kg IVB,
repeat as needed

Consider **PRBCs** 15 mL/kg IV

May require clotting factors
(FFP) and platelets in massive
bleed

(C)

Reassess hemodynamics
Repeat Hb/Hct in 2-4 hours

Consult Gastroenterology ☎

Consult General Surgery ☎

(D) Further diagnostic studies
Meckel's scan
Endoscopy
Radiolabeled red cell scan
Angiography
Laparotomy

Upper Gastrointestinal Bleeding

Kshama Daphtary

(A) Upper gastrointestinal bleeding is defined as bleeding that originates proximal to the ligament of Treitz.

Hematemesis is the passage of vomited material that is black ("coffee-grounds") or contains frank blood.
Melena is the passage of black, tarry stools.
Red guaiac-negative emesis may be seen with red Jell-O®, fruit punch, licorice, red candy or food coloring, laxatives, rifampin, beets.
Black guaiac-negative stools may be seen with bismuth (Pepto-Bismol®), iron, spinach, activated charcoal.

Determine the following:
- Is it really blood?
- Is the patient hemodynamically stable?
- Is the bleeding from the upper or lower GI tract? What is the site of the bleeding?
- Is the bleeding acute, chronic, or ongoing?

Causes of Upper Gastrointestinal Bleeding

Newborn	swallowed maternal blood, vitamin K deficiency, gastritis, duplication cysts, vascular malformations, bleeding disorders
Infant	gastritis, esophagitis, Mallory-Weiss tear, stress ulcer
Toddler	gastritis, esophagitis, peptic ulcer disease, epistaxis, Mallory-Weiss tear, esophageal varices
Child/Adolescent	esophageal varices, peptic ulcer disease, Mallory-Weiss tear

In particular, elicit history for suspected foreign body, severe gastroesophageal reflux (esophagitis), alcohol (esophageal varices, gastritis) or NSAIDS abuse (gastritis), bulimia (esophagitis). Note: stress ulcers may be seen in patients with burns, trauma, sepsis, and shock.

(B) Placement of a nasogastric tube in patients with cirrhosis facilitates the removal of blood, which could otherwise precipitate encephalopathy. It confirms the presence of bleeding and helps document ongoing blood loss. Gastric lavage can be performed, which cleans the stomach prior to endoscopy. Because acidic pH lowers the sensitivity of the guaiac test, use specific cards adjusted for testing for heme in gastric aspirates.

(C) *Apt-Downey Test*
Mix one part vomitus/stool with five parts water. Centrifuge at 2000 rpm x 2 min, and mix the 5 parts supernatant to one part 0.1N NaOH. Fetal hemoglobin, which is more resistant to alkali denaturation than adult hemoglobin, remains pink whereas maternal hemoglobin turns brown.

(D) Consider endotracheal intubation to protect the airway and assist ventilation in patients with:
- respiratory insufficiency
- altered mental status
- ongoing hematemesis
- prior to balloon tamponade of esophageal varices

(E) Consider **PRBC transfusion** to maintain hematocrit > 30% in either the presence of ongoing blood loss or excessive blood loss. Consider transfusing patients with preexisting heart or lung disease early in their presentation.

(F) In patients with chronic liver disease, melena or a sentinel bleed may precede sudden hematemesis and shock. Significant bleeding with hypotension often precipitates further liver dysfunction and the development of ascites and encephalopathy. Hepatic encephalopathy must be anticipated; treat with **lactulose**. β-blockers, which are often used for GI bleed prophylaxis, may mask signs of hemodynamic instability.

Common side effects of splanchnic vasoactive agents: skin pallor, abdominal colic, chest pain, water retention and hyponatremia, seizures, hypotension.

(A) **Clinical Manifestations**

SKIN	pallor, jaundice, ecchymosis, spider hemangiomata, prominent vessels over abdomen
HEENT	nasopharyngeal erythema/oozing/clots, tonsillar enlargement or bleeding, mucosal pigmentation
CVS	tachycardia, orthostatic hypotension, hypotension, back pain
GI	organomegaly, masses, ascites, tenderness, perianal fissure/fistula/induration, rectal tenderness or gross blood
EXT	soft tissue lesions, bone tumors

Diagnostics

Blood	CBC, differential, PT, PTT, type and cross match, peripheral smear, BUN, creatinine, consider ESR, LFTs, GGT, albumin, total protein
Imaging	abdominal radiograph
Other	consider endoscopy

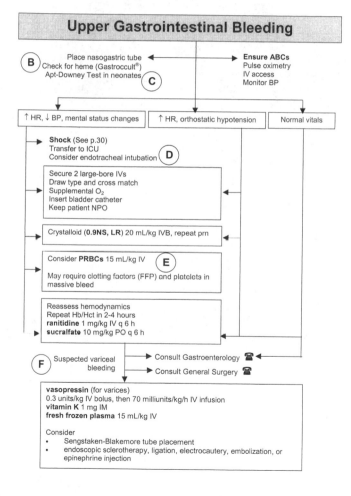

Upper Gastrointestinal Bleeding

(B) Place nasogastric tube
Check for heme (Gastroccult®)
Apt-Downey Test in neonates (C)

Ensure ABCs
Pulse oximetry
IV access
Monitor BP

↑ HR, ↓ BP, mental status changes	↑ HR, orthostatic hypotension	Normal vitals

Shock (See p.30)
Transfer to ICU
Consider endotracheal intubation (D)

Secure 2 large-bore IVs
Draw type and cross match
Supplemental O$_2$
Insert bladder catheter
Keep patient NPO

Crystalloid (**0.9NS, LR**) 20 mL/kg IVB, repeat prn

Consider **PRBCs** 15 mL/kg IV (E)

May require clotting factors (FFP) and platelets in massive bleed

Reassess hemodynamics
Repeat Hb/Hct in 2-4 hours
ranitidine 1 mg/kg IV q 6 h
sucralfate 10 mg/kg PO q 6 h

(F) Suspected variceal bleeding
→ Consult Gastroenterology ☎
→ Consult General Surgery ☎

vasopressin (for varices)
0.3 units/kg IV bolus, then 70 milliunits/kg/h IV infusion
vitamin K 1 mg IM
fresh frozen plasma 15 mL/kg IV

Consider
- Sengstaken-Blakemore tube placement
- endoscopic sclerotherapy, ligation, electrocautery, embolization, or epinephrine injection

Gastrointestinal Obstruction

Mustafa H. Kabeer and Michael Klein

> The gastrointestinal tract is a flexible, compliant, motile tube. Clinical observation is based on signs and symptoms resulting from the point of obstruction of this tube. Obstruction can be structural (e.g., atresia, adhesions) or functional (e.g., dysmotility, Hirschsprung's). Distention will occur proximal to the point of obstruction, and will be more pronounced with distal obstruction.
> In general, surgery is indicated in the presence of a double bubble sign or with clinical signs of obstruction and loops of bowel that can be counted. Obtain contrast study with obstruction if bowel loops are too numerous to count.

A

Differential Diagnosis Based on Level of GI Obstruction

Level	Nonbilious, Nondistended	Bilious, Nondistended	Bilious, Distended	Nonbilious, Distended
Esophageal				
TEF				
Gastric				
GERD				
Pyloric stenosis				
Small bowel				
Duodenal atresia				
Malrotation				
Jejunal atresia				
Ileal atresia				
Adhesive band				
Hernia				
Intussusception				
Neoplasm				
Colon				
Hirschsprung				
Meconium ileus				
Small left colon				
Meconium plug				
Colonic atresia				
NEC stricture				
Neoplasm				
Rectal				
Imperforate anus				

Note that systemic and localized inflammatory processes can produce ileus and resemble obstruction. These conditions may require both medical and surgical treatment (e.g., appendicitis, Crohn disease).

B

Blood chemistries should be obtained to detect electrolyte imbalances that result from emesis and dehydration.

Leucocytosis and thrombocytopenia may suggest infection/sepsis.

Urinalysis may be helpful in diagnosis of sepsis and imperforate anus.

Imaging should include 3 views of the abdomen, one of which should be a prone view, to help in visualizing colonic gas. Use hyperosmolar contrast medium if suspecting meconium ileus, barium for Hirschsprung's disease, and air contrast for intussusception.

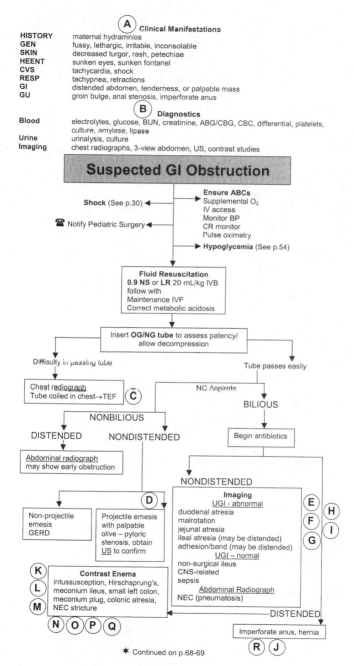

(A) **Clinical Manifestations**

HISTORY	maternal hydramnios
GEN	fussy, lethargic, irritable, inconsolable
SKIN	decreased turgor, rash, petechiae
HEENT	sunken eyes, sunken fontanel
CVS	tachycardia, shock
RESP	tachypnea, retractions
GI	distended abdomen, tenderness, or palpable mass
GU	groin bulge, anal stenosis, imperforate anus

(B) **Diagnostics**

Blood	electrolytes, glucose, BUN, creatinine, ABG/CBG, CBC, differential, platelets, culture, amylase, lipase
Urine	urinalysis, culture
Imaging	chest radiographs, 3-view abdomen, US, contrast studies

Suspected GI Obstruction

Ensure ABCs
Supplemental O₂
IV access
Monitor BP
CR monitor
Pulse oximetry

Shock (See p.30)

☎ Notify Pediatric Surgery

➤ **Hypoglycemia** (See p.54)

Fluid Resuscitation
0.9 NS or **LR** 20 mL/kg IVB
follow with
Maintenance IVF
Correct metabolic acidosis

Insert **OG/NG tube** to assess patency/
allow decompression

Difficulty in passing tube

Chest radiograph
Tube coiled in chest→TEF (C)

Tube passes easily

NG Aspirate

BILIOUS

NONBILIOUS

DISTENDED   **NONDISTENDED**

Abdominal radiograph
may show early obstruction

Begin antibiotics

NONDISTENDED
Imaging
UGI - abnormal
duodenal atresia
malrotation
jejunal atresia
ileal atresia (may be distended)
adhesion/band (may be distended)
UGI – normal
non-surgical ileus
CNS-related
sepsis
Abdominal Radiograph
NEC (pneumatosis)

(E) (H)
(F) (I)
(G)

Non-projectile
emesis
GERD

(D) Projectile emesis
with palpable
olive – pyloric
stenosis, obtain
US to confirm

(K) (L) (M) **Contrast Enema**
intussusception, Hirschsprung's,
meconium ileus, small left colon,
meconium plug, colonic atresia,
NEC stricture

(N) (O) (P) (Q)

DISTENDED

Imperforate anus, hernia

(R) (J)

✱ Continued on p.68-69

Gastrointestinal Obstruction in Infants and Children

	Lesion	Clinical Presentation	Association	Diagnosis	Management	Cautions
(C)	Esophageal atresia, T-E fistula	excessive salivation, coughing, gagging, pneumonia	VACTERL (25%), cardiac (35%), GI (24%) – duodenal atresia, imperforate anus	pass NG, chest and abdominal radiograph, pouchogram, bronchoscopy, esoph atresia→gasless abdomen	drain proximal pouch, surgery: divide fistula, esophagoesophagostomy	Keep HOB ↑ 30-45° to minimize aspiration
(D)	Pyloric stenosis	projectile nonbilious emesis, palpable olive	family history, certain ABO groups	history/physical exam, UGI/US, electrolytes ($\downarrow Cl^-$, $\downarrow K^+$ metab alkalosis)	NPO, correct electrolytes surgery: pyloromyotomy	pre-operative resuscitation
(E)	Duodenal atresia	bilious emesis usual (85% distal to ampulla) maternal oligohydramnios	annular pancreas, malrotation, Down syndrome (30%), prematurity (25-50%)	abdominal radiograph – double bubble sign	NPO, NG, IV fluids, antibiotics, surgery: duodenoduodenostomy	rule out malrotation and volvulus
(F)	Malrotation	bilious emesis	diaphragmatic hernia, abdominal wall defects, CHD, heterotaxia, duodenal atresia	UGI or BE, abdominal radiograph – double bubble sign	NPO, NG, IV fluids, antibiotics, surgery: Ladd procedure and appendectomy	**Risk for midgut volvulus, treat immediately**
(G)	Jejunal atresia	bilious emesis, mild distention, jaundice	multiple atresia (6-20%), malrotation (10%), Hirschsprung's disease (15%)	UGI or BE	NPO, NG, IV fluids, antibiotics, surgery: bowel resection and anastomosis	apple peel or Christmas tree variant – familial, premature (50%), malrotation (50%)
(H)	Ileal atresia	bilious emesis, distention, jaundice		abdominal radiograph: air fluid levels, calcium=meconium peritonitis (10%), BE		higher mortality with multiple atresias, meconium ileus and peritonitis due to antenatal perforation
(I)	Post-op adhesions	pain, anorexia, nausea, vomiting, distention	previous intra-abdominal surgery or infection	abdominal radiograph, UGI, consider CT scan	NPO, NG, IV fluids, antibiotics, surgery: adhesiolysis	beware of internal hernias and closed loop obstruction
(J)	Hernia	palpable mass in the groin, pain, emesis	mainly in boys (6:1), usually right sided (60%)	physical examination	sedation and reduction, surgery: herniorrhaphy	high risk of incarceration in premies < 1y, may contain ovaries (risk of torsion) in females
(K)	Intussusception	well nourished, sudden intermittent pain (81%), emesis, bloody stools (58%), RUQ mass (57%)	HSP, hemophilia, lymphoma, CF	physical examination, abdominal radiograph, contrast enema	NPO, NG, IV fluids, contrast enema (air reduction 95% successful), surgery: reduction and resection	be aware of pathologic lead points in 2-8%, and post-op intussusception

	Presentation	Associations	Diagnosis	Treatment	Notes
(L) Hirschsprung	bilious emesis, distention, failure to pass meconium, alternating obstipation and diarrhea	familial, Down syndrome (10%)	BE, suction rectal biopsy	NPO, NG, IV fluids, antibiotics, surgery: resection and pull-through	prone to enterocolitis (50%), suction biopsy must be done above dentate line
(M) Meconium ileus	bilious emesis, distention, failure to pass meconium	CF (20%), volvulus/atresia/perforation (25%)	abdominal radiograph: ground glass/soap bubble, calcium indicates antenatal perforation, contrast enema	uncomplicated: N-acetylcysteine or hyperosmolar enema or operate, irrigate and close; complicated: operate, irrigate and close or stomas in select cases	genetic studies and sweat test to check to CF
(N) Colonic atresia	bilious emesis, distention	skeletal anomalies, small bowel atresia, ocular defects, Hirschsprung, diaphragmatic hernia	abdominal radiograph, BE	NPO, NG, IV fluids, surgery: resection and stoma or anastomosis	prone to perforate at: transverse colon
(O) Meconium plug syndrome	bilious emesis, distention, failure to pass meconium	Hirschsprung (10%)	contrast enema	contrast enema	consider sweat test, suction rectal biopsy to rule out Hirschsprung
(P) Small left colon	bilious emesis, distention, failure to pass meconium	diabetic mothers, use of magnesium during labor	contrast enema	contrast enema and time	
(Q) NEC stricture	emesis, distention, prematurity, feeding intolerance, NEC	umbilical lines, hyperosmolar formula, prematurity, use of indomethacin	abdominal radiograph, BE	NPO, NG, IV fluids, antibiotics, surgery: resection and anastomosis	should fully evaluate the colon before surgery
(R) Imperforate anus	usually boys, improperly placed anus, absent anus	VACTERL, CHD, GI – duodenal atresia, TEF	physical examination, abdominal radiograph (include prone and cross table lateral views), US, urinalysis	dilate anal stenosis, surgery (for imperforate anus): colostomy and staged pull-through	need to determine if high or low lesion

Chapter 5 ♣ Hematological and Oncologic Disorders

Anemia

K. Jane Lee and Michael Fiore

> Anemia is a decrease in hemoglobin concentration 2 SD below the mean expected for age, sex and physiologic state.

LOWER LIMIT FOR HEMOGLOBIN (g/dl)	
> 36 weeks gestation	13
6 months to 4 years	11
5 to 7 years	11.5
8 to 11 years	12
12 to 14 years	
female	12
male	12.5
15 to 17 years	
female	12
male	13

PHYSIOLOGIC ANEMIA

Term infants by 8 to 12 weeks of age 9.4 g/dl
Pre-term infants by 3 to 6 weeks of age 7.0 g/dl

Mean Corpuscular Volume (MCV)

2 to 10 years	lower limit	70 + age in years
> 1 year	upper limit	84 + .6 (age in years)
Adults	upper limit	96

Mentzer Index = MCV/RBC in millions

Thalassemia	< 11
Iron deficiency	> 13

A Clinical manifestations depend on the severity and the rapidity of drop in hemoglobin. Significant acute blood loss can result in hemodynamic instability and/or shock. Chronic anemia may produce a picture related to a chronic decrease in O_2 carrying capacity with resultant high output CHF.

B Indicators of hemolysis: (1) ↑ reticulocyte count, (2) ↑ serum bilirubin (extravascular hemolysis), (3) ↑ LDH, (4) ↓ haptoglobin and hempexin (intravascular hemolysis), (5) schistocytes in peripheral smear

Other Laboratory Tests

Condition	Type of Tube	Amount of Blood
Folate deficiency	EDTA (purple top)	3 mL
Cobalamine deficiency	Plain (red top)	3 mL
All membrane defects e.g., spherocytosis	ACD (yellow top)	5 mL in infants 5-10 mL in older children
Enzyme defects	ACD (yellow top) if not available use buffered sodium citrate (light blue top)	2 mL MIN
Hemoglobinopathies	EDTA (purple top)	3 mL

C Severe anemia accompanied by hemodynamic instability is usually due to acute and significant blood loss (> 5% of total blood volume) or pooling.

D

Microcytic

	Clinical Manifestations	Etiology	Diagnostic Evaluation	Management
Iron Deficiency	• Most common cause of microcytic anemia • Pallor, irritability, pica	• ↓ dietary intake (especially infants drinking excessive amounts of whole milk) • Low birthweight • Blood loss	• Microcytosis, hypochromia, poikilocytosis • Mentzer index (MCV/RBC) > 13.5 • ↑ RDW • Trial of iron • ↑ FEP	• Elemental iron 3-6 mg/kg/day x 3-6 months • Reticulocytosis peaks in 5-7 days of treatment
Alpha Thalassemia	• May be asymptomatic • Severe form - transfusion dependent	• Quantitative disorder of α - globin synthesis	• Tear drop cells, target cells • May see intracellular inclusions • Mentzer index < 11.5 • Normal RDW • Hemoglobin electrophoresis	• Dependent on severity of disease
Beta Thalassemia Trait	• Mild anemia • Usually asymptomatic • Often misdiagnosed as iron deficiency anemia	• Heterozygous gene expression for β globulin chain	• Microcytosis, hypochromia, poikilocytosis • ↓ MCV, ↓ MCH • Mentzer index < 11.5	• None

✱ Continued on page 72

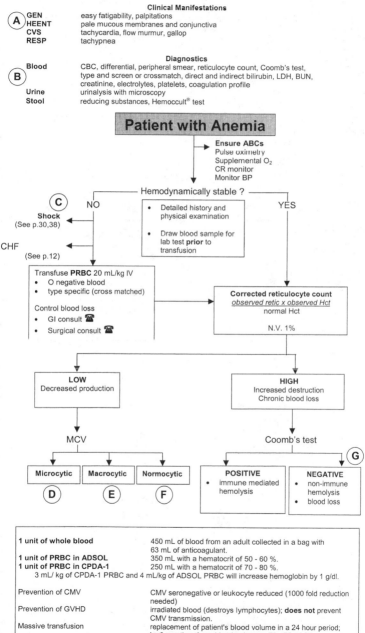

Clinical Manifestations

(A)
GEN	easy fatigability, palpitations
HEENT	pale mucous membranes and conjunctiva
CVS	tachycardia, flow murmur, gallop
RESP	tachypnea

Diagnostics

(B)
Blood	CBC, differential, peripheral smear, reticulocyte count, Coomb's test, type and screen or crossmatch, direct and indirect bilirubin, LDH, BUN, creatinine, electrolytes, platelets, coagulation profile
Urine	urinalysis with microscopy
Stool	reducing substances, Hemoccult® test

Patient with Anemia

Ensure ABCs
Pulse oximetry
Supplemental O₂
CR monitor
Monitor BP

Hemodynamically stable ?

NO — YES

(C) **Shock** (See p.30,38)

CHF (See p.12)

Detailed history and physical examination

Draw blood sample for lab test **prior** to transfusion

Transfuse **PRBC** 20 mL/kg IV
- O negative blood
- type specific (cross matched)

Control blood loss
- GI consult ☎
- Surgical consult ☎

Corrected reticulocyte count
observed retic x observed Hct
normal Hct

N.V. 1%

LOW Decreased production

HIGH Increased destruction Chronic blood loss

MCV

Microcytic	Macrocytic	Normocytic
(D)	(E)	(F)

Coomb's test (G)

POSITIVE
- immune mediated hemolysis

NEGATIVE
- non-immune hemolysis
- blood loss

1 unit of whole blood	450 mL of blood from an adult collected in a bag with 63 mL of anticoagulant.
1 unit of PRBC in ADSOL	350 mL with a hematocrit of 50 - 60 %.
1 unit of PRBC in CPDA-1	250 mL with a hematocrit of 70 - 80 %.

3 mL/ kg of CPDA-1 PRBC and 4 mL/kg of ADSOL PRBC will increase hemoglobin by 1 g/dl.

Prevention of CMV	CMV seronegative or leukocyte reduced (1000 fold reduction needed)
Prevention of GVHD	irradiated blood (destroys lymphocytes); **does not** prevent CMV transmission.
Massive transfusion	replacement of patient's blood volume in a 24 hour period; by 3 months of age blood volume = 70 - 75 mL/kg.

✳ Continued from p.70

E

Macrocytic

	Clinical Manifestations	Etiology	Diagnostic Evaluation	Management
Folate Deficiency	• Fatigue • Glossitis • Neuropsychiatric disorders	• Anticonvulsants • Congenital malabsorption	• Serum folate • Neutrophils - hypersegmented nuclei	• **Folic acid**
Vitamin B_{12} Deficiency	• Fatigue • Glossitis • Peripheral neuropathy • Ataxia • Coma	• Pernicious anemia • Transcobalamin deficiency • B_{12} malabsorption	• Serum B_{12} • Basophilic stippling • Pancytopenia often seen	• **Vitamin B_{12}**
Diamond-Blackfan Syndrome	• Pallor • 1/3 associated with congenital anomalies	• Autosomal recessive or dominant in 15%	• Macrocytosis, normochromic • ↑ Folic acid • ↑ Hb F, i antigen • ↑ ADA	• **Steroids** (2mg/kg/d)
Normal Newborn			• Macrocytic but not anemic	• None

F

Normocytic

	Clinical Manifestations	Etiology	Diagnostic Evaluation	Management
Acute Blood Loss	• Dizziness • Syncope • Orthostatic changes • Tachycardia • Hypotension • Shock	• Meckel's diverticulum • Trauma • GI bleed • Hemoptysis • Menorrhagia • Splenic sequestration	• Examine for obvious and occult causes of bleeding • Smear may be normal	• Blood transfusion if symptomatic • Treat underlying cause • Maintain intravascular volume
Chronic Renal Failure	• May be asymptomatic • Signs and symptoms of renal failure	• ↓ erythropoietin production	• Creatinine BUN • Schistocytes, burr cells	• Treat renal failure • Erythropoietin
Anemia Of Chronic Inflammation	• Frequently asymptomatic	• Any chronic inflammatory condition	• Normal reticulocyte count, target cells, schistocytes • ↑ ESR, ↑ ferritin	• Treat underlying cause
Bone Marrow Infiltration	• Bruising or bleeding • Prone to infections • Pain or pathologic fractures	• Malignancy • Osteopetrosis • Histiocytosis	• Pancytopenia • Bone marrow evaluation	• Blood transfusion if symptomatic • Treat malignancy
Physiologic Anemia Of Infancy	• Asymptomatic • Physiologic nadir at 6-8 wks of life in term infants	• Transient cessation of erythropoiesis at birth • Shortened survival of fetal RBC's • Rapid expansion of blood volume	• None required	• None
Aplastic Anemia	• Weakness • Bleeding • Bruising • Prone to infections	• Idiopathic • Viral infections (parvovirus B19) • Fanconi's anemia • Shwachman-Diamond syndrome	• Reticulocyte count • Bone marrow evaluation • Pancytopenia	• Transfusion • Immunotherapy • Bone marrow transplant
Transient Erythro-blastopenia of Childhood (TEC)	• 6 mos - 5 y age • May be asymptomatic • Pallor in previously well child	• May be associated with HHV-6 or parvovirus	• Hb F, ADA normal • MCV normal	• Transfusion if indicated • Spontaneous recovery 4-8 wks • Corticosteroids of no benefit

✳ Continued on p.73

✶ Continued from p.72

(G) <u>Causes of non-immune hemolysis</u>
Intrinsic Defects

Membrane defect	hereditary spherocytosis, hereditary elliptocytosis
Enzyme defect	G_6PD, PK, GPI, porphyrias
Hemoglobinopathies	SS, SC, S-β thalassemia, unstable hemoglobins

Extrinsic Defects
Mechanical, chemical, infections, increased phagocytosis

Disseminated Intravascular Coagulation (DIC)

Amin Alousi

> Disseminated intravascular coagulation (DIC) is an acquired disorder associated with a variety of underlying conditions (see list). This clinicopathologic syndrome occurs when the underlying disease process stimulates widespread activation of coagulation. The net result is intravascular deposition of fibrin, along with consumption of platelets and coagulation factors. This ultimately leads to bleeding and microvascular thrombosis with the potential for multi-organ failure.

A Clinical manifestation is variable, may range from prolonged bleeding at venipuncture sites and surgical sites to diffuse cutaneous and visceral hemorrhage. Patient will usually appear profoundly ill.

Diseases known to cause DIC

Infection	meningococcemia (purpura fulminans), other Gram-negative bacteria, encapsulated Gram-positive bacteria, NEC
Malignancy	ANLL (AML), metastases (neuroblastoma)
Tissue injury	shock, penetrating CNS trauma, crush injuries, fat emboli
Obstetrical complications	abruptio placentae, retained placenta or fetal tissue, sepsis, amniotic fluid emboli
Venom/toxins	snake bites, insect bites
Microangiopathic disorders	hemolytic uremic syndrome, Kasabach-Merritt syndrome (giant hemangioma)

B Fibrinogen level may fall within the normal range, as it is an acute phase reactant. Prothrombin activation fragment 1+2 and thrombin-antithrombin complexes have a high sensitivity and specificity for DIC, but are not readily available in all labs and are not usually essential.

Laboratory profile for DIC and other hematologic conditions

	DIC	Liver disease	Vitamin K deficiency/ warfarin use	Heparin use	Massive blood transfusion
PT	↑	↑	↑	↑	↑
PTT	↑	↑	↑	↑	↑
TT	↑	↑	N	↑	N/↑
Platelet count	↓	N/↓	N	N/↓	↓
Fibrinogen	↓	↓	N	N	↓
D-dimer	⊕	Negative/ weakly ⊕	Negative	Negative	Negative
Schistocytes on smear	**Yes**	Yes	No	No	No
FSP	↑	N/↑	N	N	N
Anti-thrombin III	↓	↓	N	N	↓
Factor VIII	↓	N/↑	N	N	↓
Factor V	↓	↓	N	N	↓
Factor II	↓	↓	↓	N	↓
Protein C, S	↓	↓↓	↓↓	N	↓

N = normal

Clinical Manifestations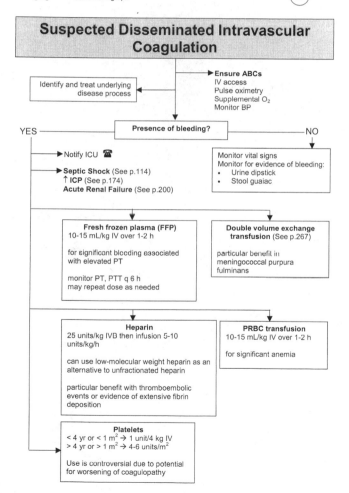

HEENT	epistaxis, mucous membrane bleeding
CVS	tachycardia, hypotension
RESP	hemoptysis, micropulmonary emboli
GI	stool occult blood, melena, hematochezia, hematemesis
GU	hematuria, renal insufficiency
CNS	increased intracranial pressure, intracranial bleed or ischemia
EXT	necrotic digits, acrocyanosis, prolonged capillary refill
SKIN	petechiae, purpura, oozing at venipuncture/surgical/gingival sites, purpura fulminans

Diagnostics

Blood	CBC, platelets, peripheral smear, PT, PTT, TT, fibrinogen, FSP/FDP, D-dimer, electrolytes, BUN, creatinine, LFTs, type and cross match, culture
Urine	urinalysis, culture
Imaging	chest radiograph

Suspected Disseminated Intravascular Coagulation

Identify and treat underlying disease process

Ensure ABCs
IV access
Pulse oximetry
Supplemental O₂
Monitor BP

Presence of bleeding?   YES ——   —— NO

NO:
Monitor vital signs
Monitor for evidence of bleeding:
- Urine dipstick
- Stool guaiac

YES:
Notify ICU ☎

Septic Shock (See p.114)
↑ **ICP** (See p.174)
Acute Renal Failure (See p.200)

Fresh frozen plasma (FFP)
10-15 mL/kg IV over 1-2 h

for significant bleeding associated with elevated PT

monitor PT, PTT q 6 h
may repeat dose as needed

Double volume exchange transfusion (See p.267)

particular benefit in meningococcal purpura fulminans

Heparin
25 units/kg IVB then infusion 5-10 units/kg/h

can use low-molecular weight heparin as an alternative to unfractionated heparin

particular benefit with thromboembolic events or evidence of extensive fibrin deposition

PRBC transfusion
10-15 mL/kg IV over 1-2 h

for significant anemia

Platelets
< 4 yr or < 1 m² → 1 unit/4 kg IV
> 4 yr or > 1 m² → 4-6 units/m²

Use is controversial due to potential for worsening of coagulopathy

Hemophilia Emergencies

Russell Clark

(A) Hemophilia is an X-linked recessive clotting factor deficiency disorder, with 20-25% of cases due to spontaneous mutation. Patients may present with:
- intracranial hemorrhage (ICH)
- intra-articular (IA) or intramuscular (IM) bleeding after minimal/occult trauma
- oral or mucosal bleeding
- post-circumcision bleeding (PCB)
- bruising in infants who crawl

Bleeding Disorders

Disorder	Deficiency	Prevalence	Diagnosis
Hemophilia A	Factor VIII:C	1/10,000, 85% of hemophiliacs	↑ PTT by Factor 8 assay
Hemophilia B (*aka* Christmas disease)	Factor IX	1/50,000, 10-15% of hemophiliacs	↑ PTT by Factor 9 assay
von Willebrand disease	Carrier protein for Factor VIII	1%, most common inherited bleeding disorder	↑ PTT, ↑ BT by vWF assay

Classification of Hemophilia

Classification	Inherent activity (%)/ Native plasma (U/dl)	Age of onset	Nature of hemorrhage	Typical initial presentation
Severe	<1	≤ 1 year	Frequent, unprovoked, IA/IM q 1-6 mos	PCB common, ICH occasional
Moderate	1 to 5	1-2 years	Often, following mild to moderate trauma	PCB common, ICH uncommon
Mild	> 5 (5-30)	2 years to adulthood	Following significant trauma or surgery, may go undiagnosed for years	Post-traumatic bleeding
Normal	50-150	N/A	N/A	N/A

Historical information to obtain in a patient with bleeding
- Is there a personal or family history of bleeding disorders?
- If the classification of hemophilia is unknown, ask about the initial presentation leading to the diagnosis. Is the hemophilia congenital or acquired?
- Did the patient bring Factor to the hospital? Has the patient ever had an allergic response to factor replacement? (Anaphylaxis is more common with Hemophilia B.)
- What is the patient's "target joint"?
- If the patient has von Willebrand's disease, is the type known?
- **Does the patient have factor inhibitors, if so, is the patient a high or low responder?**
- **Is the patient responsive to DDAVP?**

Coagulation Cascade

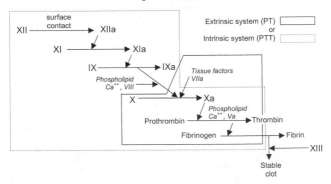

✳ Continued on p.78

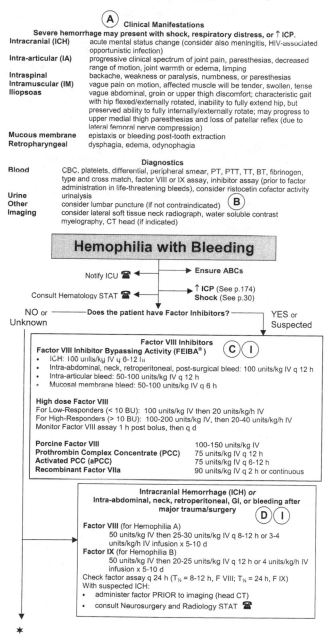

(A) Clinical Manifestations

Severe hemorrhage may present with shock, respiratory distress, or ↑ ICP.

Intracranial (ICH)	acute mental status change (consider also meningitis, HIV-associated opportunistic infection)
Intra-articular (IA)	progressive clinical spectrum of joint pain, paresthesias, decreased range of motion, joint warmth or edema, limping
Intraspinal	backache, weakness or paralysis, numbness, or paresthesias
Intramuscular (IM)	vague pain on motion, affected muscle will be tender, swollen, tense
Iliopsoas	vague abdominal, groin or upper thigh discomfort; characteristic gait with hip flexed/externally rotated, inability to fully extend hip, but preserved ability to fully internally/externally rotate; may progress to upper medial thigh paresthesias and loss of patellar reflex (due to lateral femoral nerve compression)
Mucous membrane	epistaxis or bleeding post-tooth extraction
Retropharyngeal	dysphagia, edema, odynophagia

Diagnostics

Blood	CBC, platelets, differential, peripheral smear, PT, PTT, TT, BT, fibrinogen, type and cross match, factor VIII or IX assay, inhibitor assay (prior to factor administration in life-threatening bleeds), consider ristocetin cofactor activity
Urine	urinalysis
Other	consider lumbar puncture (if not contraindicated) (B)
Imaging	consider lateral soft tissue neck radiograph, water soluble contrast myelography, CT head (if indicated)

Hemophilia with Bleeding

Notify ICU ☎ ◄──────── ► Ensure ABCs

Consult Hematology STAT ☎ ◄────── ↑ ICP (See p.174)
Shock (See p.30)

NO or ─────── Does the patient have Factor Inhibitors? ─────── YES or
Unknown   Suspected

Factor VIII Inhibitors

Factor VIII Inhibitor Bypassing Activity (FEIBA®) (C) (I)
- ICH: 100 units/kg IV q 6-12 h
- Intra-abdominal, neck, retroperitoneal, post-surgical bleed: 100 units/kg IV q 12 h
- Intra-articular bleed: 50-100 units/kg IV q 12 h
- Mucosal membrane bleed: 50-100 units/kg IV q 6 h

High dose Factor VIII
For Low-Responders (< 10 BU): 100 units/kg IV then 20 units/kg/h IV
For High-Responders (> 10 BU): 100-200 units/kg IV, then 20-40 units/kg/h IV
Monitor Factor VIII assay 1 h post bolus, then q d

Porcine Factor VIII	100-150 units/kg IV
Prothrombin Complex Concentrate (PCC)	75 units/kg IV q 12 h
Activated PCC (aPCC)	75 units/kg IV q 6-12 h
Recombinant Factor VIIa	90 units/kg IV q 2 h or continuous

Intracranial Hemorrhage (ICH) or
Intra-abdominal, neck, retroperitoneal, GI, or bleeding after
major trauma/surgery (D) (I)

Factor VIII (for Hemophilia A)
50 units/kg IV then 25-30 units/kg IV q 8-12 h or 3-4 units/kg/h IV infusion x 5-10 d
Factor IX (for Hemophilia B)
50 units/kg IV then 20-25 units/kg IV q 12 h or 4 units/kg/h IV infusion x 5-10 d
Check factor assay q 24 h (T½ = 8-12 h, F VIII; T½ = 24 h, F IX)
With suspected ICH:
- administer factor PRIOR to imaging (head CT)
- consult Neurosurgery and Radiology STAT ☎

★
Continued
on p.79

✳ Continued from p.76

B When considering lumbar puncture, raise Factor activity to at least 30% of normal prior to procedure.
Water-soluble contrast myelography is the most sensitive and definitive study for intraspinal hemorrhage.
Lateral soft tissue neck radiograph in patients with suspected retropharyngeal bleeding may be used to delineate degree of airway obstruction.

C **Factor inhibitors** are IgG antibodies that develop to the deficient factor being administered. Conduct management under the advisement of a Hematology service. Seen in 1/3 of patients with severe Hemophilia A, but only in 1-4% of those with Hemophilia B. If suspected, send blood for PTT and factor assay; a factor level of 30% should correct the PTT. Subsequent care post-stabilization should take place at a regional hemophilia center. A list of such centers is maintained by the National Hemophilia Foundation (212-328-3700, 800-42HANDI, info@hemophilia.org).

Inhibitor titers are measured in Bethesda Units (BU). Patients are classified as having a *high-responding* (>10 BU) or *low-responding* (<10 BU) anamnestic response to factor therapy.
Treatment consists of:
- **Factor VIII inhibitor bypassing activity** (FEIBA®)
  For use with either Factor VIII or IX inhibitors (long-term immune tolerance therapy required to achieve complete elimination of Factor VIII inhibitor) and in patients with an acquired Factor VIII, XI, or XIII inhibitor. Contains Factor II, activated Factor VII, Factors IX and X. From pooled human plasma, so viral transmission is possible.
- **high dose factor** replacement
- **porcine Factor VIII** therapy (Hyate®)
- **prothrombin complex concentrates** (PCCs: Bebulin VH®, Konyne 30®, Profilnine SD®, Proplex T®)
- **activated PCCs** (APPCs: Autopex T®)
- **recombinant Factor VIIa** infusion (NovoSeven®)
- plasmapheresis

D *Life-threatening hemorrhage can result from intracranial, intra-abdominal, neck, GI or retroperitoneal bleeding or following major trauma or surgery.* Mortality rates are 34% for ICH and 50% for long-term neurologic sequelae. ICH in children is usually preceded by trauma. Intracranial bleeding may be slow, with neurologic findings possibly not developing until days after a head injury. Admit for monitoring.

E *Intra-articular hemorrhage (IA)* is the most common complication in patients with hemophilia. In toddlers with a limp, IA hemorrhage is most often seen in ankles, knees, then elbows. Repeated episodes lead to synovial thickening and joint space narrowing, which predisposes to repeated traumatic synovial injury, bleeding, inflammation, remodeling, fibrosis, and contraction. A vicious cycle leads to severe chronic hemophilic arthropathy and degenerative arthritis. Prompt hip joint aspiration may reduce the risk of avascular necrosis of the femoral head. Some literature recommends **prednisone** 1 mg/kg/d PO x 5-7 d for patients with severe synovitis. *Septic arthritis* should be considered in the febrile patient, with joint findings refractory to usual factor therapy.

F *Intra-muscular hemorrhage (IM)* is the second most common hemorrhagic complication. History of trauma usually present. Most often deep and seen in the thigh, calf, forearm, and iliopsoas muscle groups. Iliopsoas hemorrhage may progress to life-threatening retroperitoneal bleed. Chronic IM bleeding may result in muscular atrophy, fibrosis, contractures, and pseudotumor formation.

G *Mucous membrane bleeding*, including epistaxis and bleeding following tooth extraction, is seen in toddlers. Although a single dose of factor may control the site of bleeding, further bleeding may be seen since mucous membranes are highly fibrinolytic, and clots easily become dislodged. Adjuvant **antifibrinolytic agents** are usually therapeutic, due to their ability to inhibit plasminogen.

H *Miscellaneous bleeding*
- Most subcutaneous ecchymosis does not require factor.
- Wounds requiring sutures should be treated the same as with post-surgical conditions.
- Up to 90% of patients with hemophilia have microscopic hematuria, and although often benign, should be admitted for monitoring. Antifibrinolytic agents are **contraindicated**, due to the risk of clot formation and obstruction of the collecting system.

✳ Continued on p.80

✶
Continued
from p.77

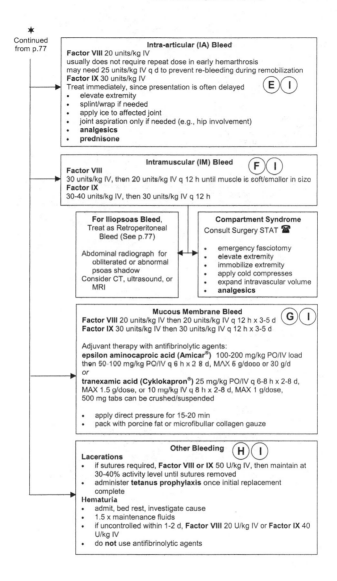

Intra-articular (IA) Bleed

Factor VIII 20 units/kg IV
usually does not require repeat dose in early hemarthrosis
may need 25 units/kg IV q d to prevent re-bleeding during remobilization
Factor IX 30 units/kg IV
Treat immediately, since presentation is often delayed   (E)(I)
- elevate extremity
- splint/wrap if needed
- apply ice to affected joint
- joint aspiration only if needed (e.g., hip involvement)
- **analgesics**
- **prednisone**

Intramuscular (IM) Bleed   (F)(I)
Factor VIII
30 units/kg IV, then 20 units/kg IV q 12 h until muscle is soft/smaller in size
Factor IX
30-40 units/kg IV, then 30 units/kg IV q 12 h

For Iliopsoas Bleed,
Treat as Retroperitoneal
Bleed (See p.77)

Abdominal radiograph for
obliterated or abnormal
psoas shadow
Consider CT, ultrasound, or
MRI

Compartment Syndrome
Consult Surgery STAT ☎

- emergency fasciotomy
- elevate extremity
- immobilize extremity
- apply cold compresses
- expand intravascular volume
- **analgesics**

Mucous Membrane Bleed   (G)(I)
Factor VIII 20 units/kg IV then 20 units/kg IV q 12 h x 3-5 d
Factor IX 30 units/kg IV then 30 units/kg IV q 12 h x 3-5 d

Adjuvant therapy with antifibrinolytic agents:
epsilon aminocaproic acid (Amicar®) 100-200 mg/kg PO/IV load
then 50-100 mg/kg PO/IV q 6 h x 2-8 d, MAX 6 g/dose or 30 g/d
or
tranexamic acid (Cyklokapron®) 25 mg/kg PO/IV q 6-8 h x 2-8 d,
MAX 1.5 g/dose, or 10 mg/kg IV q 8 h x 2-8 d, MAX 1 g/dose,
500 mg tabs can be crushed/suspended

- apply direct pressure for 15-20 min
- pack with porcine fat or microfibullar collagen gauze

Other Bleeding   (H)(I)
Lacerations
- if sutures required, **Factor VIII or IX** 50 U/kg IV, then maintain at
  30-40% activity level until sutures removed
- administer **tetanus prophylaxis** once initial replacement
  complete
Hematuria
- admit, bed rest, investigate cause
- 1.5 x maintenance fluids
- if uncontrolled within 1-2 d, **Factor VIII** 20 U/kg IV or **Factor IX** 40
  U/kg IV
- do **not** use antifibrinolytic agents

✳ Continued from p.78

Ⓘ Available products:
No cases of HIV1 transmission from clotting factor concentrates have been documented since 1986. With plasma-derived factor concentrates, there is a theoretical risk of viral contamination (hepatitis A and parvovirus, more so than hepatitis B, C, and HIV). Administer **Hepatitis B immune globulin, Hepatitis B vaccine,** and **Hepatitis A vaccine** in all previously non-immunized patients. Recombinant and monoclonal antibody purified products are preferred.

For Hemophilia A : Factor VIII-containing products
One unit factor VIII provides 2% activity.
Dose (units) = 0.5 x (% factor activity increase desired) x (weight in kg)
Maintenance dose = 25 units/kg IV q 8-12 hr or 2-3 units/kg/hr
For serious hemorrhage, always correct to 100% activity and maintain 40-50% activity for 5-7 d.
Note: there are 300 units/vial, so round dose to nearest multiple of 300.

Desmopressin (DDAVP)
0.3 mcg/kg IV diluted in 50 mL 0.9 NS given over 15-20 min, or metered dose nasal spray (1 spray or 150 mcg if < 50 kg, 2 sprays if > 50 kg)
- Use only for **mild** Hemophilia A, **not** effective for any form of Hemophilia B. Not to be used in patients < 2 yr or > 60 yr old, or in patients with ischemic heart disease.
- Increases plasma concentration of both factor VIII *and* vWF, possibly through endothelial cell degranulation (may develop tachyphylaxis).
- Monitor serum Na^+ and urine output, and restrict maintenance fluids as required. $T_{1/2}$ = 6 hr.

Cryoprecipitate (donated pool, factor VIII activity present) is generally **not** recommended due to increased transmission risk of hepatitis.

Ultra purity	Recombinant factor VIII (preferred product)	Recombinate®, Kogenate®, Bioclate®, Hexilate®
	Factor VIII concentrate	Monoclate P®, Hemophil M®, Antihemophilic factor-M® (do **not** use in previously untreated patients)
High purity	Factor VIII concentrate	Alphanate®, Koate-HP®
Intermediate purity	Factor VIII concentrate	Humate-P®, Profilate-OSD®

For Hemophilia B: Factor IX - containing products
One unit factor IX provides 1% activity.
Dose (units) = (% factor activity increase desired) x (weight in kg)
Note: there are 300 units/vial, so round dose to nearest multiple of 300.

Do **not** use cryoprecipitate (no factor IX activity).
Avoid fresh frozen plasma (not heat treated, so may not be virus-free).

High purity	Recombinant factor IX (preferred product)	Benefix®
	Factor IX concentrate	Mononine®, Alphanine SD®
Low purity	Factor IX complex concentrate (PCC)	Bebulin VH®, Konyne 80®, Profilnine SD® (do **not** use in previously untreated patients)

For von Willebrand disease
Desmopressin may increase plasma concentration of vWF in mild disease. **Contraindicated** in vWD type IIb, because it may exacerbate thrombocytopenia.

Humate P® (factor VIII concentrate) 40 units/kg IV, is preferred for more severe disease or patients with dysfunctional vWD, or **cryoprecipitate** (note associated viral transmission risks).

NOTES

Fever in the Neutropenic Patient

Amin Alousi

Neutropenia predisposes patients to a wide spectrum of bacterial and fungal infections, due to an impaired inflammatory response. Infections are commonly sinopulmonary in nature that often lack classical signs and symptoms, which then rapidly progress. Up to 2/3 of blood culture isolates remain negative. Clinical distinction between the infected neutropenic patient from a non-infected patient is extremely difficult, therefore, fever or any sign of infection, including only erythema, mandates rapid evaluation and prompt empiric treatment. Although management of infection in the non-malignant neutropenic patient has not been extensively studied, these patients are thought to be at lower risk for infection.

- *Neutropenia* (granulocytopenia) is defined as < 500 polymorphonuclear leukocytes and band forms per microliter or any count that is falling and expected to be < 500/mm^3 within 24 h.
- *Fever* is defined as a single temperature reading of > 38.4°C (po) or more than two consecutive readings of > 38°C in a 12-24 h period. All fevers, including those measured at home or during/following a blood product transfusion, mandates evaluation and treatment.

(A) Investigations should be interpreted in light of neutropenia and inability to mount inflammatory response. Examples:
- absence of radiographic infiltrates in pneumonia
- absence of pyuria in UTIs
- absence of localized pus in a catheter infection

(B) In patients with indwelling catheters, a set of blood cultures should be obtained peripherally to distinguish between central line colonization and bacteremia. In multiple lumen catheters, blood cultures should be obtained from each lumen and clearly labeled as such.

(C) A baseline chest radiograph should be obtained to compare with later films taken, as infiltrates may become more apparent when the patient's bone marrow recovers and neutrophils are "recruited" to previous occult infection sites.

(D) Causes of neutropenia

Acquired: post-infectious and drug-induced causes are most common
- Post-infectious - usually viral, transient, requires supportive care
- Drug-induced - chemotherapy, radiation therapy, other drugs (see below)
- Chronic benign neutropenia of childhood - mild, ANC> 500/mm^3, infection rare
- Neutropenia associated with immunologic disorders
- Autoimmune neutropenia - idiopathic, self-limited, anti-WBC antibodies; treat with steroids, IVIG, and manage underlying collagen vascular disease
- Isoimmune neonatal neutropenia - transient, maternal anti-WBC antibodies, normal marrow, supportive care
- Nutritional - seen with severe B12, folate, or copper deficiency; altered PMN function seen with severe phosphate or zinc deficiency

Intrinsic defects
- Cyclic neutropenia - oscillations q 3 wk, frequent stomatitis; treat with prophylactic antibiotics, G-CSF increases nadir and reduces cycle
- Chédiak-Higashi syndrome - recurrent and severe, autosomal recessive inheritance, albinism, supportive care or even marrow transplant
- Kostmann syndrome - severe infantile agranulocytosis, life-threatening infections, autosomal recessive inheritance; treat with prophylactic antibiotics, G-CSF or marrow transplant
- Schwachman-Diamond-Oski syndrome - associated with exocrine pancreatic insufficiency, autosomal recessive inheritance, may evolve into aplastic anemia or leukemia; supportive care along with pancreatic enzyme replacement, ? growth factor, marrow transplant

Drugs associated with neutropenia (partial list), other than chemotherapeutic agents
- antibiotics - amphotericin B, cephalosporins, co-trimoxazole, penicillins, sulfa, nitrofurantoin, chloramphenicol
- anticonvulsants - carbamazepine, clonazepam, ethosuximide
- anti-inflammatory agents - ibuprofen, salicylic acid and derivatives, sulfasalazine
- others - cimetidine, ACE-inhibitors

Historical information needed
- dates of past chemotherapy/radiation therapy treatments
- home medications, including the use of antipyretics
- compliance with prophylactic antibiotics
- previous febrile events, including whether a documented infection or isolate was identified
- previous blood product transfusions

✱ Continued on p.84

(A) **Clinical Manifestations**

Presence or absence of toxic appearance is not helpful in identifying the neutropenic patient at risk.

HEENT	mucositis, stomatitis, gingivitis, pharyngitis, tenderness over the sinuses, URI symptoms, recurrent otitis media
CVS	↑ HR, widened pulse pressures
RESP	findings associated with consolidation may be absent
GI	esophagitis (dysphagia, retrosternal pain), typhlitis (nausea, diarrhea, +/- RLQ pain)
GU	UTI (may be asymptomatic), perirectal abscess on visual inspection Note: digital rectal examination is **contraindicated** in the neutropenic patient due to potential for bacteremia.
EXT	tenderness over bone marrow biopsy or lumbar puncture sites, localized erythema

Diagnostics (B) (C)

Blood	CBC, differential, platelets, cultures (peripheral and from each central line lumen), reticulocyte count, electrolytes, BUN, creatinine, PT, PTT
Urine	urinalysis, culture
Imaging	baseline chest radiograph; consider sinus radiographs, abdominal radiographs, CT (sinuses, abdomen)
Other	stool studies (culture, Rotazyme®, *C. difficile* toxin), respiratory studies (throat culture, sputum Gram stain and culture, RSV-ELISA, DFA's for influenza, parainfluenza, adenovirus), wound cultures if applicable

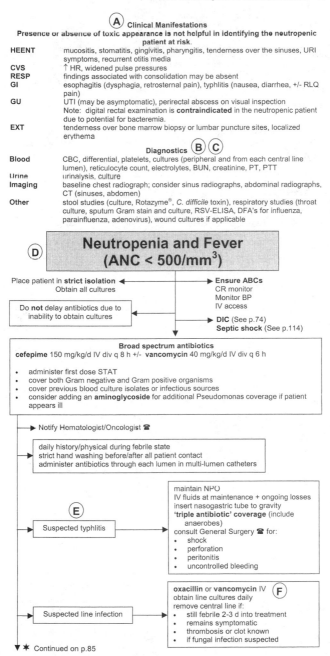

(D) **Neutropenia and Fever (ANC < 500/mm^3)**

Place patient in **strict isolation** ◀
Obtain all cultures

▶ **Ensure ABCs**
CR monitor
Monitor BP
IV access

Do **not** delay antibiotics due to inability to obtain cultures

▶ **DIC** (See p.74)
Septic shock (See p.114)

Broad spectrum antibiotics
cefepime 150 mg/kg/d IV div q 8 h +/- **vancomycin** 40 mg/kg/d IV div q 6 h

- administer first dose STAT
- cover both Gram negative and Gram positive organisms
- cover previous blood culture isolates or infectious sources
- consider adding an **aminoglycoside** for additional Pseudomonas coverage if patient appears ill

▶ Notify Hematologist/Oncologist ☎

daily history/physical during febrile state
strict hand washing before/after all patient contact
administer antibiotics through each lumen in multi-lumen catheters

(E) Suspected typhlitis ▶
maintain NPO
IV fluids at maintenance + ongoing losses
insert nasogastric tube to gravity
'triple antibiotic' coverage (include anaerobes)
consult General Surgery ☎ for:
- shock
- perforation
- peritonitis
- uncontrolled bleeding

Suspected line infection ▶
oxacillin or **vancomycin** IV (F)
obtain line cultures
remove central line if:
- still febrile 2-3 d into treatment
- remains symptomatic
- thrombosis or clot known
- if fungal infection suspected

▼ ✱ Continued on p.85

✱ Continued from p.82

(E) Typhlitis manifests as bowel wall inflammation, particularly that of the cecum, and is more commonly seen with leukemic and lymphoma patients undergoing Ara-C treatment. Patients may present with nausea, fever, diarrhea, and right lower quadrant pain, mimicking appendicitis. Abdominal radiographs may show pneumatosis, bowel wall edema, and a paucity of air, and can be confirmed with either abdominal ultrasound, CT, or MRI. All patients suspected to have typhlitis should be admitted.

(F) Minimize the use of **vancomycin** to prevent emergence of vancomycin-resistant enterococcus (VRE).

Pathogens commonly encountered in neutropenic children with fever

(G)

Gram-positive bacteria	Gram-negative bacteria	Fungi
Staphylococci Streptococci • group D • *a*-hemolytic • aerobes, anaerobes • *Clostridia spp.* • *Bacteroides spp.*	*Pseudomonas aeruginosa* *E. coli* *Klebsiella pneumoniae* *Enterobacter spp.* *Citrobacter spp.*	*Candida spp.* *Aspergillus spp.*

✻ Continued from p.83

Ⓖ

Condition	Treatment option
mucositis, gingivitis, or perirectal abscess/cellulitis	**clindamycin** or **metronidazole** (anaerobic coverage)
diffuse infiltrates on chest radiograph	**TMP/SMX** (PCP coverage) and **erythromycin** (Mycoplasma)
esophagitis	**antifungal** or **acyclovir**
diarrhea	**clindamycin** or **metronidazole** (anaerobic coverage)
fever > 7 d or new fever 4-7 d into Rx	**amphoterocin B**
fever resolves, source is identified	complete course of appropriate antibiotic continue broad spectrum Gram-negative and Gram-positive coverage until ANC > 200 and rising
fever resolves, no source identified	continue broad spectrum Gram-negative and Gram-positive coverage until ANC > 200 and rising

Sickle Cell Disease
Renato Roxas, Jr.

Sickle cell disease - a group of hemoglobinopathies characterized by the formation of sickled RBCs in response to deoxygenation.
Sickle cell anemia - sickle cell disease that results from substitution of valine for glutamic acid at the sixth amino acid position of the beta-globin molecule.
Others - HbSC, HbS-thalassemia combinations

(A)

Laboratory findings in sickle cell disease

Syndrome	Hct %	Retic %	Mean MCV	A	S	F	A$_2$	C
SS	18-28	12-25	86	0	80-95 ↑	2-20 ↑	< 3.5 ↑	0
SC	30-36	5-10	77	0	45-50 ↑	1-5	N/A	45-50 ↑
S$\beta°$	20-30	10-15	66	0	80-92 ↑	2-15 ↑	3.5-7 ↑	0
Sβ^+	30-36	3-6	70	0	65-90 ↑	2-10 ↑	3.5-6 ↑	0

(B) Pneumococcal sepsis continues to be the leading cause of death among children with sickle cell disease. If a child is febrile (T>38.6°C), management should include rapid triage, quick history and physical to exclude co-existing complications, and stat diagnostics. IV antibiotics should not be delayed to obtain cultures, and should be instituted immediately. Consider **ceftriaxone** in the persistently febrile patient, to increase Gram-negative coverage as well as cover for resistant S. pneumococcal infection. If no source of infection is found on examination, IV antibiotics should be continued until blood cultures are negative for 48 h, AND the patient is afebrile for > 24 h. Additional management includes IV hydration; monitor for signs of CHF, particularly in patients at risk for the development of cardiomyopathy.

(C) Splenic sequestration
Occurs when sickled RBCs and platelets are sequestered in the spleen, causing rapid splenic enlargement and an acute fall in Hb in excess of 2 g/dL, in spite of elevated reticulocyte counts. Signs and symptoms vary from acute pallor, lethargy, abdominal fullness, tachycardia, and tachypnea, to cardiovascular collapse. Occurs in 10-30% of children with HbSS, usually between the ages of 6 mos and 3 y. Occurs in older aged children with HbSC and sickle-beta-thal disease. Mainstay of treatment is management of shock and partial exchange transfusion.

(D) Stroke/cerebral vascular accident (CVA) is an acute, clinically apparent neurological event, which most commonly presents as hemi/monoparesis, aphasia, and seizures. It can also present as headache and mental status changes. It occurs in 7-8% of children with HbSS after the first year of life, but occurs less commonly in HbSC and sickle-beta-thal disease. Stroke has an extremely high recurrence rate. Imaging (non-contrast head CT) should be performed to rule out intracranial hemorrhage. Lumbar puncture may be indicated, if meningeal signs are present. Goal of partial exchange transfusion is to reduce Hb S quantitative level to < 30%.

(E) Acute chest syndrome
A frequent and sometimes fatal complication of sickle cell disease that occurs in up to 40% of children. See p.88.

(F) Vaso-occlusive pain crisis
Must rule out other life-threatening causes of pain! Sites are typically abdominal, long bone or back. When accompanied by other systemic signs (fever), consider osteomyelitis in the child with persistent extremity pain and cholecystitis in the child with colicky abdominal pain.

(G) Priapism is a relatively frequent complication resulting from venous pooling of blood in the corpora cavernosa. If there is no resolution within 4-6 h of initiating IV hydration and adequate pain control, partial exchange transfusion is indicated. Consult Urology.

(H) Aplastic crisis
Diagnosed when an acute fall in hemoglobin is accompanied by a markedly decreased reticulocyte count, without splenomegaly. Suppression of erythropoiesis is primarily caused by Parvovirus B19, which can be confirmed by PCR or convalescent titers, and other viruses, in the child with a history of antecedent URI. Simple PRBC transfusion is indicated in the hemodynamically unstable patient. If stable, the patient may be monitored for resolution, which typically occurs in 1-2 weeks.

Clinical Manifestations

History	Ask about: previous pain episodes, history of dactylitis, priapism, CVA, splenic sequestration, aplastic crisis, acute chest syndrome, previous ICU admissions, previous transfusions, baseline hemoglobin, type of sickle cell disease, home pain medication regimen, immunization status, use of penicillin prophylaxis, antecedent URI
GEN	fever, pain (typical or atypical)
HEENT	scleral icterus, pale conjunctiva, pharyngeal erythema
RESP	shortness of breath, cough, pleuritic chest pain
GI/GU	splenomegaly, hepatomegaly, priapism, abdominal pain
CNS	headache, altered mental status, focal neurologic deficits
EXT	hand/feet swelling, long bone pain
SKIN	jaundice, pallor

Diagnostics (A)

Blood   CBC, differential, platelet count, peripheral smear, reticulocyte count, type and cross match/hold if indicated, hemoglobin solubility or electrophoresis if indicated

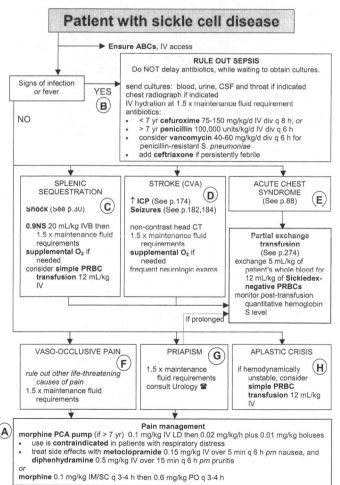

Patient with sickle cell disease

→ **Ensure ABCs**, IV access

Signs of infection or fever — **NO** / **YES (B)**

RULE OUT SEPSIS
Do NOT delay antibiotics, while waiting to obtain cultures.

send cultures: blood, urine, CSF and throat if indicated
chest radiograph if indicated
IV hydration at 1.5 x maintenance fluid requirement
antibiotics:
- < 7 yr **cefuroxime** 75-150 mg/kg/d IV div q 8 h, *or*
- > 7 yr **penicillin** 100,000 units/kg/d IV div q 6 h
- consider **vancomycin** 40-60 mg/kg/d div q 6 h for penicillin-resistant S. *pneumoniae*
- add **ceftriaxone** if persistently febrile

SPLENIC SEQUESTRATION (C)

Shock (See p.30)

0.9NS 20 mL/kg IVB then
1.5 x maintenance fluid requirements
supplemental O₂ if needed
consider **simple PRBC transfusion** 12 mL/kg IV

STROKE (CVA) (D)

↑ ICP (See p.174)
Seizures (See p.182,184)

non-contrast head CT
1.5 x maintenance fluid requirements
supplemental O₂ if needed
frequent neurologic exams

ACUTE CHEST SYNDROME (See p.88) (E)

Partial exchange transfusion (See p.274)
exchange 5 mL/kg of patient's whole blood for 12 mL/kg of **Sickledex-negative PRBCs**
monitor post-transfusion quantitative hemoglobin S level

If prolonged

VASO-OCCLUSIVE PAIN (F)

rule out other life-threatening causes of pain
1.5 x maintenance fluid requirements

PRIAPISM (G)

1.5 x maintenance fluid requirements
consult Urology ☎

APLASTIC CRISIS (H)

if hemodynamically unstable, consider **simple PRBC transfusion** 12 mL/kg IV

(A)   Pain management
morphine PCA pump (if > 7 yr) 0.1 mg/kg IV LD then 0.02 mg/kg/h plus 0.01 mg/kg boluses
- use is **contraindicated** in patients with respiratory distress
- treat side effects with **metoclopramide** 0.15 mg/kg IV over 5 min q 6 h prn nausea, and **diphenhydramine** 0.5 mg/kg IV over 15 min q 6 h prn pruritis
or
morphine 0.1 mg/kg IM/SC q 3-4 h then 0.6 mg/kg PO q 3-4 h

Acute Chest Syndrome in Sickle Cell Disease

Renato Roxas, Jr.

Acute chest syndrome is defined as a noninfectious pulmonary process, which may or may not present with abnormal chest radiographs in a patient with sickle cell disease. Pneumonia may be clinically indistinguishable from pulmonary infarction. Acute chest syndrome is a medical emergency.

(A) ABG/CBG may show hypoxemia.
On chest radiograph, pulmonary infiltrates may be seen in a single lobe or may be diffuse and bilateral. Pleural effusions are common. Chest radiograph findings may lag behind the development of pulmonary signs on physical examination.

(B) Avoid overhydration in patients with cardiomyopathies as this may lead to pulmonary edema and worsening respiratory distress.

Antibiotics must provide coverage for encapsulated organisms (*S. pneumoniae, H. influenzae*) as well as *S. aureus*. **Ampicillin/sulbactam (Unasyn®)** IV may be considered instead of cefuroxime IV. Consider adding a macrolide agent to cover Mycoplasma and/or Chlamydia.

Adequate pain control is necessary to avoid splinting of the chest, so that the patient can comply with necessary pulmonary toilet maneuvers. Excessive narcotic use may cause sedation and hypoventilation, leading to atelectasis and/or further hypoxemia. NSAIDs may be used to reduce narcotic use.

(C) Transfusions are most effective when administered early in the course of disease. Simple transfusions appear to be safe and efficacious in patients with worsening anemia and mild to moderate hypoxemia. For patients with severe hypoxemia, partial exchange transfusion is indicated.

(D) The goal of partial exchange transfusion is to reduce the Hgb S quantitative level to < 30%. Avoid hyperviscosity. Perform exchange transfusion in stages in a patient with hemodynamic instability.

Clinical Manifestations

GEN	+/- fever
RESP	cough, pleuritic chest pain, tachypnea, dyspnea, retractions, respiratory failure
GI	abdominal pain

(A) Diagnostics

Blood	ABG/CBG, CBC, differential, platelet count, culture, hemoglobin solubility, hemoglobin S quantitative, type and cross match
Imaging	chest radiograph (two-view, serial if necessary)

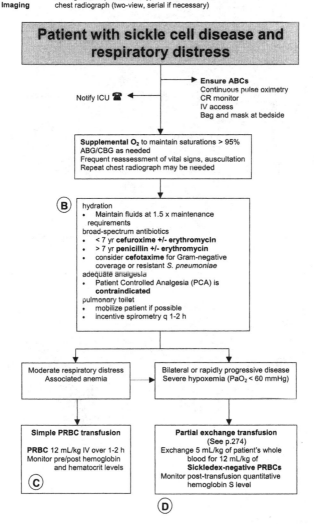

Patient with sickle cell disease and respiratory distress

Notify ICU ☎

Ensure ABCs
Continuous pulse oximetry
CR monitor
IV access
Bag and mask at bedside

Supplemental O₂ to maintain saturations > 95%
ABG/CBG as needed
Frequent reassessment of vital signs, auscultation
Repeat chest radiograph may be needed

(B) hydration
- Maintain fluids at 1.5 x maintenance requirements

broad-spectrum antibiotics
- < 7 yr **cefuroxime +/- erythromycin**
- > 7 yr **penicillin +/- erythromycin**
- consider **cefotaxime** for Gram-negative coverage or resistant *S. pneumoniae*

adequate analgesia
- Patient Controlled Analgesia (PCA) is **contraindicated**

pulmonary toilet
- mobilize patient if possible
- incentive spirometry q 1-2 h

Moderate respiratory distress
Associated anemia

Bilateral or rapidly progressive disease
Severe hypoxemia (PaO₂ < 60 mmHg)

Simple PRBC transfusion

PRBC 12 mL/kg IV over 1-2 h
Monitor pre/post hemoglobin and hematocrit levels

(C)

Partial exchange transfusion
(See p.274)
Exchange 5 mL/kg of patient's whole blood for 12 mL/kg of **Sickledex-negative PRBCs**
Monitor post-transfusion quantitative hemoglobin S level

(D)

Tumor Lysis Syndrome

Renato Roxas, Jr.

A pattern of metabolic abnormalities that includes (1) hyperkalemia, (2) hyperuricemia, and (3) hyperphosphatemia, resulting from spontaneous or treatment-related tumor necrosis or fulminant apoptosis. Common complications include hypocalcemia and secondary renal failure. Renal failure due to obstructive uropathy results from crystallization of uric acid and precipitation of $CaPO_4$. Calcium and phosphorus precipitates when the $[Ca^{++}] \times [P]$ product exceeds 58.

(A) Typically occurs prior to the initiation of therapy or up to 5 days after the start of cytotoxic treatment.

Risk factors
- large tumor burden
- malignancies with high sensitivity to chemotherapy, e.g., T-cell ALL, Burkitt's lymphoma
- elevated pre-treatment serum uric acid
- elevated LDH
- poor urine output/renal function
- particularly seen in patients with the following physical examination findings: SVC obstruction, tracheal deviation, pleural effusion, ascites, palpable kidneys, bulky abdominal disease (e.g., hepatoblastoma, stage IV neuroblastoma)

(B) Other studies to consider
- Abdominal/retroperitoneal ultrasound - for tumor involvement of the kidneys or hydronephrosis
- EKG - to assess hyperkalemia (peaked T waves, QRS widening) or hypocalcemia (prolonged QT)

(C) Hyperuricemia

Allopurinol competitively inhibits xanthine oxidase and therefore increases soluble xanthine and hypoxanthine. Can cause an erythematous maculopapular rash, which can lead to severe hypersensitivity if continued.

$NaHCO_3$ infusion to maintain urine pH 7.0-7.5 will aid in the renal excretion of uric acid. However, in patients with high uric acid loads, resultant high xanthine levels can lead to xanthine precipitation and thus renal failure at urine pH's as low as 7.0. In these situations, $NaHCO_3$ should be discontinued.

Urate oxidase is a uric acid lowering agent, but is still investigational in the US.

(D) Hypocalcemia

Symptomatic hypocalcemia warrants **calcium** supplementation, however, caution should be exercised since overzealous administration of calcium may lead to increased precipitation of $CaPO_4$. Severe alkalosis may further exacerbate $CaPO_4$ precipitation and necessitate discontinuation of $NaHCO_3$.

(E) Hyperphosphatemia

Treatment of hyperphosphatemia primarily involves enhancing renal excretion of phosphorus. Phosphorus is usually reabsorbed by the kidney, but when the reabsorption maximum is exceeded, excretion becomes dependent on GFR, thus warranting **vigorous fluid therapy** and judicious use of diuretics. **Furosemide** or **mannitol** may be used to promote urine output.

Phosphorus excretion may also be enhanced by increasing GI excretion with oral phosphate binders, such as **$Al(OH)_3$**. Results are unpredictable.

(F) Indications for dialysis
- Serum K^+ > 7 mEq/L
- Serum uric acid > 10 mg/dl
- Serum creatinine is 10X normal
- Serum P > 10 mg/dl
- If patient is uremic
- Persistent hypocalcemia
- Uncontrollable hypertension/hypervolemia

Hemodialysis is preferred due to its rapid correction of metabolic abnormalities. Chemotherapy can be re-instituted while the patient is on dialysis.

A

Clinical Manifestations

Metabolic cause	Symptoms	Signs
Hypocalcemia	anorexia, vomiting, cramps	carpopedal spasms, tetany, seizures, cardiac arrest
Hyperkalemia	weakness, paralysis, GI symptoms	ventricular arrhythmia
Hyperuricemia	• 10-15 mg/dl: nonspecific symptoms like lethargy, nausea, vomiting • ≥ 20 mg/dl: signs of renal failure, altered sensorium	↑ BP, altered sensorium
$CaPO_4$ deposition	pruritis, iritis, arthritis	joint swelling, gangrenous changes in soft tissues
Abdominal disease	abdominal pain, abdominal distension	abdominal mass
Renal involvement	dysuria, oliguria, flank pain, hematuria	renal failure

Diagnostics

Blood CBC, differential, electrolytes, CO_2, BUN, creatinine, Ca^{++}, Mg^{++}, P, uric acid
Urine urinalysis
Other abdominal/retroperitoneal ultrasound, EKG **B**

Suspected Tumor Lysis Syndrome

→ **Ensure ABCs**
CR monitor

Discontinue chemotherapy ◄

→ Consult Surgery or ICU for vascular
Hyperkalemia (See p.212) ◄   access if considering dialysis ☎

IV Hydration, Alkalinization
$D_5 0.2NS$ + 75-100 mEq $NaHCO_3$/L at
3-4X normal maintenance fluid rate

Maintain urine pH 7-7.5, Sp Gr 1.010

• Monitor for fluid overload
• Urine output should approximate fluid intake
• Assess renal function
• Monitor labs q 6-8 h

C   **E**

Hyperuricemia

allopurinol
100 mg/m^2 PO TID

repeat dose if repeat
uric acid > 7 mg/dl

Hypocalcemia

Mild: do not administer
calcium to treat elevated P

D

Severe:
calcium gluconate 10%
100-200 mg/kg/dose IV
or
calcium chloride 10%
10-30 mg/kg/dose IV over 5
minutes

Monitor for bradycardia

Hyperphosphatemia

Al(OH)$_3$ 50-150 mg/kg/d PO
div q 4-6 h

and

furosemide 1 mg/kg/dose IV
or
mannitol 0.5 g/kg/dose IV
over 15 minutes

Hypomagnesemia

MgSO$_4$ 25-50 mg/kg/dose
slow IV infusion as 10-25%
solution

Assess metabolic disturbances

Improved   Unimproved

• Continue therapy and
monitoring
• Resume chemotherapy

Dialysis
F

Chapter 6 ♣ Immunological Disorders

Anaphylaxis

Malathi Bathija

> Anaphylaxis is an immediate, life threatening, systemic reaction caused by the release of histamine and other mediators from mast cells after an IgE response to an allergen in a previously sensitized individual. The clinical spectrum varies from mild to severe reactions.

(A) Respiratory and dermatologic manifestations are the most common clinical features of anaphylaxis.

(B)

Etiology: anaphylaxis (Partial List)

Drugs	amphotericin B, **aspirin**, cephalosporins, ketoconazole, neomycin, NSAIDs, **penicillin**, sulfonamides, vancomycin
Food	bananas, beets, chocolate, citrus, egg white, fish, grains, legumes, mango, milk, nuts, **peanuts**, preservatives, **shellfish**, sunflower seeds, food additives
Plasma products	whole blood, plasma, immunoglobulins, cryoprecipitate
Foreign proteins	ACTH, antilymphocyte globulin, chymopapain, chymotrypsin, equine antivenom, insulin, protamine, streptokinase, vasopressin
Others	**Latex****, radiographic contrast material, insect stings and bites, pollen

**Suspect latex allergy in children (1) with spina bifida, (2) who have undergone multiple surgeries.

LOCAL MEASURES

When antigenic stimulant is located in extremity, e.g., bee sting, site of parenteral drug administration,

- Remove source (IV medication, blood product)
- Place extremity in dependent position
- Local ice application q 15-30 min
- Local infiltration of **epinephrine** (1:10,000) 0.1-0.2 mL SC
- Bee sting: remove by forceps or flicking. Do not squeeze soft tissue. Tourniquet may be applied *above* the site of sting to slow systemic distribution. Loosen every 5 minutes. *Remove after clinical improvement*

(C) **Diphenhydramine** causes respiratory depression, especially when given IV. Administer slowly. Steroids are used to prevent the late phase of allergic response.

(D) Split dose and administer half the dose directly in the SC tissues of the antigenic area.

(E) Rapid deterioration can occur. Monitor patients closely, even those that present with mild symptoms. Death can occur in 5-10 minutes. Continue to observe for 2-3 hours after resolution of symptoms. Discharge instructions should include instructions for EpiPen® use

(F) The most common cause of death is upper airway obstruction. Be prepared to secure/establish the airway.

(G) **Ipratropium bromide** may be nebulized with albuterol.

(H) Because of peripheral vasodilatation and increased capillary permeability, large volumes of fluid may be needed to maintain adequate circulating volume. Consider giving blood products if further boluses are needed after giving > 60 mL/kg of crystalloids within a short period of time. Monitor hemoglobin and coagulation profile.

Clinical Manifestations

HEENT	periorbital edema, lip/tongue swelling, conjunctival injection, lacrimation, rhinorrhea, sneezing
RESP	retractions, stridor, wheezing, tachypnea
CVS	hypotension, shock, arrhythmias, cardiovascular collapse
GI	nausea, vomiting, diarrhea, dysphagia
HEME	DIC
CNS	apprehension, confusion, headache
SKIN	urticaria, flushing, pruritus, sweating

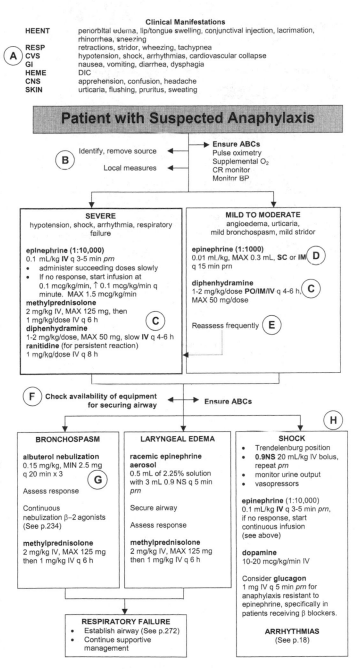

Patient with Suspected Anaphylaxis

(B) Identify, remove source ←

Local measures ←

→ **Ensure ABCs**
Pulse oximetry
Supplemental O$_2$
CR monitor
Monitor BP

SEVERE
hypotension, shock, arrhythmia, respiratory failure

epinephrine (1:10,000)
0.1 mL/kg IV q 3-5 min *prn*
- administer succeeding doses slowly
- If no response, start infusion at 0.1 mcg/kg/min, ↑ 0.1 mcg/kg/min q minute. MAX 1.5 mcg/kg/min
methylprednisolone
2 mg/kg IV, MAX 125 mg, then 1 mg/kg/dose IV q 6 h
diphenhydramine (C)
1-2 mg/kg/dose, MAX 50 mg, slow **IV** q 4-6 h
ranitidine (for persistent reaction)
1 mg/kg/dose IV q 8 h

MILD TO MODERATE
angioedema, urticaria, mild bronchospasm, mild stridor

epinephrine (1:1000)
0.01 mL/kg, MAX 0.3 mL, **SC** or **IM** (D)
q 15 min prn

diphenhydramine (C)
1-2 mg/kg/dose PO/IM/IV q 4-6 h, MAX 50 mg/dose

Reassess frequently (E)

(F) Check availability of equipment for securing airway ← → Ensure ABCs

(H)

BRONCHOSPASM

albuterol nebulization
0.15 mg/kg, MIN 2.5 mg
q 20 min x 3 (G)

Assess response

Continuous nebulization β-2 agonists (See p.234)

methylprednisolone
2 mg/kg IV, MAX 125 mg then 1 mg/kg IV q 6 h

LARYNGEAL EDEMA

racemic epinephrine aerosol
0.5 mL of 2.25% solution with 3 mL 0.9 NS q 5 min *prn*

Secure airway

Assess response

methylprednisolone
2 mg/kg IV, MAX 125 mg then 1 mg/kg IV q 6 h

SHOCK
- Trendelenburg position
- **0.9NS** 20 mL/kg IV bolus, repeat *prn*
- monitor urine output
- vasopressors

epinephrine (1:10,000)
0.1 mL/kg **IV** q 3-5 min *prn*, if no response, start continuous infusion (see above)

dopamine
10-20 mcg/kg/min IV

Consider **glucagon**
1 mg IV q 5 min *prn* for anaphylaxis resistant to epinephrine, specifically in patients receiving β blockers.

RESPIRATORY FAILURE
- Establish airway (See p.272)
- Continue supportive management

ARRHYTHMIAS
(See p.18)

Patient with AIDS and Fever

Malathi Bathija

 Proper collection and handling of specimen is important to improve yield (cultures).

COMMON BACTERIAL PATHOGENS
Blood	*Streptococcus pneumoniae*
	Haemophilus influenzae
	Salmonella sp.
GU	*Escherichia coli*
Skin/soft tissue	*Staphylococcus aureus*
	Streptococcus viridans

B Major bacterial pathogens in children with HIV are similar to immunocompetent healthy children, but the incidence of bacterial infection is greater than in those who do not have HIV.

Central line related sepsis is usually due to *Staphylococcus aureus* and *Staphylococcus epidermidis*. Catheter related infection may be treated without removal of the catheter.

OPPORTUNISTIC INFECTIONS
Bacterial	*Mycobacterium avium* complex
Fungal infections:	oral candidiasis, esophageal candidiasis, disseminated candidiasis
	Cryptococcus neoformans, Aspergillus sp., *Histoplasma capsulatum, Coccidioides immitis*
Protozoan	*Pneumocystis carinii, Toxoplasma gondii*
Viral	Herpesvirus (CMV, Varicella-Zoster)

C Infections diagnosed by clinical parameters are more common than culture positive infections. Acute pneumonia is the most common clinically diagnosed severe infection. Principles of management should be no different to that of immunocompetent patients.

D Children with HIV with nasal discharge and cough > 2 weeks should be evaluated for sinusitis.

Otitis media is a common minor infection and may be resistant to treatment. Common pathogens include *Streptococcus pneumoniae, Haemophilus influenzae*, and group A-β hemolytic streptococci.

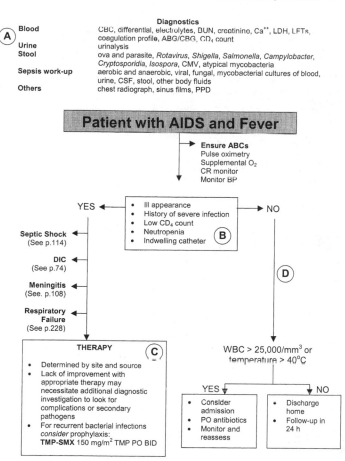

Diagnostics

Blood	CBC, differential, electrolytes, BUN, creatinine, Ca++, LDH, LFTs, coagulation profile, ABG/CBG, CD4 count
Urine	urinalysis
Stool	ova and parasite, *Rotavirus, Shigella, Salmonella, Campylobacter, Cryptosporidia, Isospora,* CMV, atypical mycobacteria
Sepsis work-up	aerobic and anaerobic, viral, fungal, mycobacterial cultures of blood, urine, CSF, stool, other body fluids
Others	chest radiograph, sinus films, PPD

Patient with AIDS and Fever

➤ Ensure ABCs
Pulse oximetry
Supplemental O_2
CR monitor
Monitor BP

YES ◄—
- Ill appearance
- History of severe infection
- Low CD_4 count
- Neutropenia
- Indwelling catheter

B

—► NO

Septic Shock ◄—
(See p.114)

DIC ◄—
(See p.74)

Meningitis ◄—
(See. p.108)

Respiratory Failure ◄—
(See p.228)

D

THERAPY **C**
• Determined by site and source • Lack of improvement with appropriate therapy may necessitate additional diagnostic investigation to look for complications or secondary pathogens • For recurrent bacterial infections *consider* prophylaxis: **TMP-SMX** 150 mg/m² TMP PO BID

WBC > 25,000/mm³ or
temperature > 40°C

YES ▼

• Consider admission • PO antibiotics • Monitor and reassess

—► NO

• Discharge home • Follow-up in 24 h

Patient with AIDS and Suspected Lung Involvement

Malathi Bathija

(A) Patients with AIDS may have respiratory symptoms due to bacterial pneumonias, viral illnesses, opportunistic infections, reactive airway disease, lymphoid interstitial pneumonitis (LIP), or cardiomyopathy. Opportunistic infections include *Pneumocystis carinii* pneumonia (PCP), *Mycobacterium-avium intracellulare* complex (MAC), aspergillosis, *Legionella*, and *Nocardia*.

(B) Always have a high index of suspicion for PCP in patients with AIDS presenting with acute respiratory distress and hypoxia (SpO$_2$ < 90% and PaO$_2$ < 60 mmHg in room air).

(C) Pathogens that may cause bacterial pneumonia include: *Streptococcus pneumoniae*, *Haemophilus influenzae* type B, Group A streptococci, *Staphylococcus aureus*, *Mycoplasma pneumoniae*, *Branhamella catarrhalis*, and Gram-negative organisms including *Pseudomonas spp.* and *Klebsiella spp.* DO NOT rely on WBC count for diagnosing infection in patients with AIDS.

(D) The most common AIDS-defining condition in infants < 1 year and opportunistic infection among HIV-infected children is *Pneumocystis carinii* (PCP) pneumonia. Most infants are infected between 4-6 months of age. Clinically they present with rapidly progressive hypoxemia. Although improved recognition and treatment of PCP have improved prognosis, it still is associated with greater risk for early death. *Patients with AIDS who present with ↑RR, hypoxia, and a normal chest radiograph should be presumed to have PCP until proven otherwise. Antibiotic therapy should be initiated immediately.*

(E) The administration of **TMP-SMX** has been associated with the following adverse effects: rash, neutropenia, thrombocytopenia, aplastic anemia, abnormal LFTs, Stevens-Johnson syndrome, and renal impairment.

Pentamidine is generally reserved for children who cannot tolerate TMP-SMX or for those who fail therapy.

(F) Bronchoalveolar lavage (BAL) is a safe and sensitive method for the diagnosis of PCP. The Wright-Giemsa stain is commonly used as a rapid screening test. Methenamine silver stain and direct immunofluorescent staining with monoclonal antibody (to detect cyst forms) are used to confirm screening results. Results may remain positive for up to 72 hours after the initiation of antibiotic therapy. A confirmatory test is important in making treatment decisions regarding secondary prophylaxis.

(G) RECOMMENDATIONS FOR THE USE OF STEROIDS IN THE TREATMENT OF PCP
Indication - moderate to severe PCP (PaO$_2$ < 70 mmHg or A-a gradient > 35 mmHg)

- > 13 years of age:
  prednisone   40 mg/dose PO BID for 5 days, then
                        40 mg PO qd for 5 days, then
                        20 mg PO qd until the end of antimicrobial therapy

- < 13 years of age:
  prednisone   2 mg/kg/d PO for 7 to 10 days, taper over the next 10 to 14 days.

NOTE: Therapy must be started within the first 72 hours of initiating antimicrobial therapy.

(H) Lymphoid interstitial pneumonitis (LIP) is a common pulmonary complication of AIDS predominantly seen in children. It is characterized by slowly progressive hypoxia with mild tachypnea, cough, and digital clubbing. It has been associated with generalized lymphadenopathy, parotid gland enlargement, and hepatosplenomegaly (chronic liver disease). The diagnosis is usually clinical with associated persistent (> 2 months) reticulonodular or interstitial findings with or without consolidation on chest radiograph or chest CT. Lung biopsy is infrequently used to determine diagnosis. BAL might be needed to rule out infectious causes. Course is usually benign.

(I) It is of extreme importance to send BAL or biopsy of specimen for susceptibility testing.

Children with advanced AIDS are at risk for disseminated infection with *Mycobacterium avium* complex (MAC), and usually present with fever, weight loss, night sweats, abdominal pain, hepatosplenomegaly, and anemia.

(J) Viral causes of pneumonia include respiratory syncytial virus (RSV), adenovirus, rubeola, varicella, and cytomegalovirus (CMV→ may cause diffuse infiltrates resembling PCP).

✳ Continued on p.98

Clinical Manifestations

GEN	fever
HEENT	parotid gland enlargement, nasal flaring, lymphadenopathy
RESP	tachypnea, rales, wheezing, rhonchi, retractions, cough
GI	hepatosplenomegaly
EXT	digital clubbing

Diagnostics

Blood	ABG/CBG (calculate A-a gradient), LDH, cold agglutinins (Mycoplasma) cultures**
BAL	cultures**, PCP
Other	chest radiograph, chest CT. Consider lung biopsy, PPD with anergy testing, RSV nasal wash
****Cultures**	bacterial (aerobic and anaerobic), viral, fungal, mycobacterial, parasitic

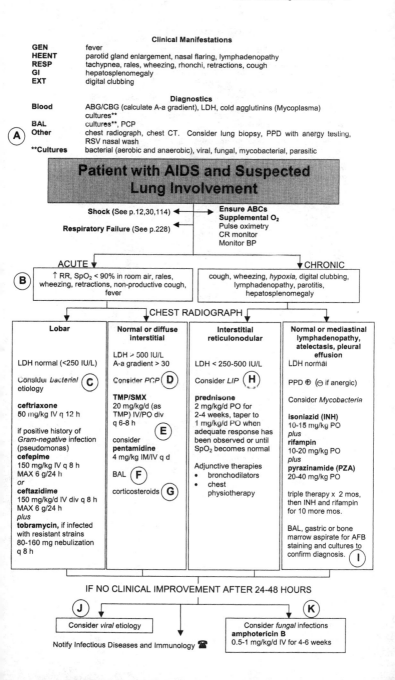

Patient with AIDS and Suspected Lung Involvement

Shock (See p.12,30,114) ← → **Ensure ABCs**
Supplemental O₂
Respiratory Failure (See p.228) ← Pulse oximetry
CR monitor
Monitor BP

ACUTE ▼

↑ RR, SpO₂ < 90% in room air, rales, wheezing, retractions, non-productive cough, fever

CHRONIC ▼

cough, wheezing, *hypoxia*, digital clubbing, lymphadenopathy, parotitis, hepatosplenomegaly

CHEST RADIOGRAPH

Lobar

LDH normal (<250 IU/L)

Consider *bacterial* etiology (C)

ceftriaxone
50 mg/kg IV q 12 h

if positive history of *Gram-negative* infection (pseudomonas)
cefepime
150 mg/kg IV q 8 h
MAX 6 g/24 h
or
ceftazidime
150 mg/kg/d IV div q 8 h
MAX 6 g/24 h
plus
tobramycin, if infected with resistant strains
80-160 mg nebulization q 8 h

Normal or diffuse interstitial

LDH > 500 IU/L
A-a gradient > 30

Consider *PCP* (D)

TMP/SMX
20 mg/kg/d (as TMP) IV/PO div q 6-8 h (E)

consider
pentamidine
4 mg/kg IM/IV q d

BAL (F)

corticosteroids (G)

Interstitial reticulonodular

LDH < 250-500 IU/L

Consider *LIP* (H)

prednisone
2 mg/kg/d PO for 2-4 weeks, taper to 1 mg/kg/d PO when adequate response has been observed or until SpO₂ becomes normal

Adjunctive therapies
• bronchodilators
• chest physiotherapy

Normal or mediastinal lymphadenopathy, atelectasis, pleural effusion

LDH normal

PPD ⊕ (⊖ if anergic)

Consider *Mycobacteria*

isoniazid (INH)
10-15 mg/kg PO
plus
rifampin
10-20 mg/kg PO
plus
pyrazinamide (PZA)
20-40 mg/kg PO

triple therapy x 2 mos, then INH and rifampin for 10 more mos.

BAL, gastric or bone marrow aspirate for AFB staining and cultures to confirm diagnosis. (I)

IF NO CLINICAL IMPROVEMENT AFTER 24-48 HOURS

(J) Consider *viral* etiology

Notify Infectious Diseases and Immunology ☎

(K) Consider *fungal* infections
amphotericin B
0.5-1 mg/kg/d IV for 4-6 weeks

(A) (B)

✴ Continued from p.96

SPECIFIC ANTIVIRAL THERAPY

Varicella	**acyclovir**	30 mg/kg IV q 8 h for 7-10 d *or* 80 mg/kg PO QID for 7-10 d
Rubeola	**acyclovir**	30 mg/kg IV q 8 h for 7-10 d
CMV	**ganciclovir**	10 mg/kg/d IV q div 12 h for 14 d, then 5 mg/kg IV q d for 5 d/week for life
Influenza A	**amantadine**	for 2-5 days < 9 y 5 mg/kg/d PO div 1-2 doses MAX 150 mg/d > 9 y and < 40 kg, 200 mg/d PO div in 1-2 doses MAX 200 mg/d > 40 kg 200 mg PO qd-BID
RSV	consider **ribavirin**	

(**K**) Consider Histoplasmosis, *Aspergillus* sp., *Candida* spp., and *Cryptococcus neoformans*. Diagnosis is confirmed by isolation of the organism.

Amphotericin B is nephrotoxic and causes liver and bone marrow suppression. Fever, hypotension and chills may also be observed. Monitor electrolytes, CBC, and LFTs.

NOTES

Immunocompromised Host with Fever

Michael Vish

A
- Immunocompromised host: an individual who has an abnormality in phagocytic, cellular or humoral immune function that predisposes him to infectious or opportunistic complications.

- Patients with loss of skin or mucous membrane integrity may also be susceptible to infectious complications.

- **Fever due to infections in an immunocompromised host represents a medical or surgical emergency.**

B Primary causes of immunocompromised states (list is not all-inclusive):
- B cell disorders
    - X-linked (Bruton) agammaglobulinemia
    - Common variable immunodeficiency
    - Selective IgA deficiency
- T cell disorders
    - DiGeorge (thymic hypoplasia)
    - X-linked immunodeficiency with hyper IgM
    - Defective cytokine production
    - T cell activation defects
- Combined B and T cell Diseases
    - Combined immunodeficiency (CID or Nezelof syndrome)
    - Cartilage hair hypoplasia
    - Severe combined immunodeficiency (SCID)
    - Wiskott-Aldrich syndrome
    - Ataxia- telangiectasia
    - Hyper IgE syndrome
- Complement system defects
- Congenital neutropenia
- Chronic granulomatous disease
- Chediak-Higashi syndrome
- Congenital asplenia

Secondary or acquired immunocompromised states:
- Splenectomy or autosplenectomy (sickle cell disease)
- Chemotherapy with resultant neutropenia (ANC < 500/mm^3)
- HIV/AIDS
- Immunosuppressive therapy (organ or bone marrow transplants)
- Malnutrition (protein calorie malnutrition)

Loss of skin or mucosal integrity
- Indwelling catheters or shunts
- Burns
- Trauma

C **Organisms Associated with Infections in Secondary Immunocompromised States**

Condition	Organism
Splenectomy, autosplenectomy, asplenia	Encapsulated organisms: *S. pneumoniae, N. meningitides, H. influenzae* Parasites: malaria
HIV/AIDS	Bacteria: *S. pneumoniae*, salmonella, pseudomonas, mycobacteria Viruses: HSV, CMV, varicella-zoster, EBV, RSV, adenovirus, parainfluenza virus Fungi: Candida (especially in children), cryptococcus, histoplasma *Pneumocystis carinii*, toxoplasma, cryptosporidia
Chemotherapy associated neutropenia	Gram-positive or Gram-negative bacteria HSV Candida, other fungi
Bone marrow transplantation	Gram-positive or Gram-negative bacteria RSV Candida *P. carinii*
Solid organ transplantation	kidney transplant – Gram-negative bacteria liver transplant – Enteric organisms including vancomycin-resistant enterococci; consider ascending cholangitis
Indwelling catheters and shunts	Gram-positive bacteria, especially coagulase-negative staphylococci

＊ Continued on page 102

Clinical Manifestations

GEN immunocompromised state: chemotherapy, immunosuppression (transplants), sickle cell disease, asplenia, chronic steroid use, congenital immunodeficiency states; fever, hypothermia, chills

SKIN petechiae, purpura, rash, discharge or induration around catheter sites

CVS tachycardia, thready pulses, decreased perfusion, hypotension is a late sign

RESP tachypnea, respiratory distress, grunting, cyanosis

GI abdominal pain, tenderness, guarding, perirectal abscess, **avoid** rectal exam – but visual inspection is necessary

Diagnostics

Blood CBC, differential, electrolytes, BUN, creatinine, glucose
cultures (aerobic and anaerobic, viral, fungal, mycobacterial) – cultures obtained from indwelling catheters must always be accompanied by simultaneous peripheral cultures

Urine urinalysis, culture, Gram stain

Others wound culture, consider lumbar puncture (See p.107), chest radiograph, Gram stain

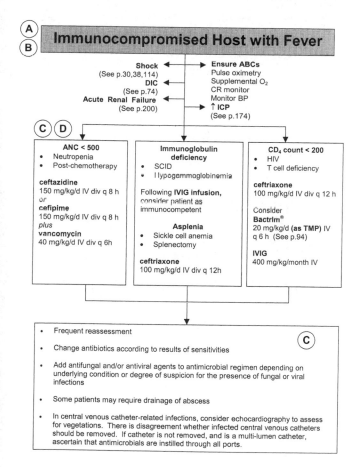

(A)
(B)

Immunocompromised Host with Fever

Shock ◄
(See p.30,38,114)
DIC ◄
(See p.74)
Acute Renal Failure ◄
(See p.200)

► **Ensure ABCs**
Pulse oximetry
Supplemental O_2
CR monitor
Monitor BP
► ↑ **ICP**
(See p.174)

(C) (D)

ANC < 500
- Neutropenia
- Post-chemotherapy

ceftazidine
150 mg/kg/d IV div q 8 h
or
cefipime
150 mg/kg/d IV div q 8 h
plus
vancomycin
40 mg/kg/d IV div q 6h

Immunoglobulin deficiency
- SCID
- Hypogammaglobinemia

Following **IVIG infusion**, consider patient as immunocompetent

Asplenia
- Sickle cell anemia
- Splenectomy

ceftriaxone
100 mg/kg/d IV div q 12h

CD$_4$ count < 200
- HIV
- T cell deficiency

ceftriaxone
100 mg/kg/d IV div q 12 h

Consider
Bactrim®
20 mg/kg/d (**as TMP**) IV
q 6 h (See p.94)

IVIG
400 mg/kg/month IV

- Frequent reassessment

- Change antibiotics according to results of sensitivities

- Add antifungal and/or antiviral agents to antimicrobial regimen depending on underlying condition or degree of suspicion for the presence of fungal or viral infections

- Some patients may require drainage of abscess

- In central venous catheter-related infections, consider echocardiography to assess for vegetations. There is disagreement whether infected central venous catheters should be removed. If catheter is not removed, and is a multi-lumen catheter, ascertain that antimicrobials are instilled through all ports.

(C)

✱ Continued from page 100

(D) Send cultures from all ports of indwelling central venous catheters. Skin abscesses and ulcers should be aspirated and sent for culture and Gram stain whenever possible. Chest radiographs should be obtained even in the absence of physical findings. Sinus imaging may be necessary as well. Abdominal findings or point tenderness over bone may necessitate imaging in search for sources of infection.

If possible, obtain blood culture prior to administration of antibiotics. However **DO NOT** delay antibiotics in order to complete diagnostic evaluation.

Gram-negative organisms generally cause the most immediately life-threatening type of infection.

Consider anaerobic infection in the presence of oral and perirectal abscess.

It is important to obtain history regarding recent use of broad-spectrum antibiotics, anti-inflammatory drugs/steroids that may predispose to opportunistic infections or resistant organisms.

NOTES

Acute Transfusion Reaction

Michael Vish

> Patients at highest risk for a transfusion reaction are those who have had multiple transfusions, previous transfusion reactions, or multiparous women. Those with suspected IgA deficiency should be given IgA deficient blood products or washed PRBC's. Patients who are immunocompromised should receive leuko-poor or irradiated, CMV-negative blood products.

(A) The following **3 systemic reaction types** present similarly and require diagnostic investigation to distinguish them.

- <u>Acute hemolytic reactions</u>: Medical emergency. Most commonly due to ABO incompatibility. Patients should be hydrated aggressively. Diuretics should be considered to maintain renal perfusion to avoid **ATN** (See p.200).

- <u>Infectious contamination</u>: Reactions vary from fevers and chills to **septic shock** (See p.114). Broad spectrum antibiotics should be considered.

- <u>Severe IgA reactions</u>: 1 in 900 have no IgA, 20% of whom make IgG against IgA. Reactions may be mild to severe. Severe systemic reactions can occur in these individuals when their own IgG reacts against donor IgA.

(B) Re-cross match donor and recipient blood STAT. Send blood for direct and indirect Coombs tests. Survey for hemoglobinuria and myoglobinuria. Donor and patient blood should be sent for Gram stain and culture.

(C) **Allergic reactions** account for approximately 1% of all transfusion reactions and include: pruritus, hives, bronchospasm/wheezing, and in extreme situations, anaphylaxis. Mild pruritus alone may be treated with diphenhydramine and careful observation. Additional symptoms mandate stopping the transfusion, close observation, treating with epinephrine and IV steroids to reverse systemic symptoms.

(D) **Nonhemolytic febrile reactions** are most commonly caused by host antibody response to donor leukocyte antigens. It may be difficult to distinguish between a simple febrile reaction and a more serious reaction. Febrile reactions are usually mild however, and are more common in multiparous women or in patients with multiple transfusion history.

Clinical Manifestations

NONSYSTEMIC	pruritus, erythema, urticaria
SYSTEMIC	chills, fever, hypotension, tachycardia, diaphoresis, bronchospasm, flushing, feeling of apprehension, mental status changes, back pain, pain at the infusion site, oozing or bleeding from wounds or IV sites, oliguria, changes in urine color

Diagnostics

Blood	repeat type and crossmatch, repeat direct and indirect Coombs, donor and recipient Gram stain/culture, PT, PTT, DIC panel
Urine	urinalysis (hemoglobin, myoglobin)

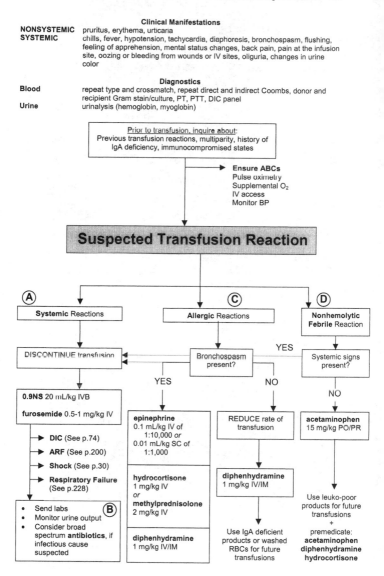

Prior to transfusion, inquire about:
Previous transfusion reactions, multiparity, history of
IgA deficiency, immunocompromised states

Ensure ABCs
Pulse oximetry
Supplemental O$_2$
IV access
Monitor BP

Suspected Transfusion Reaction

(A) Systemic Reactions

DISCONTINUE transfusion

0.9NS 20 mL/kg IVB

furosemide 0.5-1 mg/kg IV

➤ **DIC** (See p.74)
➤ **ARF** (See p.200)
➤ **Shock** (See p.30)
➤ **Respiratory Failure** (See p.228)

(B)
• Send labs
• Monitor urine output
• Consider broad spectrum **antibiotics**, if infectious cause suspected

(C) Allergic Reactions

Bronchospasm present?

YES

epinephrine
0.1 mL/kg IV of 1:10,000 or
0.01 mL/kg SC of 1:1,000

hydrocortisone
1 mg/kg IV
or
methylprednisolone
2 mg/kg IV

diphenhydramine
1 mg/kg IV/IM

NO

REDUCE rate of transfusion

diphenhydramine
1 mg/kg IV/IM

Use IgA deficient products or washed RBCs for future transfusions

(D) Nonhemolytic Febrile Reaction

Systemic signs present?

YES → DISCONTINUE transfusion

NO

acetaminophen
15 mg/kg PO/PR

Use leuko-poor products for future transfusions
+
premedicate:
**acetaminophen
diphenhydramine
hydrocortisone**

Chapter 7 ♣ Infectious Diseases

Acute Encephalitis

Maria C. Asi-Bautista

(A)

ORGANISM	CLINICAL MANIFESTATIONS	EPIDEMIOLOGY	COMMENTS
Herpes Simplex Virus (HSV) tropism for temporal lobe → aphasia, anosmia, temporal lobe seizures, focal neurologic findings	*Neonatal* (HSV type 2) disseminated → generalized encephalomalacia CNS only → bitemporal disease	transmitted most frequently through passage from an infected birth canal	> 50% suffer neurologic impairment despite therapy
	Infants and children (HSV type 1) seizures, focal neurologic findings; GCS < 6→ poor outcome irrespective of age	most common cause of non-epidemic, sporadic, focal, acute encephalitis	if untreated, mortality exceeds 70%
Rabies	*Acute neurologic phase* furious – hydrophobia paralytic – ascending symmetric paralysis	*Southeastern US:* raccoons, foxes, bats *South central US:* dogs, cattle *California:* skunks	once symptoms appear, invariably fatal
Enteroviruses	fever, URI symptoms, generalized neurologic symptoms	June to October	severe CNS involvement is rare except in neonates and immunocompromised patients.
St. Louis encephalitis (SLE)	fever, headache, lack of focal findings	central, southern, north eastern, western US	7% mortality
Western equine Encephalitis (WEE)	headache, altered consciousness, seizures; neurologic impairment common in infants	central and western US	5-15% mortality
Eastern equine Encephalitis (EEE)	fulminant disease; tropism for thalamus and basal ganglia	eastern, gulf coast, south of the US	coma and death in 1/3 of cases
West Nile virus (WNV)	fever, maculopapular rash, arthritis, lymphadenopathy, muscle weakness, meningoencephalitis	Atlantic and Gulf coast; mosquito-borne (*Culex*)	recovery is complete in survivors.
La Crosse (LAC)	seizures, focal weakness, paralysis, stupor, coma	midwestern, mid-atlantic US; mosquito-borne (*Aedes triseriatus*); summer, early fall	1% mortality
Lyme Disease (*Borrelia burgdorferi*)	erythema migrans, facial nerve palsy, arthritis. 15% to 40% may have early CNS complaints, e.g., headache, confusion, mood swings.	northeast US, upper midwest, west coast; tick-borne (*Ixodes*)	dubbed "The New Great Imitator" because of multisystem manifestation
Ehrlichiosis	Human Monocytic Ehrlichiosis (**HME**): fever, maculopapular-petechial rash, headache, myalgia, hepatosplenomegaly	south, southeastern US; tick-borne; May-July	consider in patients with febrile flu-like illness after outdoor activity in a tick-infested area.
	Human Granulocytic Ehrlichiosis (**HGE**): fever, headache, myalgia, sweats, symptoms may overlap with HME.	areas with deer ticks (*Ixodes*) (white-tailed deer); April-September	
Rocky Mountain Spotted Fever (RMSF) (*Rickettsia rickettsii*)	fever, headache, confusion, myalgias, petechial-purpuric rash	south Atlantic, south eastern, south central US; peak in early summer; tick-borne	delay (> 5 days) in diagnosis and treatment increases risk of death

(B)

OTHER LABORATORY TESTS

Organism	Source	Test	Comment
HSV type 1 & 2	CSF blood-EDTA	PCR keep sample at 4°C until assayed, TAT 2 days	CSF cultures are usually negative
St. Louis Western equine Eastern equine West Nile virus La Crosse	CSF	viral specific IgM in CSF (presence is confirmatory)	a separate specimen required for each virus being studied. call reference lab for handling.
Lyme disease	CSF blood	EIA	if EIA is ⊕ or equivocal, retest using Western immunoblot.
RMSF	CSF Blood	IFA > 1:64 IHA > 1:128	call reference lab for handling
Ehrlichiosis	CSF Blood	DNA-PCR	↑AST, ↓ platelets,↓ WBC, anemia, ↓ lymphocytes, ↓ Na⁺, ↑ BUN

PCR = polymerase chain reaction; EIA = enzyme immunoassay; IHA = indirect hemagglutination; IFA = indirect immunofluorescence antibody

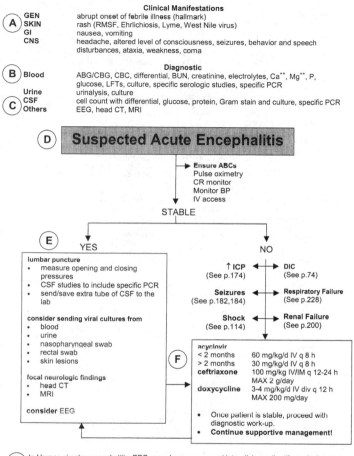

Clinical Manifestations

(A)
- **GEN** — abrupt onset of febrile illness (hallmark)
- **SKIN** — rash (RMSF, Ehrlichiosis, Lyme, West Nile virus)
- **GI** — nausea, vomiting
- **CNS** — headache, altered level of consciousness, seizures, behavior and speech disturbances, ataxia, weakness, coma

Diagnostic

(B)
- **Blood** — ABG/CBG, CBC, differential, BUN, creatinine, electrolytes, Ca^{++}, Mg^{++}, P, glucose, LFTs, culture, specific serologic studies, specific PCR
- **Urine** — urinalysis, culture

(C)
- **CSF** — cell count with differential, glucose, protein, Gram stain and culture, specific PCR
- **Others** — EEG, head CT, MRI

(D) **Suspected Acute Encephalitis**

→ **Ensure ABCs**
Pulse oximetry
CR monitor
Monitor BP
IV access

STABLE

(E) **YES**

lumbar puncture
- measure opening and closing pressures
- CSF studies to include specific PCR
- send/save extra tube of CSF to the lab

consider sending viral cultures from
- blood
- urine
- nasopharyngeal swab
- rectal swab
- skin lesions

focal neurologic findings
- head CT
- MRI

consider EEG

NO

↑ICP (See p.174) ◄──► DIC (See p.74)

Seizures (See p.182,184) ◄──► Respiratory Failure (See p.228)

Shock (See p.114) ◄──► Renal Failure (See p.200)

(F)
acyclovir
< 2 months 60 mg/kg/d IV q 8 h
> 2 months 30 mg/kg/d IV q 8 h
ceftriaxone 100 mg/kg IV/IM q 12-24 h
MAX 2 g/day
doxycycline 3-4 mg/kg/d IV div q 12 h
MAX 200 mg/day

- Once patient is stable, proceed with diagnostic work-up.
- **Continue supportive management!**

(C) In Herpes simplex encephalitis, EEG may show paroxysmal lateralizing epileptiform discharges (PLEDS). Abnormalities in the temporal lobe are best visualized by MRI.

(D) Obtain the following information: work exposure, history of tick or mosquito bite, residence or travel to an endemic area. Consider time of the year: seasonal versus nonseasonal causes.

(E) When the etiology is uncertain, it is imperative that CSF be available for specific testing, e.g., West Nile virus. Report all suspected cases to the health department.

(F) While diagnostic work-up is in progress, begin coverage with IV **acyclovir**. **Ceftriaxone** will cover most bacterial etiologic agents (meningococcemia) as well as CNS involvement in Lyme disease. If tick-borne encephalitis is suspected, begin **doxycycline**. Although tetracycline is not recommended in children < 8 years of age, the risk of dental staining is less with doxycycline. Withholding therapy can lead to a greater risk. Chloramphenicol is no longer available for use in the US.

Meningitis

Maria C. Asi-Bautista

(A) Classic triad of fever, nuchal rigidity and altered level of consciousness may not always be apparent, especially in infants and smaller children. Symptoms are usually preceded by an upper respiratory tract infection. Suspect meningitis in sick neonates < 2 months of age, because the organisms that cause bacterial infection in this age group usually infect the CNS as well.

(B) Meningitis following head trauma with CSF leaks is usually secondary to *Streptococcus pneumoniae*. *Staphylococcus epidermidis* is often the causative agent following neurosurgical procedures (e.g., VPS). In the immunocompromised host, consider HIV, *Toxoplasma gondii*, and fungal etiology.

↑ opening pressure and ↑ protein are clinically important CSF findings in bacterial meningitis. WBC is usually increased with predominance of PMNs, ↓ glucose. However, normal CSF chemistries or cell count does not rule out meningitis. Also, studies have shown that PMNs may predominate even beyond 24 hours in viral meningitis. Culture and pathogen specific PCR provide definite diagnosis. Proper specimen handling is important to ensure recovery of pathogen.

(C) INDICATIONS FOR HEAD IMAGING: (1) focal neurological exam findings, seizures, (2) increasing head circumference, (3) signs of ↑ ICP/cerebral edema, (4) lack of clinical improvement despite appropriate therapy, (5) suspected brain abscess

15% of patients with pneumococcal meningitis present in shock. Concomitant pneumonia is also a frequent finding.

(D) Cerebral blood flow (CBF) is very sensitive to blood pressure changes because of impaired autoregulation in meningitis.

(E) **Neuroimaging should be performed prior to lumbar puncture if there is (1) suspicion of a mass, (2) patients with depressed sensorium, (3) papilledema, (4) presence of focal neurological signs**
Note: increased intracranial pressure is **not** always accompanied by papilledema

CONTRAINDICATIONS TO LUMBAR PUNCTURE: (1) ↑ ICP, e.g., space occupying lesions, (2) bleeding diathesis/disorders, (3) cardiorespiratory instability, (4) DIC, (5) thrombocytopenia < 50,000/mm³, (6) infection over puncture site.
Seizures may be associated with ↑ ICP from increased metabolism and blood flow.

(F) In *Haemophilus influenzae* meningitis, the administration of **dexamethasone** prior to the first dose of antibiotics has been associated with ↓ fever, lower CSF protein, and ↓ auditory nerve damage. Dexamethasone may be considered for use in suspected *Streptococcus pneumoniae* meningitis.

EMPIRIC ANTIBIOTIC COVERAGE		
< 1 month of age: Group B Streptococcus, Listeria monocytogenes, Escherichia coli		
ampicillin	< 1 week	100-200 mg/kg/d IV div q 12 h
	> 1 week	200-400 mg/kg/d IV div q 6 h
plus		
cefotaxime	< 1 week	100 mg/kg/d IV div q 12 h
	1-4 weeks	150 mg/kg/d IV div q 8 h
or		
gentamicin	< 1 week	5.0 mg/kg/d IV div q 12h
	1-4 weeks	7.5 mg/kg/d IV div q 8h
1-3 months of age: same as above plus Streptococcus pneumoniae[☆], Neisseria meningitidis, Haemophilus influenzae		
ceftriaxone	100 mg/kg/d IV div q 12-24 h	
or		
cefotaxime	200-300 mg/kg/d IV div q 6-8 h	
plus		
ampicillin	200-400 mg/kg/d IV div q 4-6 h	
>3 months of age: Streptococcus pneumoniae[☆], Neisseria meningitidis, Haemophilus influenzae		
ceftriaxone	100 mg/kg/d IV div q 12-24 h	
or		
cefotaxime	200-300 mg/kg/d IV div q 6-8 h	
☆ If antibiotic resistant pneumococcal strain is suspected, add **vancomycin** 60 mg/kg/d IV div q 6 h until sensitivities are known		

✱ Continued on p.110

Clinical Manifestations

A **GEN** fever, hypothermia (preterm), irritability, poor feeding or change in feeding habits, anorexia, myalgias

HEENT headache, photophobia, nuchal rigidity, bulging fontanelle, ↑ head circumference

CVS bradycardia, shock

RESP respiratory distress

GI nausea and vomiting

CNS altered mental status, seizures

SKIN rash, cyanosis, petechiae

Diagnostics

B **Blood** CBC with differential, CBG/ABG, electrolytes, Ca++, glucose, BUN, creatinine, osmolality, culture. Consider PT, PTT, specific antibody titers. *Save serum for serology.*

CSF Gram stain, cell count with differential, glucose, protein, bacterial antigen, culture, etiology specific PCR. *Save CSF for future studies.*

C **Urine** culture, specific gravity, osmolality

Others Head CT, MRI, chest radiograph, strict intake and output monitoring

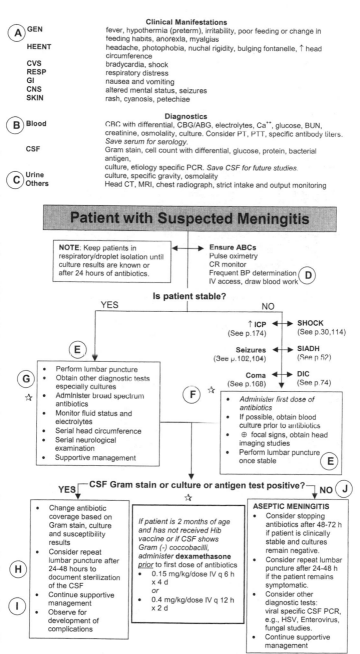

Patient with Suspected Meningitis

NOTE: Keep patients in respiratory/droplet isolation until culture results are known or after 24 hours of antibiotics.

Ensure ABCs
Pulse oximetry
CR monitor
Frequent BP determination
IV access, draw blood work **D**

Is patient stable?

YES — NO

↑ ICP (See p.174) ←→ SHOCK (See p.30,114)

Seizures (See p.102,104) ←→ SIADH (See p.52)

Coma (See p.168) ←→ DIC (See p.74)

E

G ☆
- Perform lumbar puncture
- Obtain other diagnostic tests especially cultures
- Administer broad spectrum antibiotics
- Monitor fluid status and electrolytes
- Serial head circumference
- Serial neurological examination
- Supportive management

F ☆
- *Administer first dose of antibiotics*
- If possible, obtain blood culture prior to antibiotics
- ⊕ focal signs, obtain head imaging studies
- Perform lumbar puncture once stable **E**

CSF Gram stain or culture or antigen test positive?

YES ☆ — NO **J**

H
- Change antibiotic coverage based on Gram stain, culture and susceptibility results
- Consider repeat lumbar puncture after 24-48 hours to document sterilization of the CSF

I
- Continue supportive management
- Observe for development of complications

If patient is 2 months of age and has not received Hib vaccine or if CSF shows Gram (-) coccobacilli, administer **dexamethasone** *prior to first dose of antibiotics*
- 0.15 mg/kg/dose IV q 6 h x 4 d
  or
- 0.4 mg/kg/dose IV q 12 h x 2 d

ASEPTIC MENINGITIS
- Consider stopping antibiotics after 48-72 h if patient is clinically stable and cultures remain negative.
- Consider repeat lumbar puncture after 24-48 h if the patient remains symptomatic.
- Consider other diagnostic tests: viral specific CSF PCR, e.g., HSV, Enterovirus, fungal studies.
- Continue supportive management

✳ Continued from p.108

(G) Administer fluids at maintenance. If SIADH is suspected, adjust IV rate (2/3 maintenance) and type of solution based on serum sodium and osmolality.

(H) The goal of antibiotic therapy is rapid sterilization of the CSF. Rapid sterilization has been associated with decrease in mortality and long term neurologic sequelae.

COMPLICATIONS

(I) (1) seizures, (2) ↑ ICP, (3) septic cortical vein thrombosis, (4) septic superior sagittal sinus thrombosis, (5) hydrocephalus, (6) subdural effusion, (7) SIADH, (8) DI

(J) Aseptic meningitis usually follows a benign, self-limited course from which 95% of children recover completely. Enteroviruses (Coxsackieviruses and Echoviruses) are the most common etiologic agent in viral infections in children in the summer and early fall months.

If symptoms do not resolve over a few days and CSF continues to show abnormalities, consider CSF cryptococcal antigen, AFB smear, virus-specific IgM antibodies.

OTHER CAUSES OF ASEPTIC MENINGITIS

Partially treated bacterial meningitis: persistently ↓ glucose or ↑ PMNs
Tuberculous meningitis (See p.112)
Lyme meningitis (See p.106)
Ehrlichiosis (See p.106)
Mycoplasma pneumoniae
Infective endocarditis: ↑ WBC, ↑ ESR
Post-infectious syndromes
Drugs: INH, trimethoprim-sulfamethoxazole (Bactrim®), NSAIDs, IVIG

If suspecting HSV meningitis, begin **acyclovir**   < 2 months of age   60 mg/kg/d IV div q 8 h
                                                    > 2 months of age   30 mg/kg/d IV div q 8 h

Recommended Doses of Pathogen-specific Antimicrobials in Meningitis

ORGANISM	PREFFERED DRUG	ALTERNATIVE	DURATION
Group B Streptococci	**penicillin G** < 1 week 250,000-450,000 units/kg/d IV div q 8 h > 1 week 450,000 units/kg/d IV div q 6 h	ampicillin < 1 week 100-200 mg/kg/d IV div q 12 h > 1 week 200-400 mg/kg/d IV div q 4-6 h	14 -21days
Haemophilus influenzae	**ceftriaxone** 100 mg/kg/d IV div q 12-24 h	cefotaxime 200-300 mg/kg/d IV div q 6-8 h	10 days
Listeria monocytogenes	**ampicillin** (dose as above) *plus* **gentamicin** 7.5 mg/kg/d IV div q 8 h		14-21 days
Neisseria meningitidis	**penicillin G** (dose as above)	cefotaxime or ceftriaxone (dose as above)	5-7 days
Streptococcus pneumoniae	**penicillin G** (dose as above) **ceftriaxone** (dose as above)	cefotaxime 200-300 mg/kg/d IV div q 6-8 h	10-14 days
	if MIC 0.1 **vancomycin** 60 mg/kg/d IV div q 6 h *plus* **ceftriaxone (cefotaxime)**		

NOTE: Rifampin chemoprophylaxis is recommended for contacts of index cases of *Haemophilus influenzae* and *Neisseria meningitidis* meningitis. See Red Book 2000 recommendations.

NOTES

Tuberculous Meningitis

Lawrence S. Quang

The most serious complication of pediatric tuberculosis is central nervous system disease. Tuberculous meningitis complicates 0.5% of untreated primary tuberculous infections in children. It is most common in children between the ages of 6 months and 4 years.

Rupture of caseous lesions causes release of tuberculoproteins in the subarachnoid space leading to hypersensitivity reaction → formation of exudates especially in the basal cisterns, cranial nerves and blood vessels at the base of the brain → obstructive hydrocephalus or obstruction of resorption of CSF → communicating hydrocephalus.

(A) Tuberculous meningitis can present with vague, non-specific symptoms, e.g., fever, weight loss, night sweats, malaise. A high index of suspicion is needed especially if above symptoms are associated with the presence of communicating hydrocephalus and focal neurologic signs. The most commonly affected cranial nerve is CN VI.

(B) CSF FINDINGS IN TUBERCULOUS MENINGITIS

WBC (cells/mm^3)	50-500, PMN cells early, eventually lymphocytic predominance
Glucose (mg/dL)	< 40
Protein (mg/dL)	50-500 (up to 5000 in the presence of hydrocephalus)
Gram stain	negative
AFB	sensitivity depends on volume of sample. With 10 mL, AFB stain is positive up to 30% of cases
PCR	sensitivity 54%, false positive 3-25%
Culture	75% become positive in 3-6 weeks
ELISA	IgG antibodies to purified protein derivative

OTHER TESTS

Opening pressure (lumbar puncture)	usually elevated
Head CT	basilar enhancement with communicating hydrocephalus, cerebral edema, focal infarction/ischemia, tuberculoma
Chest radiograph	normal up to 50% of cases
Tuberculin skin test	non-reactive in up to 40% of cases

HIV infected individuals will most likely have an acellular CSF response but have higher incidence of intracerebral mass lesion.

(C) In other areas of the world, the most common AIDS associated CNS infection is tuberculous meningitis.

Lumbar puncture and CSF studies for the presence of the acid fast organism should be considered in children <1 year of age who are diagnosed with tuberculous disease.

(D) Obtain neurosurgical consult for possible VP shunt placement in cases of non-communicating hydrocephalus or communicating.

(E) When resistance is suspected, use **ethambutol**.

Obtain baseline liver function test prior to initiation of anti-TB therapy.

(F) INDICATIONS FOR CORTICOSTEROIDS
- Altered consciousness
- Papilledema
- Focal neurologic symptoms
- Impending herniation
- Spinal block
- Hydrocephalus

Steroids decrease mortality and long-term neurologic sequelae by reducing vasculitis, inflammation, and intracranial pressure.

Clinical Manifestations

GEN	fever, poor feeding, anorexia, malaise, night sweats
HEENT	headache, CN III, VI, VII palsies, photophobia, bulging fontanelle, increased head circumference, nuchal rigidity, positive meningeal signs (Kernig's or Brudzinski's), anisocoria, papilledema
(A) CNS	altered level of consciousness, seizures, coma, ↑ ICP, hypertonia, change in behavior
GI	nausea, vomiting
ENDOCRINE	hyponatremia (SIADH)

Diagnostics

Blood	CBC, differential, electrolytes, BUN, creatinine, glucose, osmolality
Urine	osmolality, specific gravity
CSF	glucose, protein, cell count with differential, Gram stain, AFB stain, PCR
(B) Sepsis work up	anaerobic, aerobic, viral, fungal, mycobacterial culture of blood, urine, CSF, sputum, other body fluids
Others	chest radiograph, head CT, tuberculin skin test

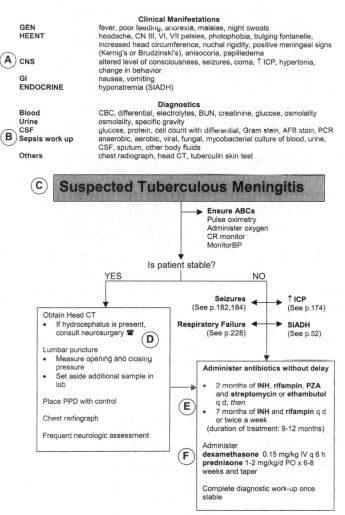

(C) **Suspected Tuberculous Meningitis**

Ensure ABCs
Pulse oximetry
Administer oxygen
CR monitor
MonitorBP

Is patient stable?

YES — NO

Seizures (See p.182,184) ←→ ↑ **ICP** (See p.174)

Respiratory Failure (See p.228) ←→ **SIADH** (See p.52)

Obtain Head CT
• If hydrocephalus is present, consult neurosurgery ☎ (D)

Lumbar puncture
• Measure opening and closing pressure
• Set aside additional sample in lab

Place PPD with control

Chest radiograph

Frequent neurologic assessment

Administer antibiotics without delay

• 2 months of **INH**, **rifampin**, **PZA** and **streptomycin** or **ethambutol** q d, *then*
• 7 months of **INH** and **rifampin** q d or twice a week
(duration of treatment: 9-12 months)

(E)

Administer
dexamethasone 0.15 mg/kg IV q 6 h
prednisone 1-2 mg/kg/d PO x 6-8 weeks and taper

(F)

Complete diagnostic work-up once stable

DRUG	DAILY DOSE (mg/kg/dose)	TWICE A WEEK DOSE (mg/kg/dose)	MAXIMUM DOSE
Isoniazid (INH)	10-15	20-30	Daily, 300 mg Twice a week, 900 mg
Rifampin	10-20	10-20	600 mg
Pyrazinamide (PZA)	20-40	50	2 g
Streptomycin	20-40	20-40	1 g
Ethambutol	15-25	50	2.5 g

Septic Shock

K. Jane Lee

> Septic shock results from dysregulation of the inflammatory response to an infectious insult. It manifests as SIRS, the systemic inflammatory response syndrome (fever, tachycardia, tachypnea, and leucocytosis) along with hypotension and hypoperfusion, and may progress to multiple organ dysfunction syndrome (MODS), including ARDS, encephalopathy, and renal failure.

(A) Patients with septic shock are initially **warm and hyperdynamic** with ↑ CO, ↓ SVR, widened pulse pressure, and warm extremities. As myocardial dysfunction progresses and the body is no longer able to compensate for ↓ SVR, the patient becomes **cold and hypodynamic** with ↓ CO, hypotension, worsening hypoperfusion, and lactic acidosis.

(B) Blood cultures may not always yield positive results. Gram stain remains a very important diagnostic tool in suspected infection, especially in patients already treated with antibiotics. In the normally sterile site, recovery of pus, positive Gram stain, or positive culture increases the likelihood of an infection. Consult with your institution's laboratory services regarding the availability of molecular biology techniques, e.g., specific PCR.

(C) **Predisposing Factors Associated with Septic Shock**

• age < 1y	• AIDS, immunodeficiency syndromes
• immunosuppressive and chemotherapeutic drugs	• malnutrition
• trauma	• prolonged use of indwelling medical devices
• burns	• functional or surgical asplenia, e.g., sickle cell disease
	• obstructive uropathy (in urosepsis)

(D) Ideally, two separate IV lines facilitate the simultaneous administration of fluids and medications.

(E) Do **not** delay giving antibiotics in order to complete diagnostic evaluation. In critically ill patients, it is prudent to obtain a blood culture prior to first dose of antibiotics. Lumbar puncture should be obtained after stabilization of the patient. (See p.108)
Antibiotic choice may vary by patient population and local susceptibility profile. Start with a third generation cephalosporin, and provide additional coverage as below for special circumstances.

Patient Population	Common Organisms	Additional Antibiotic
Infant < 8 weeks	Group B *Streptococcus*, *Listeria*, coliforms	**ampicillin**
Indwelling medical devices (VPS, CVC)	Staphylococcus, resistant Streptococcus	appropriate anti-staphylococcal coverage
Intra-abdominal source anaerobes		**metronidazole, gentamicin**
Immunosuppressed Pseudomonas fungal Herpes, varicella		**ceftazidime, tobramycin, consider cefepime amphotericin B acyclovir**
Invasive group A Streptococcus (following varicella infection)		**penicillin or clindamycin**
Herpes or varicella		**acyclovir**
Tick endemic areas (see p.106)		**doxycycline**

(F) Reassess response to volume resuscitation. Consider cardiogenic shock in differential diagnosis, e.g., myocarditis, cardiomyopathy, pericarditis, congenital heart disease.

(G) Anemia (hemoglobin < 10 g/dL or hematocrit < 30%) should be treated in order to improve oxygen delivery to the tissues.

(H) Norepinephrine should be considered in patients who (1) have persistently ↓ SVR, (2) remain hypotensive despite high doses of dopamine. Because of the small infusion volumes used in infants and children, vasoactive drugs, e.g., epinephrine, should be administered using a syringe pump. Infusion pumps may produce cyclic variations in fluid delivery rate that may cause significant changes in hemodynamic response.

(I) Dobutamine should not be used alone. It may cause worsening of hypotension in severe shock, because of its vasodilating effects. **Milrinone**, a phosphodiesterase inhibitor may be considered in cases unresponsive to adequate volume resuscitation and inotropic/vasopressor drugs.

(J) Early eradication of septic foci is essential, e.g., removal of indwelling catheters, drainage of abscesses. Antibiotic coverage should be adjusted according to sensitivity results. Adjust antibiotic dosing according to renal function.

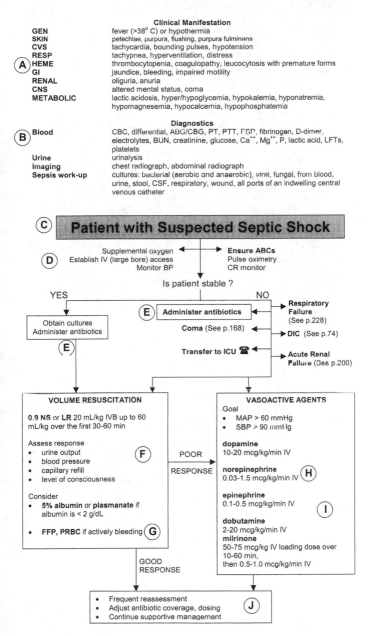

Clinical Manifestation

(A)

GEN	fever (>38° C) or hypothermia
SKIN	petechiae, purpura, flushing, purpura fulminans
CVS	tachycardia, bounding pulses, hypotension
RESP	tachypnea, hyperventilation, distress
HEME	thrombocytopenia, coagulopathy, leucocytosis with premature forms
GI	jaundice, bleeding, impaired motility
RENAL	oliguria, anuria
CNS	altered mental status, coma
METABOLIC	lactic acidosis, hyper/hypoglycemia, hypokalemia, hyponatremia, hypomagnesemia, hypocalcemia, hypophosphatemia

Diagnostics

(B)

Blood	CBC, differential, ABG/CBG, PT, PTT, FSP, fibrinogen, D-dimer, electrolytes, BUN, creatinine, glucose, Ca^{++}, Mg^{++}, P, lactic acid, LFTs, platelets
Urine	urinalysis
Imaging	chest radiograph, abdominal radiograph
Sepsis work-up	cultures: bacterial (aerobic and anaerobic), viral, fungal, from blood, urine, stool, CSF, respiratory, wound, all ports of an indwelling central venous catheter

(C) **Patient with Suspected Septic Shock**

(D) Supplemental oxygen ◀─────▶ **Ensure ABCs**
Establish IV (large bore) access   Pulse oximetry
Monitor BP   CR monitor

Is patient stable ?

YES   NO

(E) **Administer antibiotics** ◀──── **Respiratory Failure** (See p.228)

Obtain cultures
Administer antibiotics   **Coma** (See p.168) ◀──── ▶**DIC** (See p.74)

(E)   **Transfer to ICU** ☎ ◀──── **Acute Renal Failure** (See p.200)

VOLUME RESUSCITATION

0.9 NS or **LR** 20 mL/kg IVB up to 60 mL/kg over the first 30-60 min

Assess response
• urine output
• blood pressure   (F)
• capillary refill
• level of consciousness

Consider
• **5% albumin** or **plasmanate** if albumin is < 2 g/dL

• **FFP, PRBC** if actively bleeding (G)

POOR RESPONSE ─────▶

VASOACTIVE AGENTS

Goal
• MAP > 60 mmHg
• SBP > 90 mmHg

dopamine
10-20 mcg/kg/min IV

norepinephrine (H)
0.03-1.5 mcg/kg/min IV

epinephrine
0.1-0.5 mcg/kg/min IV   (I)

dobutamine
2-20 mcg/kg/min IV
milrinone
50-75 mcg/kg IV loading dose over 10-60 min,
then 0.5-1.0 mcg/kg/min IV

GOOD RESPONSE

• Frequent reassessment
• Adjust antibiotic coverage, dosing   (J)
• Continue supportive management

Chapter 8 ♣ Toxicology

General Poisoning

Randy Prescilla

(A) If osmolal gap > 10 mOsm/L, osmolal substances, e.g., alcohol may be present. Serum osmolality determination should be performed by freezing point depression method to avoid loss of volatile osmoles. Acetaminophen, salicylate, and ethanol are common co-ingestants; if not included in toxic screen panel, order specific levels.

*A **negative** screen result does **not** rule out toxic ingestion.* See page 310 for list of drugs included in most toxicology panels. (☎ Consult your local toxicology laboratory.)

(B) Suspect poisoning in cases of:
- Acute onset of symptoms that do not readily fit a specific disease entity
- Head injury/trauma
- Unexplained behavior/mental status changes, seizures
- Arrhythmia of unknown etiology
- Unexplained metabolic acidosis/alkalosis

(C)

DECONTAMINATION	
Eye Exposure	**Skin/Hair Exposure**
1. Remove contact lenses. 2. Remove solid material gently with cotton swab. 3. Irrigate eye *immediately* for **at least** 30 minutes with **0.9NS** or **LR**. 4. Do not use neutralizing solutions. 5. Perform fluorescein staining. 6. Note visual acuity before and after treatment. 7. *Alkali corneal burns are emergencies.* ☎ Consult Ophthalmology	1. Remove contaminated clothing. Leather goods are irreversibly contaminated and must be abandoned. *Note: Medical personnel must protect themselves by using impermeable gloves and gowns.* 2. Wash skin/hair with copious amounts of water for at least 30 minutes. For caustic alkali exposure, wash > 30 minutes or until "soapy" feeling is gone.

(D)

TOXIC SYNDROMES (TOXIDROMES)

Syndrome	Symptoms	Source (partial list)
Muscarinic (DUMBBELS)	**d**efecation, **u**rination, **m**iosis, **b**radycardia, **b**ronchorrhea, **e**mesis, **l**acrimation, **s**ecretions	acetylcholine, pilocarpine, mushrooms, betel nut, carbachol, organophosphates
Nicotinic	tachycardia, hypertension, muscle fasciculations, paralysis	insecticides (nicotinic), tobacco, black widow spider venom
Anticholinergic	dry skin, hyperthermia, thirst, dysphagia, mydriasis, tachycardia, urinary urgency and retention, delirium, hallucinations, respiratory failure	belladonna alkaloid, mushrooms, scopolamine, antihistamines, cyclic antidepressants, over-the-counter sleep medications
Sympathomimetic	CNS excitation, hypertension, convulsions, tachycardia	theophylline, caffeine, LSD, phencyclidine (PCP), cocaine, phenylpropanolamine, amphetamine
Narcotic	CNS depression, hypoventilation, hypotension, miosis	codeine, Lomotil®, heroin, propoxyphene (Darvon®), pentazocine (Talwin®)
Narcotic Withdrawal	diarrhea, mydriasis, goose bumps, tachycardia, lacrimation, yawning, cramps, hallucinations	alcohol, barbiturates, benzodiazepines, narcotics, chloral hydrate

✱ Continued on p.118

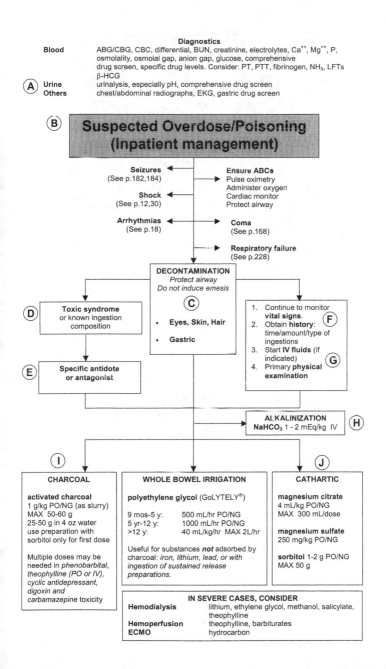

Diagnostics

(A)
- **Blood** — ABG/CBG, CBC, differential, BUN, creatinine, electrolytes, Ca^{++}, Mg^{++}, P, osmolality, osmolal gap, anion gap, glucose, comprehensive drug screen, specific drug levels. Consider: PT, PTT, fibrinogen, NH_3, LFTs, β-HCG
- **Urine** — urinalysis, especially pH, comprehensive drug screen
- **Others** — chest/abdominal radiographs, EKG, gastric drug screen

(B) **Suspected Overdose/Poisoning (Inpatient management)**

Ensure ABCs
- Pulse oximetry
- Administer oxygen
- Cardiac monitor
- Protect airway

Seizures (See p.182,184)

Shock (See p.12,30)

Arrhythmias (See p.18)

Coma (See p.168)

Respiratory failure (See p.228)

DECONTAMINATION
Protect airway
Do not induce emesis
(C)
- Eyes, Skin, Hair
- Gastric

(D) **Toxic syndrome** or known ingestion composition

(E) **Specific antidote** or antagonist

(F)
1. Continue to monitor **vital signs**.
2. Obtain **history**: time/amount/type of ingestions
3. Start **IV fluids** (if indicated) (G)
4. Primary **physical examination**

(H) **ALKALINIZATION** $NaHCO_3$ 1 - 2 mEq/kg IV

(I) **CHARCOAL**

activated charcoal
1 g/kg PO/NG (as slurry)
MAX 50-60 g
25-50 g in 4 oz water
use preparation with
sorbitol only for first dose

Multiple doses may be
needed in *phenobarbital*,
theophylline (PO or IV),
cyclic antidepressant,
digoxin and
carbamazepine toxicity

WHOLE BOWEL IRRIGATION

polyethylene glycol (GoLYTELY®)

9 mos-5 y: 500 mL/hr PO/NG
5 yr-12 y: 1000 mL/hr PO/NG
>12 y: 40 mL/kg/hr MAX 2L/hr

Useful for substances *not* adsorbed by
charcoal: *iron, lithium, lead*, or with
ingestion of sustained release
preparations.

(J) **CATHARTIC**

magnesium citrate
4 mL/kg PO/NG
MAX 300 mL/dose

magnesium sulfate
250 mg/kg PO/NG

sorbitol 1-2 g PO/NG
MAX 50 g

IN SEVERE CASES, CONSIDER

Hemodialysis	lithium, ethylene glycol, methanol, salicylate, theophylline
Hemoperfusion	theophylline, barbiturates
ECMO	hydrocarbon

✳ Continued from p.116

COMMON EMERGENCY ANTIDOTES

POISON	ANTIDOTE	DOSE	COMMENTS
Acetaminophen	N-acetylcysteine	See page 123	
Atropine	physostigmine 0.01-0.03 mg/kg/dose	0.5 mg IV over 6 sec q 20 min *prn* MAX 1 mg/min	Do not use in asthma, diabetes, urinary obstruction, or retention.
Benzodiazepines (midazolam)	flumazenil (Romazicon®) 0.01 mg/kg MAX 0.2 mg	0.2 mg (2 mL) IV over 30 sec, may repeat after 30 sec with 0.3 mg (3 mL). Further doses 0.5 mg over 30 sec. If no response in 5 min or max 5 mg, cause of sedation unlikely to be benzodiazepine	Not recommended for cyclic antidepressant poisoning, and in seizures and increased ICP
β – blockers	glucagon	100-150 mcg/kg IV push then 2.5-5 mg/hr. Taper over 5-12 hours	Effects of single dose observed in 5-10 min and lasts for 15-30 min
Calcium channel Blocker (CCB)	Ca gluconate 10% (100 mg/mL)	100-200 mg/kg/dose MAX 2-3 g slow IV Titrate to adequate response.	Monitor Ca^{++} levels. **Contraindicated** in digitalis poisoning
	glucagon	See above dose	
Carbon monoxide	O_2	100% by inhalation	In severe cases, consider hyperbaric chamber
Digoxin	Specific antibody fragments (Digibind®)	See page 142	
Ethylene glycol	fomepizole (Antizol®)	See page 124	
	ethyl alcohol 50% 1:1 in D_5W	See page 124	
Iron	deferoxamine (DFO)	See page 134	
Lead	CaEDTA BAL	See Table p.119	Level > 80 mcg/dL and/or encephalopathy is a medical emergency
Nitrite (MetHb)	methylene blue 1% solution (10 mg/mL)	1-2 mg/kg IV over 5 min MAX dose in infants: 4 mg/kg	May cause hemolysis in G6PD deficient patient.
Opiate (Darvon®, Lomotil®)	naloxone	0.1 mg/kg/dose IV *prn* (reversal of respiratory depression)	MAX effect: 2 hours Continuous IV infusion may be needed.
Organophosphate/ carbamates	atropine, pralidoxime (2-PAM)	See page 136	

Adapted in part from: Shannon MW and LM Haddad. The emergency treatment of poisoning. In: Haddad LM, Shannon MW, Winchester JF (eds). *Clinical Management of Poisoning and Drug Overdose* 3rd edition. Philadelphia: WB Saunders Co., Inc. 1998. p 4.

Agents that may be toxic or fatal in small quantities (one pill or one teaspoonful)

Benzocaine	Desipramine	Methanol
Camphor	Diphenhydramine	Methyl salicylate
Chloroquine	Diphenoxylate	Orphenadrine
Chlorpromazine	Ethylene glycol	Quinine
Clonidine	Hydroxychloroquine	Theophylline
Codeine	Imipramine	Thioridazine

Modified from Koren GK: Medications that can kill a toddler with one tablet or teaspoon. J Toxicol Clin Toxicol 1993: 31:407-413

History
- Tell family members to retrieve containers of medications or toxins whenever possible.
- Review patient's old chart if available.
  Ask about family and family history of psychiatric problems, drug addiction, alcoholism, allergies, occupational and recreational histories, chronic diseases, asthma, and sickle cell anemia.
- Inquire about possible medications at home, including relatives', friends' and visitors'.

Alkalinization
Useful in cases of salicylate, cyclic antidepressant and phenobarbital poisoning. Monitor serum pH (goal: 7.45-7.55), calcium, potassium closely.

Ⓙ **Gastric decontamination**
- The use of ipecac syrup in health care facilities is no longer recommended.
- Activated charcoal *does not* effectively adsorb iron and heavy metals, alcohol, organophosphates/carbamates, cyanide, hydrocarbons, caustics, and corrosives.
- *Gastric lavage is no longer routinely recommended.*

Ⓘ **Cathartic**
- May be given with first dose of charcoal
- Routine use is no longer recommended; do not use in trivial ingestions.
- Do not use in multiple doses in children.
- Do not use sorbitol in children <1 y, use with caution in children <3 years of age.
- Watch out for hypernatremic dehydration and cardiovascular collapse.

All cases of *accidental* toxic ingestion need:
- Poison Control consult ☎
- Social work consult ☎
- Review of old chart (if applicable)

All cases of *intentional* toxic ingestion need:
- All of the above.
- Psychiatric consult ☎
- 24-hr sitter
- Suicide precautions

Homicide/child abuse should be suspected in infants who present with poisoning. If suspected, these children will need
- All of the above (except suicide precautions)
- Restriction of parental visits

Suggested treatment of lead-induced encephalopathy and/or serum levels >70mcg/dL

Condition, [Pb] (mcg/dL)	Dose	Regimen/Comments
Encephalopathy	BAL 450 mg/m^2/d + CaNA$_2$EDTA 1500 mg/m^2 /d	75 mg/m^2 IM every 4 hours for 5 d Continuous infusion, or 2-4 divided IV doses for 5 d (start 4 h after BAL)
Symptomatic, [Pb] > 70	BAL 300-450 mg/m^2/d + CaNA$_2$EDTA 1000-1500 mg/m^2 /d	50-75 mg/m^2 IM every 4 hours for 3-5 d Continuous infusion, or 2-4 divided IV doses for 5 d (start 4 h after BAL) Base the dose and duration on [Pb] and the severity of symptoms.

Modified from Henretig FM. Lead. In *Goldfrank's Toxicologic Emergencies*, 6th edition, Stamford, CT: Appleton and Lange 1998, p 1301

Acetaminophen Toxicity

Adora Poon

Acetaminophen is an over-the-counter medication used for antipyresis and mild-moderate pain control. It is found in many different concentrations and preparations (e.g., Aceta®, APAP®, Feverall®, Genapap®, Panadol®, Pedia pap®, Tempra®, Tylenol®), including combination preparations, e.g., Tylenol® with codeine.

Overdose may be intentional with single doses exceeding 140 mg/kg or unintentional overdose from incorrect dosage or inadvertent over administration via combination preparations.

Acetaminophen is metabolized to sulfate/glucuronide (90-95%) and a cytotoxic P450 metabolite NAPQI (5-10%), which combines with glutathione to become a nontoxic metabolite. Damage to the liver (as well as kidneys and heart) in acetaminophen overdose is due to saturation of sulfate/glucuronide metabolism and glutathione depletion, resulting in excess free NAPQI.

(A)

	Stage I	Stage II	Stage III	Stage IV
Onset	0 - 24 hours	24 - 72 hours	72 - 96 hours	4 days – 2 wks
Clinical Effects	• Asymptomatic • Anorexia • Nausea • Vomiting • Pallor • Diaphoresis	• Resolution of Stage I symptoms • RUQ abdominal tenderness • Elevation of LFTs • Oliguria	• Worsening of initial stage I symptoms • Coagulopathy • Jaundice • Hepatic encephalopathy • Renal failure • Myocardial pathology • Death	• Complete resolution of hepatic dysfunction if damage in Stage III is reversible

(B) If combination preparation was ingested, observe for the development of signs and symptoms due to co-ingestants.

(C) If syrup of ipecac was given prior to arrival to the hospital, **activated charcoal** should be given 1-1 ½ hours after, in order to minimize risk of vomiting and aspiration.

Ideally, **N-acetylcysteine** should be given 1 hour after activated charcoal, since charcoal binds N-acetylcysteine, and may decrease availability.

If N-acetylcysteine dose is vomited within one hour of administration, the dose should be repeated.

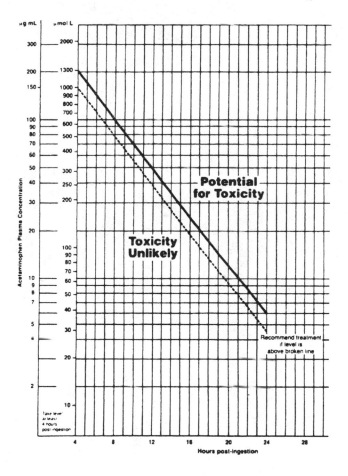

μg mL | μmol L

Acetaminophen Plasma Concentration

Potential for Toxicity

Toxicity Unlikely

Recommend treatment if level is above broken line

Take level at least 4 hours post-ingestion

Hours post-ingestion

Rumack-Matthew Nomogram.
Check units (μg/mL or μmol/L) before plotting.

Cautions for use of this chart
The time coordinates refer to time post-ingestion. Serum levels drawn before 4 hours may not represent peak levels. The graph relates only to plasma levels following a single acute overdose. The broken line, which represents a 25% allowance below the solid line, is included to allow for possible errors in acetaminophen plasma assays and estimated time from ingestion of an overdose.
Modified from Rumack BH, Matthew H. *Acetaminophen Poisoning and Toxicity.* Pediatrics 55:871-876, 1975. With permission.

NOTES

Clinical Manifestations

(A) Decreasing level of consciousness is unusual, unless a co-ingestant is present.

Diagnostics

Blood acetaminophen levels (at least 4 hours post-ingestion), LFTs, CBC with differential, BUN, creatinine, glucose, drug screen. Consider β HCG, especially in intentional ingestions. Monitor LFTs, CBC, and platelets q 24 hours x 4 days while treatment in progress.

Urine drug screen

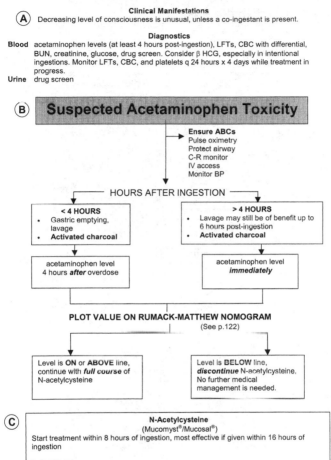

(B) ## Suspected Acetaminophen Toxicity

Ensure ABCs
Pulse oximetry
Protect airway
C-R monitor
IV access
Monitor BP

HOURS AFTER INGESTION

< 4 HOURS
- Gastric emptying, lavage
- **Activated charcoal**

> 4 HOURS
- Lavage may still be of benefit up to 6 hours post-ingestion
- **Activated charcoal**

acetaminophen level 4 hours *after* overdose

acetaminophen level *immediately*

PLOT VALUE ON RUMACK-MATTHEW NOMOGRAM
(See p.122)

Level is **ON** or **ABOVE** line, continue with *full course* of N-acetylcysteine

Level is **BELOW** line, *discontinue* N-acetylcysteine. No further medical management is needed.

(C)
N-Acetylcysteine
(Mucomyst®/Mucosal®)

Start treatment within 8 hours of ingestion, most effective if given within 16 hours of ingestion

Indications
- Serum acetaminophen level in toxic range
- Estimated ingestion more than 140 mg/kg
- Less than 24 hours since ingestion
- No levels available

Dose
140 mg/kg PO/NG, then 70 mg/kg PO/NG q 4 h x 17 doses in 1:3 dilution with juice/carbonated beverage

Alcohol Ingestions: Ethanol, Isopropanol, Methanol, Ethylene Glycol

Randy Prescilla

	CNS depression	Breath/ odor	Characteristic findings	High anion gap acidosis	Ketosis	Commercial products	Metabolites
Ethanol	+	+	alcoholic ketoacidosis not usually associated with CNS depression or ethanol in blood	+	+	solvents, beverages, cologne, mouth-washes, cough syrups	acetalde-hyde, acetic acid
Iso-propanol	++	+	hemorrhagic tracheo-bronchitis, gastritis	-	+	rubbing alcohol, solvents, lacquer, de-icers	acetone
Methanol	+	-	blindness, pink edematous optic disc	++	-	antifreeze, solvents, gasohol, denaturant, windshield wiper fluid	formaldehyde, formic acid (toxic)
Ethylene glycol	+	-	renal failure, hypocalcemia, Ca oxalate crystals in urine	++	-	antifreeze, solvents, de-icers, aircondition-ing units	oxalic acid, glycolic acid (toxic)

(B) Ethanol levels 100-150 mg/dL are consistent with intoxication. Levels as low as 50 mg/dL can produce symptoms such as hypoglycemia, hypothermia and coma in infants and toddlers. Death has been reported following ingestion of 20 oz of a mouthwash containing 10% ethanol.

POTENTIAL CONTRIBUTION OF ALCOHOLS TO THE OSMOLAR GAP

Substance	Gram molecular weight	mOsm/L (at 100 mg/dL)
methanol	32	33.7
ethanol	46	22.8
ethylene glycol	62	19.0
isopro-panol	60	17.6

ESTIMATION OF BLOOD ALCOHOL LEVELS

1. Calculate osmolal gap (Δ osmolality)

$$\Delta \text{ osmolality} = \text{measured osmolality} - \frac{\text{calculated osmolality}}{0.93}$$

where 0.93 is the percentage of water in serum

Note: measured serum osmolality must be determined by freezing point depression osmometer.

2. Predicted serum concentration (mg/dL) $= \dfrac{(\Delta \text{ osmolality})(\text{molecular weight})}{10}$

3. Example (ethylene glycol): Δ osmolality = 30

Serum concentration $= \dfrac{(30)(62)}{10} = 186$ mg/dL

Note: A normal osmolal gap **does not** rule out ingestion of a toxic alcohol.

✱ Continued on p.126

Clinical Manifestations

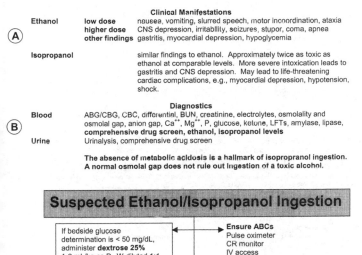

(A)	Ethanol	low dose	nausea, vomiting, slurred speech, motor incoordination, ataxia
		higher dose	CNS depression, irritability, seizures, stupor, coma, apnea
		other findings	gastritis, myocardial depression, hypoglycemia
	Isopropanol		similar findings to ethanol. Approximately twice as toxic as ethanol at comparable levels. More severe intoxication leads to gastritis and CNS depression. May lead to life-threatening cardiac complications, e.g., myocardial depression, hypotension, shock.

Diagnostics

(B)	Blood	ABG/CBG, CBC, differential, BUN, creatinine, electrolytes, osmolality and osmolal gap, anion gap, Ca^{++}, Mg^{++}, P, glucose, ketone, LFTs, amylase, lipase, **comprehensive drug screen, ethanol, isopropanol levels**
	Urine	Urinalysis, comprehensive drug screen

The absence of metabolic acidosis is a hallmark of isopropanol ingestion. A normal osmolal gap does not rule out ingestion of a toxic alcohol.

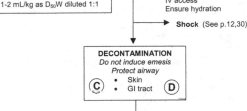

Suspected Ethanol/Isopropanol Ingestion

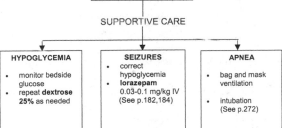

If bedside glucose determination is < 50 mg/dL, administer **dextrose 25%** 1-2 mL/kg as $D_{50}W$ diluted 1:1

Ensure ABCs
Pulse oximeter
CR monitor
IV access
Ensure hydration

Shock (See p.12,30)

DECONTAMINATION
Do not induce emesis
Protect airway
(C) • Skin
• GI tract (D)

SUPPORTIVE CARE

HYPOGLYCEMIA
• monitor bedside glucose
• repeat **dextrose 25%** as needed

SEIZURES
• correct hypoglycemia
• **lorazepam** 0.03-0.1 mg/kg IV (See p.182,184)

APNEA
• bag and mask ventilation
• intubation (See p.272)

CONSIDER HEMODIALYSIS
• hepatic failure
• hemodynamic instability
• alcohol levels 400-500 mg/dL
• in infants with osmolality > 340 mOsm/L

✳ Continued from p.123

(C) Skin decontamination is warranted due to the risk of dermal absorption and inhalation.

(D) Although **activated charcoal** has no role in the treatment of alcohol ingestions, it should be given in suspected multiple drug or toxin ingestion.

(E) Symptoms may not be apparent initially. There is a latent period of about 8-24 hours prior to development of symptoms in methanol, and about 1-4 hours in ethylene glycol ingestions. Monitor patients closely.

With methanol ingestion, blurring of vision may lead to **permanent visual loss** if not managed promptly.

(F) Both methanol and ethylene glycol ingestions result in severe metabolic acidosis with a high anion gap. However, an initial normal pH does not rule out significant ingestion/toxicity. Hypocalcemia in ethylene glycol ingestion is due to chelation of Ca^{++} by oxalate which is then excreted and crystals may be visualized in the urine. Monitor serum Ca^{++} closely and observe for signs of hypocalcemia with tetany. The fluorescent dye in radiator antifreeze is excreted in urine and can be demonstrated by a Wood's lamp examination.

(G)

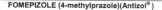

FOMEPIZOLE (4-methylprazole)(Antizol®)

Loading dose of 15 mg/kg IV followed by doses of 10 mg/kg every 12 hours for 4 doses. The dose is then increased to 15 mg/kg every 12 hours until serum ethylene glycol or methanol concentrations have decreased below 20 mg/dL.

Each dose should be administered by slow intravenous infusion over 30 minutes.

A separate dosing schedule is recommended for use during hemodialysis. Consult your regional Poison Control Center for details.

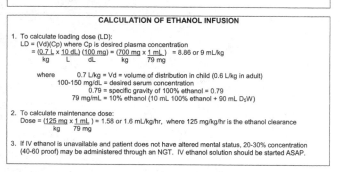

CALCULATION OF ETHANOL INFUSION

1. To calculate loading dose (LD):
   $$LD = (Vd)(Cp) \text{ where } Cp \text{ is desired plasma concentration}$$
   $$= \frac{(0.7 \text{ L}}{kg} \times \frac{10 \text{ dL})}{L} \frac{(100 \text{ mg})}{dL} = \frac{(700 \text{ mg}}{kg} \times \frac{1 \text{ mL})}{79 \text{ mg}} = 8.86 \text{ or } 9 \text{ mL/kg}$$

   where   0.7 L/kg = Vd = volume of distribution in child (0.6 L/kg in adult)
   100-150 mg/dL = desired serum concentration
   0.79 = specific gravity of 100% ethanol = 0.79
   79 mg/mL = 10% ethanol (10 mL 100% ethanol + 90 mL D_5W)

2. To calculate maintenance dose:
   $$Dose = \frac{(125 \text{ mg}}{kg} \times \frac{1 \text{ mL})}{79 \text{ mg}} = 1.58 \text{ or } 1.6 \text{ mL/kg/hr, where } 125 \text{ mg/kg/hr is the ethanol clearance}$$

3. If IV ethanol is unavailable and patient does not have altered mental status, 20-30% concentration (40-60 proof) may be administered through an NGT. IV ethanol solution should be started ASAP.

(H) If hemodialysis is initiated, the ethanol infusion should be continued at twice the usual infusion rate = 250-350 mg/kg/hour.

(I) In laboratory animals, folic acid promotes catalase-mediated metabolism of formate to CO_2 and H_2O. Whether it has the same effects on humans is unclear.

(J) Pyridoxine and thiamine are cofactors in the metabolism of ethylene glycol that lead to the formation of nontoxic metabolites.

Clinical Manifestations

Ⓔ **Methanol** nausea, vomiting, abdominal pain, GI bleeding, pancreatitis, CNS depression, irritability, headache, dizziness, stupor, coma, apnea. **Cloudy or blurred vision is characteristic and may progress to blindness.**

Ethylene Glycol

Stage 1 (4-8 hours) CNS depression, lethargy, seizures, coma, tetany, persistent vomiting, cardiac arrhythmias

Stage 2 (8-16 hours) coma, cardiopulmonary failure

Stage 3 (24-72 hours) acute tubular necrosis/renal failure

Diagnostics

Ⓑ **Blood** ABG/CBG, CBC, differential, platelets, BUN, creatinine, electrolytes, osmolality, anion gap, Ca^{++}, Mg^{++}, P, glucose, ketone, LFTs, amylase, lipase, **comprehensive drug screen, methanol, ethylene glycol levels**

Ⓕ **Urine** Urinalysis with microscopy, occult blood, comprehensive drug screen

Others EKG (QTc), Wood's lamp examination of face, chest, mouth and urine; stool for occult blood

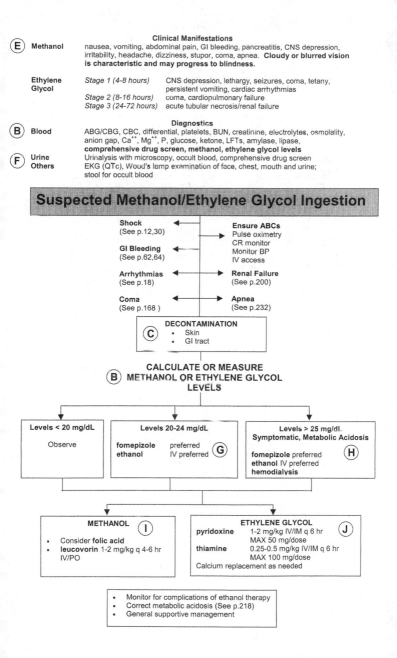

Suspected Methanol/Ethylene Glycol Ingestion

Shock (See p.12,30) ← → **Ensure ABCs** / Pulse oximetry / CR monitor / Monitor BP / IV access

GI Bleeding (See p.62,64) ←

Arrhythmias (See p.18) ← → **Renal Failure** (See p.200)

Coma (See p.168) ← → **Apnea** (See p.232)

Ⓒ **DECONTAMINATION**
- Skin
- GI tract

Ⓑ **CALCULATE OR MEASURE METHANOL OR ETHYLENE GLYCOL LEVELS**

Levels < 20 mg/dL

Observe

Levels 20-24 mg/dL

fomepizole preferred Ⓖ
ethanol IV preferred

Levels > 25 mg/dL Symptomatic, Metabolic Acidosis

fomepizole preferred Ⓗ
ethanol IV preferred
hemodialysis

METHANOL Ⓘ
- Consider **folic acid**
- **leucovorin** 1-2 mg/kg q 4-6 hr IV/PO

ETHYLENE GLYCOL Ⓙ
pyridoxine 1-2 mg/kg IV/IM q 6 hr MAX 50 mg/dose
thiamine 0.25-0.5 mg/kg IV/IM q 6 hr MAX 100 mg/dose
Calcium replacement as needed

- Monitor for complications of ethanol therapy
- Correct metabolic acidosis (See p.218)
- General supportive management

Caustic Ingestion/Exposure

Adora Poon

> Acids and alkaline agents are caustic chemicals that can cause direct tissue damage. **Alkalis** cause deep penetrating liquefaction necrosis that can result in GI perforation, usually in the esophagus. **Acids** produce superficial coagulation necrosis and eschar formation.

Alkaline Agents	Acidic Agents
bleaches (NaOH), denture cleaners, KOH, NaHCO$_3$, drain cleaners, Liquid Plumber®, lye, oven cleaners, ammonia, and monophosphate	toilet bowl cleaners, swimming pool products, battery fluid, chlorine bleach, HCl, acetic acid, carbolic acid, phenyl, iodine, silver nitrate

(A) *Serious esophageal injury may be present even in the absence of oral burns.* Look for other associated injuries, especially if suspecting child abuse.

(B) Consider comprehensive drug screens in patients with intentional/multiple drug ingestion. Esophagogram is not reliable and, therefore, is not indicated in the acute phase of caustic ingestion.

(C) Determine: (1) amount/type of ingestion, (2) product concentration, (3) time of ingestion. If possible, have a family member bring the suspected poison in its original container.

(D) **An alkali burn to the cornea is always an emergency.** Consult Ophthalmology ☎

(E) Caustics in liquid form (strong base) are more commonly associated with strictures of the esophagus. Barium swallow or esophagogram is recommended 10-20 days following injury.

(F) Respiratory symptoms can develop following ingestion or inhalation of laundry detergents and oven cleaners (NaOH). Observe for worsening of respiratory symptoms due to airway obstruction secondary to airway edema

(G)

Grading of esophageal burns	I	II		III
		IIa	IIb	
Endoscopic exam	Mucosal erythema and edema; no ulcers	Submucosal lesions and ulcers		Deep ulcers and necrosis involving periesophageal tissues
		Non-circumferential	Circumferential	
Prognosis	No risk of stricture	Strictures rare	Strictures common (≈75%)	Strictures invariable, high risk of perforation
Management	May discharge home once able to eat and drink	Observe, advance soft diet as tolerated, consider NG	Steroids/stents for strictures; Observe for complications; Oral feeds contraindicated if risk for perforation	Strictures are steroid-resistant; Close observation with follow up exams (endoscopy, CT, contrast radiography)

Clinical Manifestations

(A)

HEENT	erythema, inflammation, and burns of the cornea, face, lips, mouth
	hoarseness, aphonia, drooling
CVS	shock
RESP	dyspnea, respiratory distress, stridor, cough
GI	dysphagia, vomiting, GI bleeding, epigastric pain, retrosternal pain, peritoneal
	signs
CNS	altered level of consciousness
OTHERS	metabolic acidosis

Diagnostics

(B)

Blood	ABG/CBG, CBC, differential, type and crossmatch, electrolytes, BUN,
	creatinine, Ca^{++}, Mg^{++}, P, glucose, LFTs, PT, PTT, amylase, drug screen
Urine	drug screen, urinalysis
Others	chest and abdominal radiographs, pH of tears and saliva, endoscopy

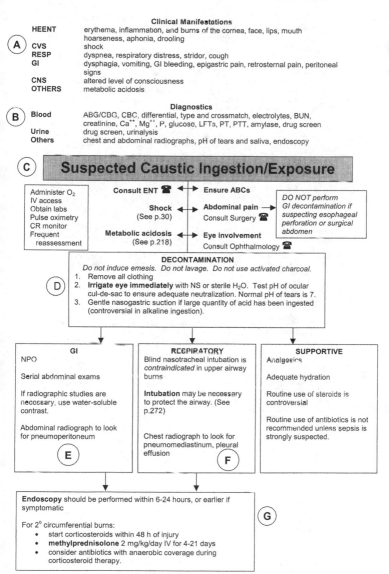

(C) ## Suspected Caustic Ingestion/Exposure

Administer O_2
IV access
Obtain labs
Pulse oximetry
CR monitor
Frequent
 reassessment

Consult ENT ☎ ◄► **Ensure ABCs**

Shock ◄► **Abdominal pain** →
(See p.30) Consult Surgery ☎

Metabolic acidosis ◄► **Eye involvement**
(See p.218) Consult Ophthalmology ☎

DO NOT perform GI decontamination if suspecting esophageal perforation or surgical abdomen

DECONTAMINATION

(D)

Do not induce emesis. Do not lavage. Do not use activated charcoal.
1. Remove all clothing
2. **Irrigate eye immediately** with NS or sterile H_2O. Test pH of ocular cul-de-sac to ensure adequate neutralization. Normal pH of tears is 7.
3. Gentle nasogastric suction if large quantity of acid has been ingested (controversial in alkaline ingestion).

GI

(E)

NPO

Serial abdominal exams

If radiographic studies are necessary, use water-soluble contrast.

Abdominal radiograph to look for pneumoperitoneum

RESPIRATORY

(F)

Blind nasotracheal intubation is *contraindicated* in upper airway burns

Intubation may be necessary to protect the airway. (See p.272)

Chest radiograph to look for pneumomediastinum, pleural effusion

SUPPORTIVE

Analgesics

Adequate hydration

Routine use of steroids is controversial

Routine use of antibiotics is not recommended unless sepsis is strongly suspected.

(G)

Endoscopy should be performed within 6-24 hours, or earlier if symptomatic

For 2° circumferential burns:
- start corticosteroids within 48 h of injury
- **methylprednisolone** 2 mg/kg/day IV for 4-21 days
- consider antibiotics with anaerobic coverage during corticosteroid therapy.

Cyclic Antidepressant Overdose

Lee Benjamin

Cyclic antidepressants (CAs) are known to have significant CVS and CNS effects because of their anticholinergic, adrenergic, and quinidine-like properties. Uses of CAs in children include ADHD, enuresis, OCD, chronic pain, and depression. High index of suspicion is necessary to quickly treat and prevent complications of **seizures**, **arrhythmias**, and the most common cause of death, **refractory hypotension**. *Even in therapeutic doses, EKG changes can occur, and torsade de pointes and sudden death have been reported.*

(A) **Signs and symptoms** usually present within the 4-6 hours of ingestion. The anticholinergic toxidrome is typically present, with depressed mental status, hyperthermia, mydriasis, decreased bowel sounds, and dry, flushed skin and urinary retention. Cardiovascular effects of arrhythmias and hypotension are frequent, as are seizures.
Mnemonic for anticholinergic overdose:
"**Hot** as a hare
Blind as a bat
Red as a beet
Dry as a bone
Mad as a hatter"

(B) EKG is essential in diagnosis and management. CA levels are not useful in initial assessment, but qualitative drug screens are useful to indicate presence of drug.

(C) Treatment of overdose requires rapid recognition. Be persistent in asking about medication lists of patient, relatives, and friends. Multiple drug overdoses are common. Obtain medication bottles, if available.

(D) GI decontamination: Gastric lavage followed by **activated charcoal** administration is indicated even several hours after ingestion, as anticholinergic properties delay gastric emptying and intestinal transit. Repeated charcoal administration without cathartic may be effective.

(E) 12 lead ECG findings: Maximal **QRS > 100 milliseconds** in limb leads is the best indicator for severity of overdose and predicts the development of seizures and arrhythmias. Axis deviation > 120 degrees of terminal 40 milliseconds of QRS may be helpful as well, especially in adolescents.

(F) Arrhythmias: Sinus tachycardia is most common. Supraventricular, junctional rhythms, idioventricular rhythms and bradycardia with conduction blocks have been noted. Wide complex tachycardias are associated with major morbidity and mortality. Therapeutic agents may include **NaHCO₃** and **lidocaine**. Use of phenytoin is controversial, and is not currently recommended.

(G) Seizures: Benzodiazepines are the mainstay of treatment. Barbiturates may worsen hypotension, and phenytoin interferes with conduction anomalies. General anesthesia may be needed.

(H) Hypotension: **0.9 NS** IV bolus for intravascular volume expansion. With persistent hypotension, begin inotropic support including **dopamine + norepinephrine** or **dobutamine + norepinephrine**. CAs block reuptake of norepinephrine at the neuromuscular junction. Inotropic agents such as dopamine, which in part rely on norepinephrine release from storage vesicles, may be ineffective when used alone. In refractory hypotension, ECMO and cardiopulmonary bypass have been used. Cyclic antidepressant antibodies are not currently recommended for use.

(I) Alkalinization: **NaHCO₃** loading and alkalinization of the blood decrease cellular effects of CAs. Indications include QRS duration > 100 ms, hypotension, and wide complex tachycardia. Utility in seizures is unknown, however seizures represent serious toxicity, and cardiovascular manifestations are likely. Run fluids at 1.5 times maintenance. There are no criteria for discontinuing the infusion, however, clinical and EKG improvements should be used to guide therapy. Monitor pH, potassium, and calcium closely.

(J) Hyperventilation: efficacy is not equal to alkalinization with NaHCO₃ loading. When combined with NaHCO₃ administration, severe alkalosis may occur, which may lead to seizures and arrhythmias.

Clinical Manifestations

(A)

HEENT	mydriasis, dry mucous membranes
CVS	sinus tachycardia, bradycardia possible, ventricular tachycardia, conduction block, sudden death, hyper/hypotension
RESP	decreased effort
GI	decreased bowel sounds
SKIN	flushed, dry as evidenced by lack of axillary moisture
CNS	confusion, hallucinations, lethargy, myoclonus, coma, seizure
Others	hyperthermia, urinary retention

Diagnostics

(B)

Blood	electrolytes, glucose, BUN, creatinine, Ca^{++}, CBC, drug screen
Urine	drug screen, urinalysis
Others	12 lead EKG with rhythm strip, consider acetaminophen, aspirin levels

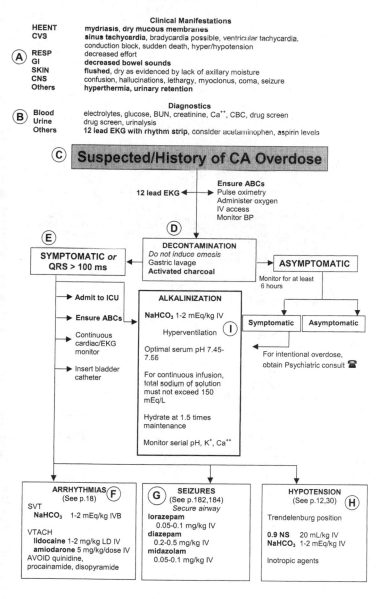

(C) **Suspected/History of CA Overdose**

Ensure ABCs
12 lead EKG ← → Pulse oximetry
Administer oxygen
IV access
Monitor BP

(D) **DECONTAMINATION**
Do not induce emesis
Gastric lavage
Activated charcoal

(E) **SYMPTOMATIC or QRS > 100 ms**

ASYMPTOMATIC
Monitor for at least 6 hours

→ Admit to ICU

→ Ensure ABCs

→ Continuous cardiac/EKG monitor

→ Insert bladder catheter

ALKALINIZATION

NaHCO$_3$ 1-2 mEq/kg IV

Hyperventilation

(I)

Optimal serum pH 7.45-7.55

For continuous infusion, total sodium of solution must not exceed 150 mEq/L

Hydrate at 1.5 times maintenance

Monitor serial pH, K$^+$, Ca^{++}

Symptomatic   Asymptomatic

For intentional overdose, obtain Psychiatric consult ☎

ARRHYTHMIAS (F)
(See p.18)
SVT
NaHCO$_3$ 1-2 mEq/kg IVB

VTACH
lidocaine 1-2 mg/kg LD IV
amiodarone 5 mg/kg/dose IV
AVOID quinidine, procainamide, disopyramide

SEIZURES (G)
(See p.182,184)
Secure airway
lorazepam
0.05-0.1 mg/kg IV
diazepam
0.2-0.5 mg/kg IV
midazolam
0.05-0.1 mg/kg IV

HYPOTENSION (H)
(See p.12,30)

Trendelenburg position

0.9 NS 20 mL/kg IV
NaHCO$_3$ 1-2 mEq/kg IV

Inotropic agents

Hydrocarbon Exposure

Kshama Daphtary

HOUSEHOLD PRODUCTS CONTAINING HYDROCARBONS

Adhesives (glues)	Kitchen wax	Motor oils	Solvents
Baby oil	Lacquers	Naphtha	Stain removers
Car wax	Laxatives	Paint removers	Stoddard solvent
Cod liver oil	Lighter fluid	Paint thinner	Typewriter correction fluid
Contact cement	Liquid solder	Paraffin	Varnish removers
Furniture polish	Mineral oil	Paste waxes	Gasoline
Insecticides	Mineral seal oil	Pesticides	
Kerosene	Mothballs	Petroleum jelly	

Refer to standard toxicology reference for specific properties of each hydrocarbon and their toxic profile.

(A) Aspiration pneumonitis following **ingestion** is a common presentation. Following **inhalation**, cardiovascular and neurologic toxicities are major concerns, especially in cases of substance abuse, e.g., "huffing" or "bagging" of glue solvents, gasoline, etc. Persistent cough generally indicates aspiration.

(B) Radiographic evidence of pneumonitis may be seen as early as 15 minutes or as late as 24 hours. Pneumothoraces, pneumomediastinum, pneumatocoeles, and pleural effusion may be seen.

(C) Hydrocarbons may be used as a solvent for insecticides. Anticipate cholinergic crisis secondary to organophospate poisoning (See p.136).

(D) Hypoglycemia and concomitant opiod abuse may complicate clinical picture.

(E) Consider gastric evacuation in:
- Large volume ingestions (> 30 mL)
- Intentional ingestions
- Hydrocarbon with inherent toxicity (CHAMP)
  - **C**amphor
  - **H**alogenated hydrocarbons
  - **A**romatic hydrocarbons
  - Hydrocarbons associated with
  - **M**etals
  - Hydrocarbons associated with
  - **P**esticides

(F) CNS depression is due to hypoxia rather than the direct toxic effect of hydrocarbons absorbed systemically. Co-ingestants may complicate clinical picture.

(G) In general, risk for aspiration following ingestion is greatest with hydrocarbons with low viscosity and surface tension.

(H) Fever within 24 hours is usually related to direct tissue toxicity and not infection. Leucocytosis may be secondary to chemical pneumonitis.

(I) The myocardium develops an increased sensitivity to catecholamines (used as bronchodilators) that may lead to arrhythmias.

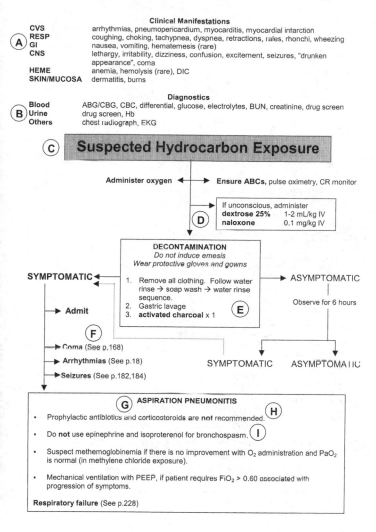

Clinical Manifestations

(A)
CVS	arrhythmias, pneumopericardium, myocarditis, myocardial infarction
RESP	coughing, choking, tachypnea, dyspnea, retractions, rales, rhonchi, wheezing
GI	nausea, vomiting, hematemesis (rare)
CNS	lethargy, irritability, dizziness, confusion, excitement, seizures, "drunken appearance", coma
HEME	anemia, hemolysis (rare), DIC
SKIN/MUCOSA	dermatitis, burns

Diagnostics

(B)
Blood	ABG/CBG, CBC, differential, glucose, electrolytes, BUN, creatinine, drug screen
Urine	drug screen, Hb
Others	chest radiograph, EKG

(C) ## Suspected Hydrocarbon Exposure

Administer oxygen ◄───► Ensure ABCs, pulse oximetry, CR monitor

(D)
If unconscious, administer
dextrose 25% 1-2 mL/kg IV
naloxone 0.1 mg/kg IV

DECONTAMINATION
Do not induce emesis
Wear protective gloves and gowns

SYMPTOMATIC ◄

(E)
1. Remove all clothing. Follow water rinse → soap wash → water rinse sequence.
2. Gastric lavage
3. **activated charcoal** x 1

► **ASYMPTOMATIC**

Observe for 6 hours

► Admit

(F)
► Coma (See p.168)
► Arrhythmias (See p.18)
► Seizures (See p.182,184)

SYMPTOMATIC   ASYMPTOMATIC

(G) **ASPIRATION PNEUMONITIS** (H)

- Prophylactic antibiotics and corticosteroids are **not** recommended.

- Do **not** use epinephrine and isoproterenol for bronchospasm. (I)

- Suspect methemoglobinemia if there is no improvement with O_2 administration and PaO_2 is normal (in methylene chloride exposure).

- Mechanical ventilation with PEEP, if patient requires $FiO_2 > 0.60$ associated with progression of symptoms.

Respiratory failure (See p.228)

Iron Poisoning

Jacqueline Spaulding

Toxicity may be seen following ingestion of > 20 mg/kg of elemental iron. Increasing incidence of toxicity is seen as a result of easy availability, high doses of iron in prenatal vitamins, and brightly colored, sugarcoated iron pills that resemble candy. When inquiring about medications available in the household, specifically ask about iron pills. Some people do not consider "vitamins" as medication.

(A)

Clinical Stages of Iron Toxicity

Stage I *< 6 hours post–ingestion*
Signs and symptoms related to GI injury: nausea, vomiting, gastroenteritis, abdominal pain, coagulopathy, lethargy, hematemesis, hematochezia

Stage II *Latent period 6-24 hours*
Transition between resolution of symptoms and appearance of overt systemic toxicity. Deceptive improvement. Observe closely.

Stage III *Systemic toxicity 4-40 hours*
Multiple organ failure: cerebral dysfunction, coma, myocardial depression, renal and hepatic failure.

Stage IV *7-10 days*
Hepatic and renal failure possible

Stage V *Late complications*
GI obstruction secondary to scarring and strictures (pyloric, antral, intestinal)

Elemental Iron Equivalents

Ferrous sulfate (hydrate)	20%
Ferrous sulfate (dried)	37%
Ferrous gluconate	12%
Ferrous lactate	19%
Ferrous chloride	28%
Ferrous fumarate	33%
Ferric phosphate	37%
Ferrous pyrophosphate	12%

Example: $FeSO_4$

325 mg x 0.2 = 65 mg of elemental Fe

(B) Use heparinized tube for serum iron determinations. Levels are more useful 3-4 hours post-ingestion for liquids/tablets. **Notify laboratory if child is on DFO, because DFO alters serum levels of iron.**

(C) **Do not** use activated charcoal. **Do not** use syrup of ipecac because the persistent emesis induced by syrup of ipecac may mask vomiting produced by iron, which may lead to underestimation of the severity of iron toxicity. **Gastric lavage** is considered to be procedure of choice when gastric decontamination is warranted.

(D) Use **GoLYTELY®** PO or per NGT in children at 40 mL/kg/hr; in adults use 2 L/hr until rectal effluent is clear.

(E) *Yersinia enterocolitica* septicemia has been described in previously healthy children being treated for iron overdose with **deferoxamine**.

Indications for starting deferoxamine
(1) Serum iron > 300 mcg/dL
(2) All symptomatic patients with more than transient minor symptoms
(3) Lethargy, significant abdominal pain, hypovolemia, or acidosis
(4) Positive abdominal radiograph

Clinical Manifestations

(A) Major   stupor, shock, acidosis, hematemesis, bloody diarrhea, coma
    Minor   vomiting, diarrhea, lethargy, hyperglycemia, hypoglycemia

Diagnostics

(B) Blood   serum iron (SI), total iron binding capacity (TIBC), comprehensive drug screen,
             ABG/CBG, CBC with differential, platelets, type and cross-match, electrolytes, glucose,
             BUN, creatinine, PT, PTT, LFTs
    Urine   drug screen
    Other   chest and abdominal radiographs

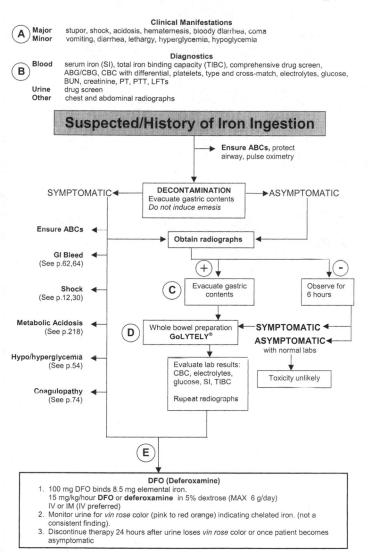

Suspected/History of Iron Ingestion

Ensure ABCs, protect airway, pulse oximetry

SYMPTOMATIC ◄ **DECONTAMINATION**
Evacuate gastric contents
Do not induce emesis ► ASYMPTOMATIC

Ensure ABCs ◄

GI Bleed ◄
(See p.62,64)

Obtain radiographs ◄

(+)   (−)

(C) Evacuate gastric contents   Observe for 6 hours

Shock ◄
(See p.12,30)

Metabolic Acidosis ◄
(See p.218)

(D) Whole bowel preparation GoLYTELY® ◄ **SYMPTOMATIC** ◄

ASYMPTOMATIC ◄
with normal labs

Hypo/hyperglycemia ◄
(See p.54)

Evaluate lab results:
CBC, electrolytes,
glucose, SI, TIBC

Repeat radiographs

Toxicity unlikely

Coagulopathy ◄
(See p.74)

(E)

DFO (Deferoxamine)

1. 100 mg DFO binds 8.5 mg elemental iron.
   15 mg/kg/hour **DFO** or **deferoxamine** in 5% dextrose (MAX 6 g/day)
   IV or IM (IV preferred)
2. Monitor urine for *vin rose* color (pink to red orange) indicating chelated iron. (not a
   consistent finding).
3. Discontinue therapy 24 hours after urine loses *vin rose* color or once patient becomes
   asymptomatic

Organophosphate/Carbamate Poisoning

Varsha Gharpure

Organophosphates/carbamates are used as insecticides, miticides, and aphicides. Children can be exposed to these agents from intentional or unintentional misuse. These agents are also potent chemical warfare agents. The 1995 terrorist attack in a Japanese subway involved the nerve gas sarin.

(A) Organophosphates/carbamates inhibit the action of acetylcholinesterase (AChE) leading to accumulation of acetylcholine at parasympathetic, sympathetic and somatic synapses. Organophosphates and carbamates produce identical symptomatology. However, symptomatology related to carbamate ingestion is generally limited to a 1–2 day course because the carbamoyl-AChE bond is more readily hydrolyzed. Carbamates penetrate CNS poorly and hence have limited CNS toxicity. Pulmonary edema and respiratory failure are also rare with carbamates.

Absorption: skin (slowest), conjunctiva, across GI and GU mucosa and through inhalation (most rapid). Toxicity usually occurs within 4 to 12 hours, and may not manifest until after 24 hours. Nerve gases can cause respiratory arrest within 5 minutes.

Hydrocarbons (See p.132) or methyl alcohol (See p.124) are occasionally used as a vehicle for insecticides/pesticides.

(B) Erythrocyte AChE and plasma chE activity should be measured to document toxicity. Plasma ChE is a more sensitive indicator of exposure. Erythrocyte AChE better correlates with clinical effects. Ideally, a drop in enzyme activity by 50% from baseline value is suggestive of severe toxicity. Demonstration of rising ChE levels with treatment is often necessary since pre-morbid levels are unavailable in most patients. Erythrocyte AChE should be monitored once 2-PAM therapy is started. Levels are not helpful in carbamate ingestion.

Blood for erythrocyte AChE levels should be collected in EDTA tubes (lavender top). Plasma ChE levels collected in lavender or red top. Do not collect blood in fluoride containing tubes since enzyme will be inactivated. If test cannot be performed immediately, specimen should be centrifuged, and frozen. **Treatment should be started without waiting for results.**

Elevated pancreatic isoamylase activity and prolongation of QT interval including torsade de pointes can occur with severe ingestion.

(C) Duration of action of drugs metabolized by pseudocholinesterase such as opioids, succinylcholine, mivacurium, ester anesthetics (cocaine and tetracaine) and esmolol, can be prolonged, and should be avoided or used with caution. Avoid parasympathomimetic agents like pyridostigmine. Phenothiazines and antihistamines have cholinergic effects and may enhance organophosphate toxicity.

(D) **Atropine** (antimuscarinic) may be administered by SC, IO or ET route. It has no effects on nicotinic receptors. Pupillary dilatation is an early response to atropine, but the end point of treatment is reversal of cholinergic symptoms. Tachycardia is not a contraindication to the use of atropine.

(E) **Pralidoxime** (2-PAM) restores acetylcholinesterase activity by regenerating the phosphorylated AChE. Even though it is most useful before irreversible inactivation of ChE occurs (24 to 48 hours), **patients presenting late may still benefit from this medication.** It may also function as a free organophosphate scavenger. Any patient needing atropine for cholinergic signs and symptoms must also receive 2-PAM regardless of the absence of nicotinic or CNS manifestations. Respiratory and cardiac arrest, hypertension, dizziness and blurred vision are reported side effects of rapid IV bolus. It should be administered with caution in the presence of renal failure. It is **not** useful for pure carbamate ingestions. **Obidoxime** is the alternative oxime available in some countries. Obidoxime has no advantage over pralidoxime.

Clinical Manifestations
Associated with petroleum or garlic odor

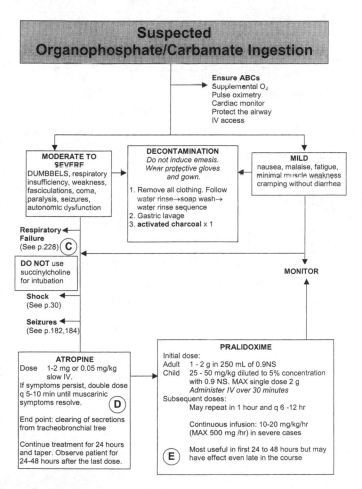

(A) MUSCARINIC Diarrhea, Urination, Miosis, Bradycardia, Bronchorrhea, Emesis, Lacrimation, Salivation (DUMBBELS)

NICOTINIC Muscle weakness and fasciculations, Mydriasis, Adrenal medulla activity increase, Tachycardia, Cramping of skeletal muscles, and Hypertension (MMATCH)

CENTRAL Dizziness, alteration in level of consciousness, seizures, coma and death

Diagnostics

(B) BLOOD ABG/CBG, CBC, differential, BUN, creatinine, electrolytes, glucose, LFTs, erythrocyte acetyl cholinesterase (AChE), plasma pseudocholinesterase (plasma chE), pancreatic isoamylase levels

URINE drug screen
IMAGING chest radiograph
OTHER 12 lead EKG

Suspected Organophosphate/Carbamate Ingestion

Ensure ABCs
Supplemental O_2
Pulse oximetry
Cardiac monitor
Protect the airway
IV access

MODERATE TO SEVERE
DUMBBELS, respiratory insufficiency, weakness, fasciculations, coma, paralysis, seizures, autonomic dysfunction

DECONTAMINATION
*Do not induce emesis.
Wear protective gloves and gown.*
1. Remove all clothing. Follow water rinse→soap wash→ water rinse sequence
2. Gastric lavage
3. **activated charcoal** x 1

MILD
nausea, malaise, fatigue, minimal muscle weakness cramping without diarrhea

Respiratory Failure
(See p.228) (C)

DO NOT use succinylcholine for intubation

Shock
(See p.30)

Seizures
(See p.182,184)

MONITOR

ATROPINE
Dose 1-2 mg or 0.05 mg/kg slow IV.
If symptoms persist, double dose q 5-10 min until muscarinic symptoms resolve. (D)

End point: clearing of secretions from tracheobronchial tree

Continue treatment for 24 hours and taper. Observe patient for 24-48 hours after the last dose.

PRALIDOXIME
Initial dose:
Adult   1 - 2 g in 250 mL of 0.9NS
Child   25 - 50 mg/kg diluted to 5% concentration with 0.9 NS. MAX single dose 2 g
Administer IV over 30 minutes

Subsequent doses:
May repeat in 1 hour and q 6 -12 hr

Continuous infusion: 10-20 mg/kg/hr (MAX 500 mg /hr) in severe cases

(E) Most useful in first 24 to 48 hours but may have effect even late in the course

Theophylline Toxicity

Bulent Ozgonenel

Consider theophylline toxicity if:
- Patient received > 10 mg/kg theophylline/aminophylline
- Theophylline level > 20 mcg/mL
- Patients have symptoms of toxicity despite therapeutic levels of theophylline (10-20 mcg/mL)

Suspect theophylline toxicity in the following patients :
- Asthmatics on theophylline at home or receiving IV theophylline in the hospital
- Children with access to theophylline, e.g., accidental ingestions
- Children with hepatic or cardiac disease treated with theophylline

---

Time to achieve peak serum levels	Therapeutic conditions	Overdose conditions
Immediate-release theophylline	2 hr	6 hr
Sustained-release theophylline	6 hr	12 hr

(A) Severity of **hypokalemia** is proportional to peak serum theophylline levels.
Monitor serum theophylline levels regardless of an initial low value, especially with slow-release preparations.

(B) **Activated charcoal:** administer sorbitol or magnesium citrate only with the first dose. Administer charcoal even after IV overdose. **GoLYTELY®** 40 mL/kg/hr PO or per NGT, MAX 2 L/hr

(C) Infants are at a greater risk for arrhythmias.

(D) **Seizures** can be generalized tonic-clonic, but occasionally are focal and resistant to therapy.

Drugs known to inhibit theophylline metabolism (partial list)	
allopurinol	furosemide
cimetidine	nifedipine
ciprofloxacin	propranolol
erythromycin	verapamil

Factors that decrease theophylline metabolism
COPD
congestive heart failure
liver failure
Influenza, pneumonia

Clinical Manifestations

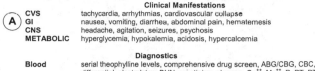

(A)	CVS	tachycardia, arrhythmias, cardiovascular collapse
	GI	nausea, vomiting, diarrhea, abdominal pain, hematemesis
	CNS	headache, agitation, seizures, psychosis
	METABOLIC	hyperglycemia, hypokalemia, acidosis, hypercalcemia

Diagnostics

Blood	serial theophylline levels, comprehensive drug screen, ABG/CBG, CBC, differential, electrolytes, BUN, creatinine, glucose, Ca^{++}, Mg^{++}, P, PT, PTT
Urine	comprehensive drug screen
Others	EKG

Suspected Theophylline Poisoning

Discontinue theophylline ◄──────► **Ensure ABCs**
Pulse oximetry
EKG monitoring

(B)

SYMPTOMATIC ◄── **DECONTAMINATION**
Do not induce emesis
Gastric lavage
activated charcoal 1.0 g/kg PO
repeat q 4-6 h or more frequently
for 18-24 h ──► ASYMPTOMATIC
WITH LEVELS
> 20 mcg/mL

ENSURE HYDRATION
0.9 **NS** 20 mL/kg IV
bolus, then 2500
mL/m²/day maintenance
of D_5 .45 NS + KCl

Ensure ABCs ◄──

(C) **Arrhythmias**
(See p.18) ──────────────► Serial levels q 4 h

(D) **Seizures**
(See p.182,184)

Hypotension/
Shock ──► Consider treatment of
(See p.30)   vomiting if protracted

GI Bleeding
(See p.62,64) ──────────────► Observe until levels
≤therapeutic

HEMOPERFUSION/HEMODIALYSIS
Consult Nephrology ☎
1. Theophylline level > 80 mcg/mL
   (for chronic toxicity > 40 mcg/mL)
2. Symptoms are severe: seizures, refractory hypotension,
   ventricular dysrhythmias, protracted vomiting

Clonidine Toxicity

Jacqueline Spaulding

> Clonidine may be used as an antihypertensive agent, in the therapy of ADHD, in the management of opioid, alcohol and nicotine withdrawal, in autism, and in Tourette's syndrome. It is available as a tablet, transdermal patch, or as apraclonidine eyedrops.
> *As little as 0.1 mg of drug has produced signs and symptoms of toxicity in children.*
> - Peak effect (oral)   30-60 minutes (antihypertensive effect)
> - Plasma T ½ life   8.5 hours
> - Duration of effect (oral)   6-24 hours (hypotensive effect)

(A) Clonidine is an imidazoline compound. It is a potent α_2 adrenergic agonist that acts centrally and peripherally. It also binds central α_2 adrenergic receptors in the brainstem which results in a central inhibitory effect of norepinephrine release, causing decreased sympathetic outflow, bradycardia, sedation, and hypotension.

(B) Clonidine is not routinely detected in comprehensive drug screens. No specific laboratory test needs to be obtained unless patients have other symptoms (i.e., vomiting, fever). A baseline EKG may be helpful in the initial management.

(C) If ingestion of a large amount of liquid or pills occurred within 60 minutes of arrival to the hospital, perform gastric lavage prior to giving activated charcoal. In cases of ingestion of the clonidine patch, activated charcoal followed by whole bowel irrigation may help prevent absorption of clonidine. Ingestion of apraclonidine eyedrops produces similar symptoms.

(D) Hypotension is secondary to inhibition of central sympathetic outflow. Blood pressure usually returns to normal within 24 hours. Paradoxical hypertension may be observed and is usually transient, but if there is imminent end-organ compromise, only use short acting antihypertensive agents.

(E) Arrhythmias may occur and therefore, evaluation with a baseline EKG and ongoing cardiac monitoring is necessary. A-V block usually responds to discontinuation of the drug.

(F) Improvement in level of consciousness or sensorium is generally observed within 24-36 hours, however, intubation with mechanical ventilation may be required.

(G) Seizures, although rare have been associated with clonidine toxicity. The mechanism for these seizures is unknown.

(H) **Naloxone** administration has been shown by some studies to reverse the effects of clonidine on blood pressure.

Clinical Manifestations

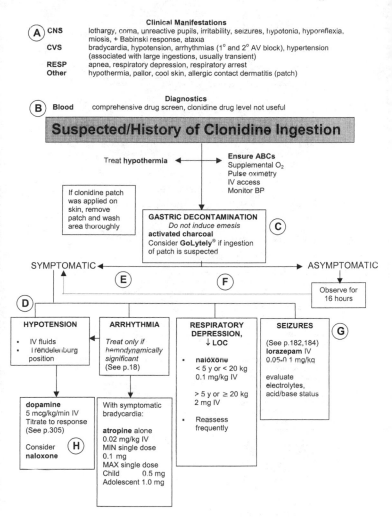

(A) CNS lethargy, coma, unreactive pupils, irritability, seizures, hypotonia, hyporeflexia, miosis, + Babinski response, ataxia

CVS bradycardia, hypotension, arrhythmias (1° and 2° AV block), hypertension (associated with large ingestions, usually transient)

RESP apnea, respiratory depression, respiratory arrest

Other hypothermia, pallor, cool skin, allergic contact dermatitis (patch)

Diagnostics

(B) Blood comprehensive drug screen, clonidine drug level not useful

Suspected/History of Clonidine Ingestion

Treat **hypothermia** ◄——— **Ensure ABCs**
Supplemental O_2
Pulse oximetry
IV access
Monitor BP

If clonidine patch was applied on skin, remove patch and wash area thoroughly

GASTRIC DECONTAMINATION (C)
Do not induce emesis
activated charcoal
Consider **GoLytely®** if ingestion of patch is suspected

SYMPTOMATIC ◄——————————————————————————► ASYMPTOMATIC

(E)   (F)

Observe for 16 hours

(D)

HYPOTENSION	**ARRHYTHMIA**	**RESPIRATORY DEPRESSION, ↓ LOC**	**SEIZURES** (G)
• IV fluids • Trendelenburg position	*Treat only if hemodynamically significant* (See p.18)	• **naloxone** < 5 y or < 20 kg 0.1 mg/kg IV > 5 y or ≥ 20 kg 2 mg IV • Reassess frequently	(See p.182,184) **lorazepam** IV 0.05–0.1 mg/kg evaluate electrolytes, acid/base status
dopamine 5 mcg/kg/min IV Titrate to response (See p.305) Consider (H) **naloxone**	With symptomatic bradycardia: **atropine** alone 0.02 mg/kg IV MIN single dose 0.1 mg MAX single dose Child 0.5 mg Adolescent 1.0 mg		

Digoxin Toxicity

Shilpa Sangvai

Digoxin is a commonly used cardiac glycoside. Other sources of digitalis include: digitoxin, ouabain, lanotoside C, deslanoside, and gitalin. Plant sources include foxglove, oleander, red squill, lilly of the valley. Skin secretions of certain toads may also contain digitalis.

Mechanisms of action: (a) enhances cardiac contractility by inhibiting the Na-K-ATPase pump which increases intracellular calcium; (b) delays A-V node conduction by enhancing vagal tone at therapeutic levels and prolongs refractory period at supratherapeutic levels.

Serum T ½ life	36 hours	Elimination	renal
Bioavailability	80%	Therapeutic level	0.8-2.0 ng/mL
Initial effect (oral)	30 minutes	Toxic level	> 2 ng/mL
Peak effect (oral)	2-6 hr (may persist > 24 hr)	Severe toxicity	> 5 ng/mL

Drugs that affect digoxin concentration	
INCREASE	DECREASE
amiodarone, calcium channel blockers, indomethacin, macrolide antibiotics, quinidine	cholestyramine, hydralazine, neomycin, nitroprusside

(A) In children, common presenting symptoms include GI complaints, sinus bradycardia and 1° A-V block. However, CNS symptoms may appear before cardiac and GI symptoms.

(B) Levels obtained > six hours after ingestion reflect clinical severity more accurately.

(C) Digitalis toxicity can occur even with therapeutic levels when associated with hypokalemia (from concurrent use of diuretics) and hypomagnesemia. Correct hypokalemia with **KCI** 0.25-0.5 mEq/kg IV over 1 hour. Repeat as needed. Monitor EKG.

(D) Consider **atropine** if bradycardia occurs.

(E) Pacemaker (external or transvenous) should be considered when arrhythmia is not responsive to conventional medical management and **Digibind®** is not immediately available. Cathecolamines may aggravate digitalis-induced arrhythmias.

(F) Degree of hyperkalemia correlates with mortality. The preferred first line of treatment is Digibind®. If not immediately available, glucose-insulin solution, $NaHCO_3$ may be used. Monitor serial potassium levels.

(G) Hypokalemia may occur after Digibind® administration. Signs and symptoms generally improve in ≤ 30 minutes. If toxicity recurs or persists, consider repeating dose. **Toxicity from other drugs should be considered.** NOTE: Use the higher dose if results of the two calculations are significantly different.

INDICATIONS FOR DIGIBIND®
1. Ventricular arrhythmia
2. Progressive bradyarrhythmia
3. 2° to 3° block not responsive to atropine
4. Hyperkalemia
5. Increased risk for arrest: ingestion of > 4 mg (child), level > 10 ng/mL (6-8 hr post-ingestion)

Infants and Small Children Dose Estimates of DIGIBIND® (in mg) from Steady-State Serum Digoxin Concentration

Wgt in kg	Serum Digoxin Concentration (ng/mL)						
	1	2	4	8	12	16	20
1	0.4 mg*	1 mg*	1.5 mg*	3 mg*	5 mg	6 mg	8 mg
3	1 mg*	2 mg*	5 mg	9 mg	14 mg	18 mg	23 mg
5	2 mg*	4 mg	8 mg	15 mg	23 mg	30 mg	38 mg
10	4 mg	8 mg	15 mg	30 mg	46 mg	61 mg	76 mg
20	8 mg	15 mg	30 mg	61 mg	91 mg	122 mg	152 mg

* Dilution of reconstituted vial to 1 mg/mL may be desirable

Clinical Manifestations

CVS — (EKG) sinus bradycardia, AV block, supraventricular tachyarrhythmias, ventricular tachyarrhythmias

GI — anorexia, nausea, vomiting, abdominal pain

CNS — lethargy, weakness, restlessness, fatigue, drowsiness, confusion, altered mental status, hallucinations, visual changes

METABOLIC — hyperkalemia

Diagnostics

12 lead EKG with rhythm strip, serial serum electrolytes, Ca^{++}, Mg^{++}, BUN, creatinine, digoxin level, consider ABG, drug screen if multiple ingestions suspected

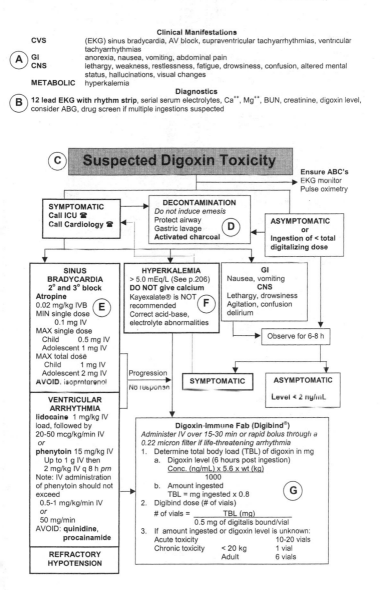

Suspected Digoxin Toxicity

Ensure ABC's
EKG monitor
Pulse oximetry

SYMPTOMATIC
Call ICU ☎
Call Cardiology ☎

DECONTAMINATION
Do not induce emesis
Protect airway
Gastric lavage
Activated charcoal

ASYMPTOMATIC
or
Ingestion of < total digitalizing dose

SINUS BRADYCARDIA
2° and 3° block
Atropine
0.02 mg/kg IVB
MIN single dose
0.1 mg IV
MAX single dose
Child   0.5 mg IV
Adolescent 1 mg IV
MAX total dose
Child   1 mg IV
Adolescent 2 mg IV
AVOID isoproterenol

HYPERKALEMIA
> 5.0 mEq/L (See p.206)
DO NOT give calcium
Kayexalate® is NOT recommended
Correct acid-base, electrolyte abnormalities

GI
Nausea, vomiting
CNS
Lethargy, drowsiness
Agitation, confusion
delirium

Observe for 6-8 h

VENTRICULAR ARRHYTHMIA
lidocaine 1 mg/kg IV load, followed by 20-50 mcg/kg/min IV
or
phenytoin 15 mg/kg IV
Up to 1 g IV then
2 mg/kg IV q 8 h *prn*
Note: IV administration of phenytoin should not exceed
0.5-1 mg/kg/min IV
or
50 mg/min
AVOID: quinidine, procainamide

Progression

No response

SYMPTOMATIC

ASYMPTOMATIC
Level < 2 ng/mL

Digoxin-Immune Fab (Digibind®)
Administer IV over 15-30 min or rapid bolus through a 0.22 micron filter if life-threatening arrhythmia
1. Determine total body load (TBL) of digoxin in mg
   a. Digoxin level (6 hours post ingestion)
   $$\frac{\text{Conc. (ng/mL)} \times 5.6 \times \text{wt (kg)}}{1000}$$
   b. Amount ingested
      TBL = mg ingested x 0.8
2. Digibind dose (# of vials)
   $$\text{\# of vials} = \frac{\text{TBL (mg)}}{0.5 \text{ mg of digitalis bound/vial}}$$
3. If amount ingested or digoxin level is unknown:
   Acute toxicity   10-20 vials
   Chronic toxicity   < 20 kg   1 vial
                              Adult   6 vials

REFRACTORY HYPOTENSION

Antiepileptic Drug Overdose:
Phenobarbital, Carbamazepine, Phenytoin

Maria C. Asi-Bautista

AED = Antiepileptic drug

(A) **Carbamazepine (CBZ)** is structurally related to imipramine. Anticholinergic effects such as delayed gastric emptying and urinary retention may be observed. SIADH may also develop as a late complication of therapy. Hematopoietic toxicity may be seen following therapeutic doses and in chronic use.

Phenytoin (PHT) cardiotoxicity is attributed to the diluent, propylene glycol. **Do not administer IV phenytoin faster than 1 mg/kg/min, MAX 50 mg/min.** Extravasation into subcutaneous tissues can lead to tissue necrosis. **Fosphenytoin** is a water-soluble prodrug form of phenytoin. It can be administered up to 150 phenytoin-equivalents/minute IV, or in the absence of IV access, intramuscularly. However, hypotension, bradycardia and asystole have resulted from IV overdose of fosphenytoin. Cardiotoxicity has not been reported in oral overdose. Cerebellar atrophy may develop following severe overdose.

Phenobarbital can be given IM when venous access is limited. When given with other sedative/hypnotic drugs such as benzodiazepines, additive respiratory depressant effect can be seen. Be prepared to establish the airway with endotracheal intubation in the event of respiratory arrest.

(B) Monitor serial drug levels. With CBZ, obtain abdominal radiographs to look for concretions if symptoms develop late or when levels continue to rise despite discontinuation of drug.

(C) Consider multiple drug overdoses. Children may develop symptoms of toxicity at lower levels.

(D) Monitor patients for at least 24 hours. Frequent reassessment.

(E) Seizures secondary to AED overdose is more common in **carbamazepine** ingestion. For seizures not responsive to benzodiazepines, **phenobarbital** is the drug of choice for toxin-induced seizures. Evaluate electrolytes, glucose, and blood gas measurements.

(F) Phenobarbital level > 80 mcg/mL is usually associated with coma. Consider other toxic causes of coma: opioids, ethanol, benzodiazepines, phenothiazines, sedative-hypnotics, cyclic antidepressants. **Do not** use flumazenil especially in the presence of cyclic antidepressants co-ingestion.

(G) Alkalinization is **not** routinely recommended in the management of rhabdomyolysis. However, in severe phenobarbital toxicity, urine alkalinization (pH 7.5) may aid in drug elimination. Monitor blood and urine pH, potassium and calcium closely.

ANTICONVULSANT-DRUG INTERACTIONS

Carbamazepine		
Decreases serum levels of:	Serum levels are **increased** by:	Serum levels are **decreased** by:
doxycycline haloperidol warfarin phenytoin valproic acid lamotrigine primidone	diltiazem erythromycin isoniazid nicotine propoxyphene verapamil	carbamazepine (auto induction), benzodiazepines, phenobarbital, phenytoin, primidone, succinimide, valproic acid,
Phenytoin		
Increases serum levels of:	**Decreases** serum levels of:	Serum levels are **increased** by:
acetaminophen toxic metabolite (NAPQI) oral anticoagulants primidone	amiodarone carbamazepine corticosteroids cyclosporine doxycycline furosemide theophylline valproic acid	cimetidine, ethosuximide, fluconazole, isoniazid, oral anticoagulants, trimethoprim, valproic acid, amiodarone, sulfonamides

Modified from Table 41-4 Drug interactions of common anticonvulsants, p. 697, Goldfrank's Toxicologic Emergencies, 6th ed., 1998, Appleton and Lange.

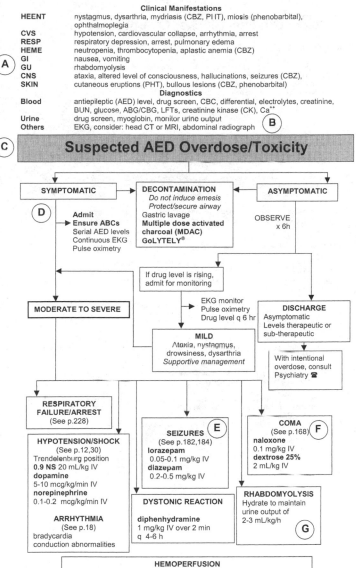

Clinical Manifestations

HEENT	nystagmus, dysarthria, mydriasis (CBZ, PHT), miosis (phenobarbital), ophthalmoplegia
CVS	hypotension, cardiovascular collapse, arrhythmia, arrest
RESP	respiratory depression, arrest, pulmonary edema
HEME	neutropenia, thrombocytopenia, aplastic anemia (CBZ)
GI	nausea, vomiting
GU	rhabdomyolysis
CNS	ataxia, altered level of consciousness, hallucinations, seizures (CBZ),
SKIN	cutaneous eruptions (PHT), bullous lesions (CBZ, phenobarbital)

Diagnostics

Blood	antiepileptic (AED) level, drug screen, CBC, differential, electrolytes, creatinine, BUN, glucose, ABG/CBG, LFTs, creatinine kinase (CK), Ca++
Urine	drug screen, myoglobin, monitor urine output
Others	EKG, consider: head CT or MRI, abdominal radiograph

Ⓐ Ⓑ Ⓒ

Suspected AED Overdose/Toxicity

SYMPTOMATIC → **DECONTAMINATION** ← **ASYMPTOMATIC**

Ⓓ

DECONTAMINATION
Do not induce emesis
Protect/secure airway
Gastric lavage
Multiple dose activated charcoal (MDAC)
GoLYTELY®

SYMPTOMATIC
Admit
Ensure ABCs
Serial AED levels
Continuous EKG
Pulse oximetry

ASYMPTOMATIC
OBSERVE
x 6h

If drug level is rising, admit for monitoring

EKG monitor
Pulse oximetry
Drug level q 6 hr

MODERATE TO SEVERE

DISCHARGE
Asymptomatic
Levels therapeutic or
sub-therapeutic

MILD
Ataxia, nystagmus,
drowsiness, dysarthria
Supportive management

With intentional
overdose, consult
Psychiatry ☎

**RESPIRATORY
FAILURE/ARREST**
(See p.228)

SEIZURES Ⓔ
(See p.182,184)
lorazepam
0.05-0.1 mg/kg IV
diazepam
0.2-0.5 mg/kg IV

COMA Ⓕ
(See p.168)
naloxone
0.1 mg/kg IV
dextrose 25%
2 mL/kg IV

HYPOTENSION/SHOCK
(See p.12,30)
Trendelenburg position
0.9 NS 20 mL/kg IV
dopamine
5-10 mcg/kg/min IV
norepinephrine
0.1-0.2 mcg/kg/min IV

ARRHYTHMIA
(See p.18)
bradycardia
conduction abnormalities

DYSTONIC REACTION

diphenhydramine
1 mg/kg IV over 2 min
q 4-6 h

RHABDOMYOLYSIS
Hydrate to maintain
urine output of
2-3 mL/kg/h

Ⓖ

HEMOPERFUSION
Continued deterioration despite maximized supportive management in
phenobarbital and **carbamazepine** overdose.

Calcium Channel Blocker Overdose

Matthew N. Denenberg

> Calcium channel blockers (CCBs) are one of the most commonly prescribed classes of cardiovascular medications. Currently, they are the leading cause of death from cardiovascular drug overdose. They are used in the management of SVT, angina and hypertension. Common calcium channel blocker preparations include **verapamil, diltiazem, nifedipine,** nicardipine, nimodipine, isradipine and felodipine. **Be aware of sustained release preparations**.

(A) CCBs decrease calcium influx into cardiac muscle and vascular smooth muscle. This directly results in the clinical manifestations through decreased AV and SA nodal conduction, decreased cardiac contractility (decreased cardiac output), and smooth muscle dilatation (decreased SVR). **Nifedipine** can cause a significant reflex tachycardia secondary to its effect on vascular smooth muscle. **Verapamil** can cause hyperglycemia secondary to insulin suppression.

(B) Laboratory findings are nonspecific and should be directed at ruling out other causes for the patient's clinical presentation. CCB levels are available in some toxicology laboratories, but the actual serum concentrations are not predictive and only confirm the presence of the drug.

EKG findings include normal sinus rhythm, **bradyarrhythmias,** various degrees of **AV block,** QRS prolongation, inverted P-waves, nonspecific ST-T wave changes, and asystole.

(C) Assess for suicide attempt versus accidental ingestion. Always consider multi-drug ingestion in any patient who presents with a drug overdose.

(D) Gastric lavage is indicated if the patient presents within 1 to 2 hours of ingestion. If sustained-release preparations are suspected, consider lavage for as long as 4 to 6 hours post ingestion followed by whole bowel irrigation. **Do not induce emesis,** as these patients can decompensate very rapidly and without warning.

(E) **Calcium** has been shown to reverse the negative inotropic effects of CCBs. Both formulations are equally effective. **Calcium chloride** has more calcium per volume than **calcium gluconate,** but may worsen the metabolic acidosis associated with CCB overdose.

(F) **Glucagon,** when administered with calcium, has been reported to reverse the effects of CCB overdose by increasing cyclic AMP, thereby improving cardiac contractility. Use of **milrinone** has also been reported to improve outcome. Higher doses of pressor agents (**dopamine, epinephrine,** and **norepinephrine**) may be required in patients with refractory hypotension/bradycardia. Dobutamine may worsen the effects of CCBs through peripheral vasodilatation, and is therefore **not** indicated.

(G) These treatments have been effective in a few case reports and may be tried in refractory cases. **Aminopyridine** is not currently available in the USA, but has been shown to increase Ca^{++} influx.

(H) Consider discharge if asymptomatic after 6 to 8 hours of observation. Admit all patients to a monitored bed if symptomatic or if sustained release medications are ingested. Deaths have been reported in children with ingestion of a single sustained release tablet.

Clinical Manifestations

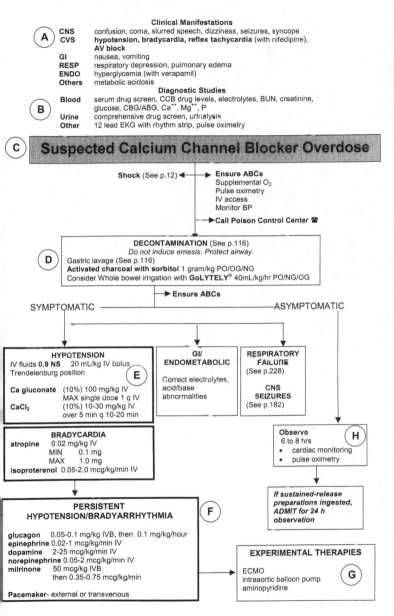

(A)
CNS	confusion, coma, slurred speech, dizziness, seizures, syncope
CVS	**hypotension, bradycardia, reflex tachycardia** (with nifedipine), **AV block**
GI	nausea, vomiting
RESP	respiratory depression, pulmonary edema
ENDO	hyperglycemia (with verapamil)
Others	metabolic acidosis

Diagnostic Studies

(B)
Blood	serum drug screen, CCB drug levels, electrolytes, BUN, creatinine, glucose, CBG/ABG, Ca^{++}, Mg^{++}, P
Urine	comprehensive drug screen, urinalysis
Other	12 lead EKG with rhythm strip, pulse oximetry

(C) ## Suspected Calcium Channel Blocker Overdose

Shock (See p.12) ◄──► **Ensure ABCs**
Supplemental O$_2$
Pulse oximetry
IV access
Monitor BP

──► **Call Poison Control Center** ☎

(D) **DECONTAMINATION** (See p.116)
Do not induce emesis. Protect airway.
Gastric lavage (See p.116)
Activated charcoal with sorbitol 1 gram/kg PO/OG/NG
Consider Whole bowel irrigation with **GoLYTELY®** 40mL/kg/hr PO/NG/OG

──► **Ensure ABCs**

SYMPTOMATIC ─────────────────────────────── ASYMPTOMATIC

(E)
HYPOTENSION
IV fluids **0.9 NS** 20 mL/kg IV bolus
Trendelenburg position

Ca gluconate	(10%) 100 mg/kg IV MAX single dose 1 g IV
CaCl$_2$	(10%) 10-30 mg/kg IV over 5 min q 10-20 min

GI/ ENDOMETABOLIC

Correct electrolytes, acid/base abnormalities

RESPIRATORY FAILURE
(See p.228)

CNS SEIZURES
(See p.182)

(H) **Observe**
6 to 8 hrs
• cardiac monitoring
• pulse oximetry

If sustained-release preparations ingested, ADMIT for 24 h observation

BRADYCARDIA
atropine	0.02 mg/kg IV
	MIN 0.1 mg
	MAX 1.0 mg
isoproterenol	0.05-2.0 mcg/kg/min IV

(F) **PERSISTENT HYPOTENSION/BRADYARRHYTHMIA**

glucagon	0.05-0.1 mg/kg IVB, then 0.1 mg/kg/hour
epinephrine	0.02-1 mcg/kg/min IV
dopamine	2-25 mcg/kg/min IV
norepinephrine	0.05-2 mcg/kg/min IV
milrinone	50 mcg/kg IVB then 0.35-0.75 mcg/kg/min

Pacemaker- external or transvenous

(G) **EXPERIMENTAL THERAPIES**

ECMO
intraaortic balloon pump
aminopyridine

Methemoglobinemia

Vera Borzova

Methemoglobinemia is defined as the presence of > 1-2% methemoglobin in the blood. Methemoglobin is the oxidized (ferric) form of hemoglobin that is unable to carry O_2, producing functional anemia. It also shifts the oxygen-hemoglobin dissociation curve to the left and interferes with oxygen delivery to the tissues. Methemoglobinemia can be congenital or acquired.

A Suspect methemoglobinemia in patients who present with marked cyanosis not responsive to 100% oxygen. Other causes of cyanosis must also be considered: cardiac and pulmonary disease, G6PD deficiency (administration of methylene blue can cause acute hemolysis in G6PD deficiency).

B Anemic patients may become symptomatic at lower levels and should be treated with methylene blue accordingly.

PO_2 is normal even in the presence of severe methemoglobinemia. PO_2 is a measure of the partial pressure of oxygen in *plasma*, not oxygen bound to hemoglobin. Use measured oxyhemoglobin (by co-oximetry) to help guide therapy. A difference will be noticed between the measured (co-oximetry) and calculated (standard blood gas machine) oxygen saturation.

RAPID BEDSIDE TEST
Place a few drops of patient's blood on filter paper or white paper towel. Compare with normal control. Chocolate-colored blood due to methemoglobin does not brighten after exposure to air.

C Gastric lavage is performed to prevent further absorption of oxidizing agents.

OXIDIZING AGENTS/TOXINS
Local anesthetics	benzocaine, lidocaine
Antimicrobials	chloroquine, dapsone, primaquine, sulfonamides
Analgesics	phenazopyridine, phenacetin
Nitrite and nitrates	amyl nitrite, butyl nitrite, isobutyl nitrite, sodium nitrite, nitroglycerin, nitric oxide
Others	metoclopramide, aniline dyes, phenytoin, well water

Methemoglobinemia has been observed in infants with infectious diarrhea, where nitrite and nitrates may be released.

D Cumulative doses of methylene blue > 7 mg/kg can cause dyspnea, chest pain, tremor, cyanosis, hemolytic anemia.

E NADH reductase deficiency requires treatment only for cosmetic purpose: **methylene blue** 3-5 mg/kg PO once daily is non-toxic and prevents cyanosis. **Ascorbic acid** 200-500 mg PO in divided doses every day can also be used.

There is no treatment for methemoglobinemia due to M hemoglobin.

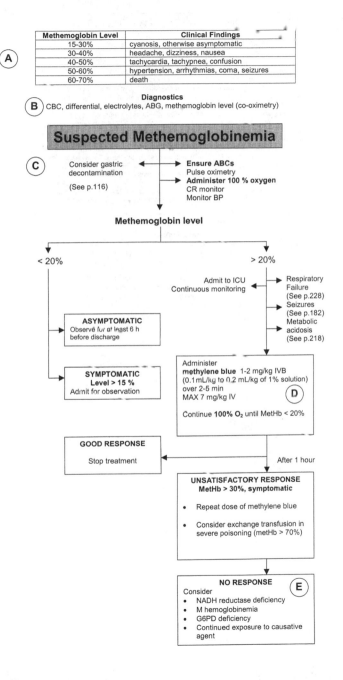

A

Methemoglobin Level	Clinical Findings
15-30%	cyanosis, otherwise asymptomatic
30-40%	headache, dizziness, nausea
40-50%	tachycardia, tachypnea, confusion
50-60%	hypertension, arrhythmias, coma, seizures
60-70%	death

Diagnostics

B CBC, differential, electrolytes, ABG, methemoglobin level (co-oximetry)

Suspected Methemoglobinemia

C Consider gastric decontamination

(See p.116)

Ensure ABCs
Pulse oximetry
Administer 100 % oxygen
CR monitor
Monitor BP

Methemoglobin level

< 20%

> 20%

Admit to ICU
Continuous monitoring

Respiratory Failure
(See p.228)
Seizures
(See p.182)
Metabolic acidosis
(See p.218)

ASYMPTOMATIC
Observe for at least 6 h before discharge

SYMPTOMATIC
Level > 15 %
Admit for observation

Administer
methylene blue 1-2 mg/kg IVB
(0.1 mL/kg to 0.2 mL/kg of 1% solution)
over 2-5 min
MAX 7 mg/kg IV

D

Continue **100% O$_2$** until MetHb < 20%

GOOD RESPONSE

Stop treatment

After 1 hour

UNSATISFACTORY RESPONSE
MetHb > 30%, symptomatic

- Repeat dose of methylene blue

- Consider exchange transfusion in severe poisoning (metHb > 70%)

NO RESPONSE E
Consider
- NADH reductase deficiency
- M hemoglobinemia
- G6PD deficiency
- Continued exposure to causative agent

Envenomations: Spiders, Scorpions

Bulent Ozgonenel

Spiders only bite once, so more than one bite rules out arachnidism. Few spiders have fangs long or strong enough to penetrate the human epidermis.
- The **Black Widow spider** (*Latrodectus mactans*) is a neurotoxic species that can be found in warm, dark, dry places, and bites only when disturbed. While the male is clinically insignificant, the female is approximately 1.5 cm in length and has a characteristic red hourglass spot on its belly, with its venomous potential greatest in the summer. Action: its proteins release acetylcholine and norepinephrine, causing a range of symptoms from cramps to paralysis, and systemic hypertension.
- The **Brown Recluse spider** (*Loxosceles reclusa*) is a dermonecrotic species that can also be found in warm, dark, dry places, but more specifically in southern and central USA. Only 9-12 mm in length, the brown recluse has a characteristic violin-like mark on its cephalothorax. Action: sphingomyelinase D causes RBC membrane lysis, activates platelets predisposing to thrombosis, and activates complement.

The **sculptured or bark scorpion** (*Centruroides*) is the only species to cause serious envenomation and is primarily found in Arizona, as well as Texas, New Mexico, and Nevada. Action: opens sodium channels and releases acetylcholine and norepinephrine.

Clinical Manifestations: Local

(A)

Black Widow (neurotoxic)	• initial prickling fades → radiating pain along extremity within 30 min • tender regional lymphadenopathy, minimal edema • "target" or "halo" at bite spot fades after 12 h
Brown Recluse (dermonecrotic)	• often unnoticed, painless bite → localized erythema, pain 1-8 h after bite • "target" or "bull's eye" lesions: central vesicle with ischemic ring and erythematous ring due to extravasated blood • subcutaneous discoloration, bleeding within 24 h, formation of eschar, sloughing with tissue defect • regional lymphadenopathy
Sculptured Scorpion	• extreme localized pain with hyperesthesia • no local erythema or swelling at site • lymphangitis with regional lymphadenopathy

(B) The only available scorpion antivenin in the USA is produced from goat serum in Antivenom Production Laboratory of Arizona State University, and does not have FDA approval. Its use is restricted to the state of Arizona, and its transport across state lines is prohibited.

(A) Systemic Clinical Manifestations
Black Widow (neurotoxic)

HEENT facial grimace or swelling
CVS conduction abnormalities
RESP severe chest pain, respiratory failure (with bite to upper extremities)
GI severe abdominal pain/rigidity without palpable tenderness (with bite to lower extremities)
CNS *motor:* muscle cramping within 1-12 h, paralysis, seizures
autonomic: nausea, vomiting, malaise, diaphoresis (only upper lip or nose), ↑SBP and DBP, ↑ HR, dysphoria

Brown Recluse (dermonecrotic)

GEN infrequent, "loxoscelism" may occur 1-2 d after bite: ever, chills, sweats, malaise, arthralgias, morbilliform rash
GI/GU nausea, vomiting, renal failure
HEME hemolysis, jaundice, DIC, thrombocytopenia

Sculptured Scorpion

GEN 12-48 h, agitation, restlessness
HEENT nystagmus, roving eye movements, diplopia
CVS arrhythmias
RESP respiratory compromise due to motor activity
CNS *motor:* involuntary jerking movements, fasciculations (peripheral muscles, tongue), facial twitching, rarely seizures
autonomic: ↑ HR, ↑ BP, salivation, diaphoresis

Diagnostics

Laboratory studies are **not** helpful in Black Widow spider or scorpion bites.
For Brown Recluse spiders: CBC, platelets, differential, PT, PTT, BUN, creatinine, urinalysis

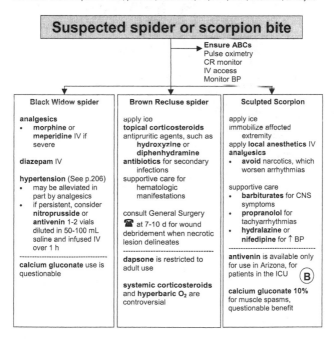

Suspected spider or scorpion bite

→ Ensure ABCs
Pulse oximetry
CR monitor
IV access
Monitor BP

Black Widow spider	Brown Recluse spider	Sculpted Scorpion
analgesics • **morphine** or **meperidine** IV if severe **diazepam** IV **hypertension** (See p.206) • may be alleviated in part by analgesics • if persistent, consider **nitroprusside** or **antivenin** 1-2 vials diluted in 50-100 mL saline and infused IV over 1 h ------ **calcium gluconate** use is questionable	apply ice **topical corticosteroids** antipruritic agents, such as **hydroxyzine** or **diphenhydramine** **antibiotics** for secondary infections supportive care for hematologic manifestations consult General Surgery ☎ at 7-10 d for wound debridement when necrotic lesion delineates ------ **dapsone** is restricted to adult use **systemic corticosteroids** and **hyperbaric O₂** are controversial	apply ice immobilize affected extremity apply **local anesthetics** IV **analgesics** • avoid narcotics, which worsen arrhythmias supportive care • **barbiturates** for CNS symptoms • **propranolol** for tachyarrhythmias • **hydralazine** or **nifedipine** for ↑ BP ------ **antivenin** is available only for use in Arizona, for patients in the ICU (B) **calcium gluconate 10%** for muscle spasms, questionable benefit

Snake Bites

Bulent Ozgonenel

Only 10% of snake species in the US are venomous, and most bites do not result in envenomation. 90% of bites occur between April and October, since snakes are poikilothermic. 80% of bites occur on hands and/or fingers. 50% of bite victims are young adult males, commonly associated with alcohol intoxication, with 40% of bites rendered non-accidental or due to careless handling.

Two families of venomous snakes
- **Crotalidae** or **pit vipers** include rattlesnakes, cottonmouths (have white mouths), and copperheads.
- **Elapidae** include only the **coral snake**; accounts for < 1% of all snake bites, bites only when handled. The coral snake is found in Arizona and other southern Gulf states.

Exercise caution when handling a snake brought to the ED to avoid being bitten by the snake which might make repeated attempts to do so.

Snake identification

Venomous pit viper	Nonvenomous pit viper	Coral snake
vertical, elliptical ("cat's eyes") pupils	round pupils	round pupils
triangular-shaped head	double row of subcaudal scales	black snout
two movable recurved fangs	no fangs, only teeth (multiple)	short, fixed maxillary fangs
indentation or pit between eye and nostril		yellow rings adjacent to red rings (vs. that of the nonvenomous king snake in which yellow and red rings are separated by black rings): *"Red on yellow kills a fellow, red on black venom lack"*

(A) Historical factors needed to determine severity of snake envenomation
- size and species of the snake (relative toxicity)
- amount of venom injected, number of bites, location/depth of bite (those to the head and trunk tend to be more severe than those to extremities)
- time elapsed before treatment (interval)
- age, size, and underlying medical condition of the victim
- victim's individual susceptibility to the venom

(B) Crotalidae bites
- peptide action → microangiopathic vascular permeability, edema, and hemorrhage
- enzymatic action → hemolysis, necrosis, and defibrination (fibrin lysis)

Coral snake bites: result in primarily neurological signs and symptoms.

(C) Antivenin is seldom indicated if > 12-24 h since bite.

(D) Cryotherapy has been associated with worsened extremity necrosis and limb amputations. Fasciotomy is rarely indicated, since proteolytic enzyme activity in these envenomations is not generally associated with an ↑ in intracompartmental pressures.

(E) If the skin testing is highly positive, suggesting enhanced risk with proposed antivenin treatment, proceed with guidance by your regional Toxicology center ☎, which may be able to advise on premedication and modified therapy, as well as assess the likelihood of needing antivenin treatment.

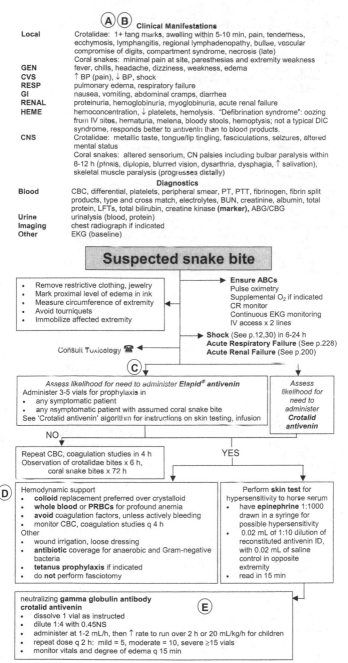

(A)(B) Clinical Manifestations

Local	Crotalidae: 1+ fang marks, swelling within 5-10 min, pain, tenderness, ecchymosis, lymphangitis, regional lymphadenopathy, bullae, vascular compromise of digits, compartment syndrome, necrosis (late)
	Coral snakes: minimal pain at site, paresthesias and extremity weakness
GEN	fever, chills, headache, dizziness, weakness, edema
CVS	↑ BP (pain), ↓ BP, shock
RESP	pulmonary edema, respiratory failure
GI	nausea, vomiting, abdominal cramps, diarrhea
RENAL	proteinuria, hemoglobinuria, myoglobinuria, acute renal failure
HEME	hemoconcentration, ↓ platelets, hemolysis. "Defibrination syndrome": oozing from IV sites, hematuria, melena, bloody stools, hemoptysis; not a typical DIC syndrome, responds better to antivenin than to blood products.
CNS	Crotalidae: metallic taste, tongue/lip tingling, fasciculations, seizures, altered mental status
	Coral snakes: altered sensorium, CN palsies including bulbar paralysis within 8-12 h (ptosis, diplopia, blurred vision, dysarthria, dysphagia, ↑ salivation), skeletal muscle paralysis (progresses distally)

Diagnostics

Blood	CBC, differential, platelets, peripheral smear, PT, PTT, fibrinogen, fibrin split products, type and cross match, electrolytes, BUN, creatinine, albumin, total protein, LFTs, total bilirubin, creatine kinase **(marker)**, ABG/CBG
Urine	urinalysis (blood, protein)
Imaging	chest radiograph if indicated
Other	EKG (baseline)

Suspected snake bite

- Remove restrictive clothing, jewelry
- Mark proximal level of edema in ink
- Measure circumference of extremity
- Avoid tourniquets
- Immobilize affected extremity

Ensure ABCs
Pulse oximetry
Supplemental O₂ if indicated
CR monitor
Continuous EKG monitoring
IV access x 2 lines

Shock (See p.12,30) in 6-24 h
Acute Respiratory Failure (See p.228)
Acute Renal Failure (See p.200)

Consult Toxicology ☎

(C)

*Assess likelihood for need to administer **Elapid®** antivenin*
Administer 3-5 vials for prophylaxis in
- any symptomatic patient
- any asymptomatic patient with assumed coral snake bite
See 'Crotalid antivenin' algorithm for instructions on skin testing, infusion

*Assess likelihood for need to administer **Crotalid antivenin***

NO

Repeat CBC, coagulation studies in 4 h
Observation of crotalidae bites x 6 h,
coral snake bites x 72 h

YES

(D) Hemodynamic support
- **colloid** replacement preferred over crystalloid
- **whole blood** or **PRBCs** for profound anemia
- **avoid** coagulation factors, unless actively bleeding
- monitor CBC, coagulation studies q 4 h

Other
- wound irrigation, loose dressing
- **antibiotic** coverage for anaerobic and Gram-negative bacteria
- **tetanus prophylaxis** if indicated
- do **not** perform fasciotomy

Perform **skin test** for hypersensitivity to horse serum
- have **epinephrine** 1:1000 drawn in a syringe for possible hypersensitivity
- 0.02 mL of 1:10 dilution of reconstituted antivenin ID, with 0.02 mL of saline control in opposite extremity
- read in 15 min

neutralizing **gamma globulin antibody**
crotalid antivenin   (E)
- dissolve 1 vial as instructed
- dilute 1:4 with 0.45NS
- administer at 1-2 mL/h, then ↑ rate to run over 2 h or 20 mL/kg/h for children
- repeat dose q 2 h: mild = 5, moderate = 10, severe ≥15 vials
- monitor vitals and degree of edema q 15 min

Mushroom Poisoning
Girija Natarajan

> The time for onset of symptoms following ingestion of mushrooms is crucial in predicting toxicity. Rapid onset of GI symptoms are generally due to non-toxic ingestions. Mortality in amanita (cyclopeptides, Group 1) poisoning approaches 10-50%, accounting for 90-95% of all mushroom poisoning deaths.

(A) Mushroom identification
In most instances, contact with the regional Toxicology center will be needed to obtain consultation from a mycologist in identification of the suspected mushroom ingested. If the mushroom is available, consider taking a spore print on white and black paper. Consultants may need to store immature spores in formaldehyde for staining Meixner stain, to identify amanita species. Suspicious mushrooms are often white capped with white gills, with either little brown, large brown, or red boletes, warts or scales on the cap, an upper ring around the upper stem, or a lower ring around the lower stem. Cyclopeptide (Group 1, amanita) toxicity is readily identifiable by the resulting clinical phases and accounts for 90-95% of all deaths from mushroom poisoning.

General Plant Poisoning

> 80% of cases of plant poisoning occur in children under 6 years of age. More than 80% are asymptomatic, with < 7% requiring a visit to a health care facility. Your regional Poison Control can provide a list of poisonous and nonpoisonous common household and garden plants.

(B)

General Plant Poisoning

Group	Plant	Toxin	Mechanism	Presentation
GI irritants	dieffenbachia (dumbcane), parlor ivy, caladium, arisaema triphyllum (jack in the pulpit)	calcium oxalate crystals	trypsin, resorcinol, bradykinin, histamine	oropharyngeal swelling, dysphagia, dysarthria, respiratory compromise
	daffodil, pokeweed, baneberry, yew	oxalates, phytolaccine, pokeweed mitogen	locally and centrally mediated emesis	mucosal irritation, diaphoresis, delirium, arrhythmia, seizures
	Lectin group: abrus, ricinus	abrin, ricin	inhibits protein synthesis	CNS, liver, renal dysfunction, cardiac arrhythmias
	Solanine group: potato, black nightshade	solanine alkaloids	anticholinesterase effects	CNS and peripheral cholinergic effects
	Colchicine group: autumn crocus	colchicine	antimitotic	GI irritation, marrow suppression, ascending paralysis, hepatotoxicity, hematuria
	Diverse sx: mayapple, bloodroot	sanguinarine	antimitotic, purgative	GI irritation, liver and renal failure, pancytopenia, polyneuropathy
Cardiac glycosides	digitalis: foxglove, oleander	digoxin, oleandrin	inhibits Na-K ATP-ase	gastric irritation, cardiac arrhythmias, hypotension, seizures, ataxia, weakness, paresthesias, liver dysfunction
	aconitine: monkshood	diterpine, norditerpine alkaloids	inhibits Na-K ATP-ase and ventricular automaticity	
	veratrum: veratrum viride			
	grayanotoxin: rhododendron	grayanotoxin, andromedotoxin	↑ Na channel permeability (cardiac)	

✱ Continued on p.155

✳ Continued from p.154

Nicotine-like action	poison hemlock, tobacco	nicotine, conine anabasine		salivation, diaphoresis, tremors, hypotension, respiratory depression
CNS acting convulsants and hallucinogens	water hemlock, nutmeg, mace	cicutoxin	stimulates central cholinergic receptors	vomiting, abdominal pain, status epilepticus, long term cognitive loss
Cyanogenic group	apple, apricot, cherry, tapioca	amygdalin		(delayed onset) hypotension, metabolic acidosis, seizures, coma, altered respirations, bitter almond smell
Belladonna group	atropa belladonna, datura	atropine, hyoscyamine	ACh receptor antagonist in heart, smooth muscle, and glands	anticholinergic effects, seizures
Hepatotoxic group	akee, comfrey	hypoglycin, b methylene cyclopropyl	inhibits fatty acid oxidation, G6Pase activity	↓ glucose, liver dysfunction
Christmas plants	holly, poinsettia	polyphenols		GI irritation
Plant dermatitis	dumbcane, philodendron	antigenic proteins	allergic contact dermatitis	urticaria

Clinical Manifestations

Group 1: Cyclopeptides	delayed GI and hepatic sx	Phase 0 (0-6 h): latent, asymptomatic Phase 1 (6-12 h): vomiting, profuse diarrhea Phase 2 (12-24 h): ↓ symptoms, ↑ liver enzymes, acidosis, electrolyte abnormalities, hypoglycemia Phase 3 (>24 h): jaundice, shock, hepatic coma, renal failure
Group 1a: Cortinarius orellanus	delayed renal sx	24-48 h: mild gastritis 2-21 d: tubulointerstitial nephritis (oliguria, polyuria, vomiting, flank pain, fever, chills, night sweats, intense burning)
Group 2: Amanita muscura	CNS and peripheral anticholinergic sx	½-3 h: alternating lethargy and confusion, psychosis, seizures, vomiting, diarrhea, visual hallucinations, urinary retention, constipation, flushing, mydriasis
Group 3: Gyrometra	delayed GI sx then predominant CNS sx	6-24 h: vomiting, diarrhea, abdominal cramps 24-48 h: seizures, CNS depression, intravascular hemolysis, methemoglobinemia, hepatorenal failure
Group 4: Clitocybe and Boletus	rapid cholinergic sx	½-2 h: diaphoresis, salivation, urination, defecation, bronchorrhea, bronchospasm, bradycardia, seizures (subsides in 6-24 h)
Group 5: Coprinus	disulfiram reaction	Up to 1 wk: vomiting, flushing, tachycardia, ↓ BP
Group 6: Psilocybe	LSD-like effects	⅓ h: visual hallucinations, ataxia, altered perception, vomiting, weakness, seizures, fever, tachycardia, mydriasis (subsides in 6 h)
Group 7: GI irritants	rapid GI sx	½-2 h: vomiting, diarrhea, headache (subsides in 24 h)

Diagnostics

Blood   electrolytes, glucose, BUN, creatinine, protein, calcium, bilirubin, LFTs, alkaline phosphatase, PT, PTT, fibrinogen, T3, T4, methemoglobin level
Urine   urinalysis (RBCs, WBCs)
Other   HPLC and RIA for amanitotoxins in gastroduodenal fluid, serum, urine and stool

Suspected Mushroom Poisoning

(A) Identify mushroom group
Consult Poison Control ☎

→ Ensure ABCs
Pulse oximetry
Monitor BP
IV access

IV hydration, correct fluid deficits and/or hypoglycemia
GI decontamination
- **syrup of Ipecac**, provided mental and respiratory status are stable, and in the absence of a disulfiram reaction:
  10 mL PO < 1 y age, 15 mL for 1-12 y, 30 mL > 12 y
- **activated charcoal**
  1 g/kg (10-30 g) PO q 2-4 h/ continuous nasogastric infusion
24 h observation

Specific Treatment by Group

Group 1	delayed GI and hepatic sx	Forced diuresis GI decontamination **High dose penicillin** (inhibits liver uptake of amanitotoxin)
Group 1a	delayed renal sx	Alkaline diuresis **Multiple dose activated charcoal (without sorbitol)** Hemodialysis, peritoneal dialysis, hemoperfusion
Group 2	CNS and peripheral anticholinergic sx	Seizures → **diazepam** CNS effects → **physostigmine** 0.02 mg/kg IV
Group 3	delayed GI sx then predominant CNS sx	Seizures → **pyridoxine** 25 mg/kg IV Hemoglobin M → **PRBC** transfusion, **methylene blue** IV **Folic acid** Methemoglobinemia → dialysis
Group 4	rapid cholinergic sx	**Atropine** 0.1-1.0 mg/kg IV
Group 5	disulfiram reaction	Tachycardia → **propranolol** PO
Group 6	LSD-like effects	**Diazepam**
Group 7	rapid GI sx	Anti-emetic

✴ Continued on p.157

✱ Continued from p.156

Clinical Manifestations

GEN	pain
HEENT	ocular pain, conjunctivitis, corneal abrasions, oropharyngeal bullae, dysphagia, dysarthria
CVS	arrhythmias, blocks, ↓ BP
RESP	respiratory distress
GI/GU	vomiting, diarrhea, melena, abdominal pain, liver dysfunction, renal dysfunction
CNS	altered mental status, delirium, seizures
	Cholinergic effects: salivation, blurred vision (miosis), ↓ HR, diaphoresis
	Anticholinergic effects: mydriasis, dry skin, ↑ HR, urinary retention, hallucinations
EXT	edema
SKIN	contact dermatitis

Diagnostics

Blood	CBC, platelets, LFTs, bilirubin, alkaline phosphatase, PT, PTT, BUN, creatinine, electrolytes, ABG/CBG, digoxin level if indicated, methemoglobin level if indicated
Urine	methylene cyclo propyl acetic acid if indicated
Other	EKG

General Plant Poisoning

Identify plant (B) ——————→ **Ensure ABCs**
Consult Poison Control Center ☎

———→ **Shock** (See p.12,30)
Seizures (See p.182,184)
Arrhythmias (See p.18)

Skin/eye exposure
- copious local irrigation
- local/systemic analgesics as needed
- notify Ophthalmology if indicated ☎

IV hydration, correct fluid deficits, prevent myoglobinuria

GI decontamination (See p.116)
- **syrup of ipecac,** provided mental and respiratory status are stable
  10 mL PO < 1 yr age, 15 mL for 1-12 yr, 30 mL > 12 yr
- gastric lavage
- **activated charcoal**
  1 g/kg (10-30 g) PO/NG q 2-4 h/ continuous nasogastric infusion
- **propylethylene glycol** (Go-LYTELY®)
- cathartic for whole bowel irrigation (**magnesium citrate, magnesium sulfate, sorbitol**)

supportive: cold milk/ice cream as demulcent

Specific Antidotes

For cardiac glycoside group	**Digibind®** (See p.142)
For belladonna alkaloid group	**physostigmine** 0.02 mg slow IV for high fever, hypotension, arrhythmias, CNS symptoms
For cyanogenic group (methemoglobinemia)	**amyl nitrite** 1 crush ampule inhalation **sodium nitrite 3% solution** 0.33 mL/kg IV **sodium thiosulfate 25% solution** 1.6 mL/kg IV, repeat in 30-60 min, MAX 50 mL/dose
For hepatotoxic group	**L-carnitine**

Chapter 9 ♣ Metabolic Disorders

Acute Neonatal Hyperammonemia

Amit Sarnaik

> Acute neonatal hyperammonemia (serum ammonia > 200 mmol/L) results from failure of detoxification of ammonia, produced from catabolism of amino acids because of deficiencies of urea cycle enzymes or inhibition of urea cycle enzymes due to organic acidemias. Hyperammonemia with or without metabolic acidosis is the characteristic biochemical manifestation of these disorders. The clinical manifestations result from the toxic effects of ammonia on the CNS.

(A) Blood for serum ammonia should be obtained as a free-flowing sample without using a tourniquet. Specimen should immediately be placed into a green-top heparinized tube on ice and transported to the laboratory.

(B) *Transient hyperammonemia of the newborn* is seen in premature infants with low birth weight, with slight elevation of serum ammonia levels (40-50 mmol/L). Infants are generally asymptomatic, and ammonia levels return to baseline within 6-8 weeks without known neurologic sequelae.

(C) Treatment goals:
1. Reduction of serum ammonia levels by facilitating excretion.
2. Reduction of ammonia production by preventing further catabolism of endogenous proteins.
3. Facilitating detoxification of ammonia by providing arginine in urea cycle defects, with the exception of arginase deficiency.

Sodium benzoate forms hippuric acid with endogenous glycine, which is cleared by the kidneys at 5 times the GFR. 1 mole of benzoate removes 1 mole of ammonia as glycine.

Sodium phenylacetate conjugates with glutamine to form phenylacetylglutamine, which is excreted by the kidneys. 1 mole of phenylacetate removes 2 moles of ammonia as glutamine.

Arginine serves as a source of ornithine molecules to keep the urea cycle operating, facilitating detoxification of ammonia.

(D) Disorders of organic acidemias can interfere with the urea cycle enzymes, causing hyperammonemia with high anion gap metabolic acidosis. However, regardless of anion gap, urine organic acids must still be obtained on all patients with hyperammonemia.

Urea cycle enzyme deficiency	<ul><li>carbamyl phosphate synthetase (CPS)</li><li>N-acetylglutamate synthetase</li><li>ornithine transcarbamylase (OTC)</li><li>argininosuccinate synthetase, argininosuccinate lyase,</li><li>arginase</li></ul>
Organic acidemias	<ul><li>propionic acidemias</li><li>methylmalonic acidemias</li><li>isovaleric acidemias</li><li>fatty acid acyl CoA dehydrogenase deficiency</li></ul>
Transient hyperammonemia of the newborn	

Clinical Manifestations

GEN	newborn infant with irritability, hypotonia, lethargy, decreased feeds, hypothermia
CVS	tachycardia, bradycardia, dehydration, hypotension, shock
RESP	central hyperventilation, grunting, apnea
GI	vomiting (may be severe)
CNS	hypotonia, irritability, seizures, opisthotonus, lethargy

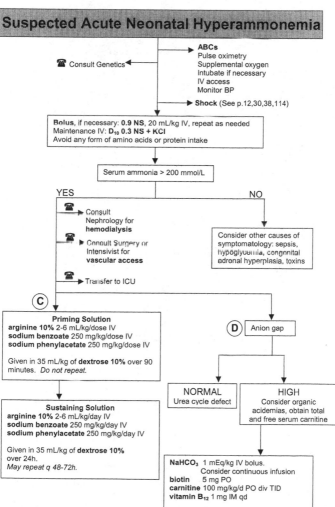

(A) Diagnostics

Blood	ammonia, AST, ALT, electrolytes, ABG/CBG, Ca^{++}, anion gap, BUN, creatinine
	save 7 mL of blood in a green-top heparinized tube for plasma amino acid quantitation (send to appropriate laboratory)
Urine	urinalysis, organic acids
	freeze 10-15 mL for further testing

(B) Suspected Acute Neonatal Hyperammonemia

☎ Consult Genetics ◄

ABCs
Pulse oximetry
Supplemental oxygen
Intubate if necessary
IV access
Monitor BP

► **Shock** (See p.12,30,38,114)

Bolus, if necessary: 0.9 NS, 20 mL/kg IV, repeat as needed
Maintenance IV: D$_{10}$ **0.3 NS + KCl**
Avoid any form of amino acids or protein intake

Serum ammonia > 200 mmol/L

YES | **NO**

☎ ► Consult
Nephrology for
hemodialysis

☎ ► Consult Surgery or
Intensivist for
vascular access

☎ ► Transfer to ICU

Consider other causes of
symptomatology: sepsis,
hypoglycemia, congenital
adrenal hyperplasia, toxins

(C)
Priming Solution
arginine 10% 2-6 mL/kg/dose IV
sodium benzoate 250 mg/kg/dose IV
sodium phenylacetate 250 mg/kg/dose IV

Given in 35 mL/kg of **dextrose 10%** over 90
minutes. *Do not repeat.*

(D) Anion gap

NORMAL
Urea cycle defect

HIGH
Consider organic
acidemias, obtain total
and free serum carnitine

Sustaining Solution
arginine 10% 2-6 mL/kg/day IV
sodium benzoate 250 mg/kg/day IV
sodium phenylacetate 250 mg/kg/day IV

Given in 35 mL/kg of **dextrose 10%**
over 24h.
May repeat q 48-72h.

NaHCO$_3$ 1 mEq/kg IV bolus.
Consider continuous infusion
biotin 5 mg PO
carnitine 100 mg/kg/d PO div TID
vitamin B$_{12}$ 1 mg IM qd

Interpretation of Blood Gases

Hrishikesh Dingankar

Henderson-Hesselbach equation: $pH = pK + \log(HCO_3/\text{dissolved } CO_2)$
- For the bicarbonate buffering system:
  $pK = 6.1$, normal $HCO_3 = 24$, normal $PCO_2 = 40 \rightarrow$ dissolved $CO_2 = 40 \times 0.003 = 1.2$
  therefore, $pH = 6.1 + \log(24/1.2) = 6.1 + 1.3 = 7.4$
- By rearranging the Henderson-Hesselbach equation,
  $[H^+] = 24 \times PCO_2/HCO_3$
  $24 \times 40/24 = 40$ nM/L
- Balance between HCO_3 and dissolved CO_2 in arterial blood is maintained at 20:1 with H^+ concentration of 40 nM/L and a pH of 7.4
- Plasma bicarbonate has 2 components:
1. Metabolic component (MC)
2. Respiratory component (RC)
   $CO_2 + H_2O \rightarrow H_2CO_3 \rightarrow H^+ + HCO_3$
   Acute $\uparrow$ in $PaCO_2$ of 1 mmHg above 40 will $\uparrow$ RC by 0.068 mEq/L
   Acute $\downarrow$ in $PaCO_2$ of 1 mmHg below 40 will $\downarrow$ RC by 0.2 mEq/L
   e.g. $PaCO_2 = 60$ mmHg $\rightarrow$ RC=$(60-40) \times 0.067 = (+)1.34$ mEq/L
   $PaCO_2 = 20$ mmHg $\rightarrow$ RC=$(20-40) \times 0.2 = (-)4$ mEq/L
   MC = plasma HCO_3 – RC (when $PCO_2 > 40$)
   MC = plasma HCO_3 + RC (when $PCO_2 < 40$)
   Normal MC = 22-26 mEq/L
   MC > 26 implies excess base, MC < 22 implies deficient base

- Alveolar gas equation
1. $PiO_2 = FiO_2 \times (P_{atm} - P_{H2O})$ PiO_2 = partial pressure of O_2 in the conducting airway
   P_{atm} = barometric pressure (760 mmHg at sea level)
   P_{H2O} = water vapor pressure (47 mmHg at 37° C)
2. $PAO_2 = PiO_2 - PACO_2/R$ PAO_2 = partial pressure of O_2 in the alveoli
   $PACO_2$ = partial pressure of CO_2 in the alveoli
   R = respiratory quotient – amount of CO_2 produced/O_2 consumed (normal = 0.8)
3. PaO_2 = partial pressure of oxygen in blood
- At sea level, PaO_2 of 80-100 is considered normal when breathing room air

- Definitions:
1. Acidemia – increase in H^+ concentration
2. Alkalosis – decrease in H^+ concentration

Classification

Disorder	pH	Underlying Abnormality	Compensation	Examples of Clinical Situations
Respiratory acidosis	$\downarrow$	$\uparrow PCO_2$	$\uparrow HCO_3$	Airway obstruction e.g., asthma
Respiratory alkalosis	$\uparrow$	$\downarrow PCO_2$	$\downarrow HCO_3$	Central hyperventilation e.g., early aspirin poisoning
Metabolic acidosis	$\downarrow$	$\downarrow HCO_3$	$\downarrow PCO_2$	Diabetic ketoacidosis
Metabolic alkalosis	$\uparrow$	$\uparrow HCO_3$	$\uparrow PCO_2$	Chloride losing states e.g., pyloric stenosis

Note: in a simple acid-base disorder with accompanying compensation, PCO_2 and HCO_3 *always* move in the same direction.

Compensatory Changes

Acid-Base Status	Abnormality	Compensation
Respiratory acidosis	alveolar ventilation insufficient	$\uparrow$ renal HCO_3 reabsorption which $\uparrow$ serum HCO_3 concentration
Respiratory alkalosis	alveolar ventilation excessive	$\downarrow$ renal HCO_3 reabsorption with $\downarrow$ serum bicarbonate concentration
Metabolic acidosis	gain of strong acid or primary loss of HCO_3	stimulates chemoreceptors which result in $\uparrow$ ventilation and $\downarrow PCO_2$
Metabolic alkalosis	primary gain of a strong base or loss of a strong acid	inhibits the chemoreceptors with resultant hypoventilation and $\uparrow PCO_2$

Note: it may be impossible to distinguish the primary acid-base disorder simply by looking at a blood gas measurement when the pH is normal. Additional tests are needed.
For example: pH 7.0, PCO_2 30, HCO_3 18 may represent chronic respiratory alkalosis with metabolic compensation, or chronic metabolic acidosis with respiratory compensation.

✳ Continued on p.162

Interpretation of Blood Gases

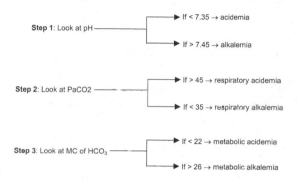

Step 1: Look at pH
→ If < 7.35 → acidemia
→ If > 7.45 → alkalemia

Step 2: Look at PaCO2
→ If > 45 → respiratory acidemia
→ If < 35 → respiratory alkalemia

Step 3: Look at MC of HCO_3
→ If < 22 → metabolic acidemia
→ If > 26 → metabolic alkalemia

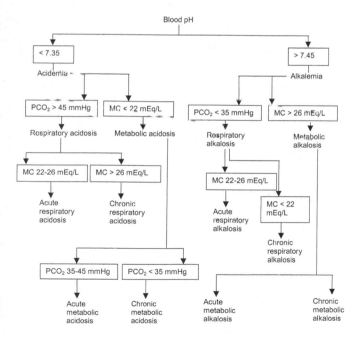

✳ Continued from p.160

Expected Changes in pH and Compensatory Responses in Acid Base Disorders

Disorder	Expected Changes
For every ↑ PCO_2 by 1 mmHg	*Acute* (hours): pH ↓ by 0.008 units and HCO_3 ↑ by 0.1 mEq/L *Chronic* (days): pH ↓ by 0.0025 units and HCO_3 ↑ by 0.4 mEq/L
↓ PCO_2 by 1 mmHg	*Acute*: pH ↑ by 0.007 units and HCO_3 ↓ by 0.25 mEq/L *Chronic*: pH ↑ by 0.003 units and HCO_3 ↓ by 0.5 mEq/L
↓ HCO_3 by 1 mEq/L	pH ↓ by 0.012 units and PCO_2 ↓ by 1.25 mmHg
↑ HCO_3 by 1 mEq/L	pH ↑ by 0.003-0.008 units and PCO_2 ↓ by 0.2-0.9 units

Winter's formula: provides an estimate of adequacy of the compensatory ventilatory response to metabolic acidosis. Whether or not PCO_2 has been lowered enough by increased respiratory rate can serve as a rough indicator of whether the ability of the CNS to compensate has been compromised, e.g., a diabetic with DKA and severe metabolic acidosis, and has developed cerebral edema may not have an appropriately low PCO_2

Expected PCO_2 = [1.5 x HCO_3] + 8 [± 2]

Capillary blood gas sampling:
1. Correlation with arterial sample best for pH, moderate for PCO_2, worst for PO_2
2. Correlation with PO_2 poor because of arteriovenous mixing during sampling, arterial and venous blood have slightly different pH and PCO_2 but very different PO_2

	Arterial	Venous
pH	7.35 – 7.45	0.04 units < arterial pH
PCO_2	35 – 45 mmHg	5 – 7 mmHg > arterial
PO_2	95 mmHg	40 mmHg
SaO_2	97%	75%

Pitfalls of capillary sampling for blood gases:
1. Improperly warmed capillary bed ↓ accuracy
2. Squeezing the soft tissue to collect blood can distort results
3. Prolonged period required for collection (slow bleeding) allows the sample to equilibrate with air resulting in falsely ↑ PO_2 and falsely ↓ PCO_2

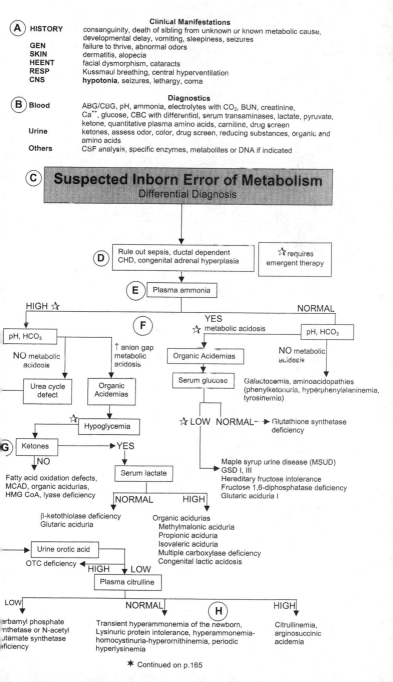

Clinical Manifestations

(A) HISTORY consanguinity, death of sibling from unknown or known metabolic cause, developmental delay, vomiting, sleepiness, seizures
GEN failure to thrive, abnormal odors
SKIN dermatitis, alopecia
HEENT facial dysmorphism, cataracts
RESP Kussmaul breathing, central hyperventilation
CNS **hypotonia**, seizures, lethargy, coma

Diagnostics

(B) Blood ABG/CBG, pH, ammonia, electrolytes with CO_2, BUN, creatinine, Ca^{++}, glucose, CBC with differential, serum transaminases, lactate, pyruvate, ketone, quantitative plasma amino acids, carnitine, drug screen
Urine ketones, assess odor, color, drug screen, reducing substances, organic and amino acids
Others CSF analysis, specific enzymes, metabolites or DNA if indicated

(C) **Suspected Inborn Error of Metabolism**
Differential Diagnosis

(D) Rule out sepsis, ductal dependent CHD, congenital adrenal hyperplasia

☆ requires emergent therapy

(E) Plasma ammonia

HIGH ☆   NORMAL

(F)   YES
☆ metabolic acidosis

pH, HCO_3 pH, HCO_3

NO metabolic acidosis   ↑ anion gap metabolic acidosis   Organic Acidemias   NO metabolic acidosis

Urea cycle defect   Organic Acidemias   Serum glucose   Galactosemia, aminoacidopathies (phenylketonuria, hyperphenylalaninemia, tyrosinemia)

☆ Hypoglycemia   ☆ LOW   NORMAL → Glutathione synthetase deficiency

(G) Ketones → YES

NO   Serum lactate   Maple syrup urine disease (MSUD) GSD I, III Hereditary fructose intolerance Fructose 1,6-diphosphatase deficiency Glutaric aciduria I

Fatty acid oxidation defects, MCAD, organic acidurias, HMG CoA, lyase deficiency

NORMAL   HIGH

β-ketothiolase deficiency
Glutaric aciduria   Organic acidurias
Methylmalonic aciduria
Propionic aciduria
Isovaleric aciduria
Multiple carboxylase deficiency
Congenital lactic acidosis

Urine orotic acid
OTC deficiency   HIGH   LOW
Plasma citrulline

LOW   NORMAL   (H)   HIGH

arbamyl phosphate
nthetase or N-acetyl
utamate synthetase
eficiency   Transient hyperammonemia of the newborn, Lysinuric protein intolerance, hyperammonemia-homocystinuria-hyperornithinemia, periodic hyperlysinemia   Citrullinemia, arginosuccinic acidemia

＊ Continued on p.165

Inborn Errors of Metabolism

Michael Fiore

(A) Inborn errors of metabolism are caused by gene mutations, usually transmitted in an autosomal recessive or x-linked recessive pattern, resulting in alterations in specific protein structures (enzymes, transport proteins, receptors, and structural elements), involved in the metabolism of amino acids, carbohydrates, organic acids, nitrogen, or fatty acids. Clinical manifestations range from asymptomatic to severe lethal mutations.

Relatively uncommon disorders, but require prompt diagnosis and treatment to prevent poor outcome. Even if survival is unlikely, all attempts should be made to confirm the diagnosis in order to provide information for genetic counseling.

(B) Inborn Errors of Metabolism Associated with Abnormal Odors

Disease	Urine Odors
Maple Syrup Urine Disease	Maple syrup
Isovaleric aciduria	Sweaty feet
Hypermethionemia	Cooked cabbage
Tyrosinemia	Cooked cabbage
Multiple carboxylase deficiency	Cat urine
Phenylketonuria	Musty
Trimethylaminuria	Rotting fish
Oasthouse urine disease	Hops
Glutaric acidemia type II	Sweaty feet

(C) Infants typically present with a normal prenatal and immediate post-natal course, then a few days after discharge, may present with poor feeding, hypotonia, or irritability. Occasionally, they may remain well until a catabolic state is induced by an intercurrent illness such as a viral infection, or poor nutrition, when they become much more symptomatic.

(D) Differential diagnosis:
- sepsis
- CNS infections
- congenital adrenal hyperplasia
- PDA closure in ductal-dependent cardiac lesion with shock
- hypoglycemia
- hypocalcemia
- pyloric stenosis
- gastroenteritis

(E) Factors that lead to false elevation of serum ammonia levels:
- Capillary blood specimen
- Prolonged standing of specimen in room temperature
- Specimen collected in ammonium-heparin tube
- Mixed with air bubbles during collection
- Ammonia-contaminated reagent water
- Improper laboratory standardization according to patient's age

(F) Prevention measures: Avoid catabolism. Many of the biochemical pathways that are affected are those that are involved in the breakdown of fats or protein. This occurs at times when glucose is not available as a preferred substrate for ATP production.
- Aggressive nutrition
- Immunizations to avoid preventable viral/bacterial disease
- Continuous infusion of dextrose (10% or 15% dextrose) during illness or periods of fasting

(G) Ketosis is a biochemical hallmark of fat breakdown

(H) Transient hyperammonemia of the newborn rarely persists after 24 hours of age

✳ Continued from p.163

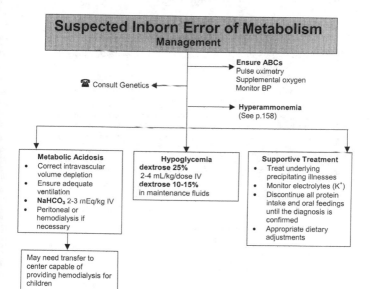

Suspected Inborn Error of Metabolism
Management

☎ Consult Genetics ◄

Ensure ABCs
Pulse oximetry
Supplemental oxygen
Monitor BP

Hyperammonemia
(See p.158)

Metabolic Acidosis
- Correct intravascular volume depletion
- Ensure adequate ventilation
- **NaHCO₃** 2-3 mEq/kg IV
- Peritoneal or hemodialysis if necessary

May need transfer to center capable of providing hemodialysis for children

Hypoglycemia
dextrose 25%
2-4 mL/kg/dose IV
dextrose 10-15%
in maintenance fluids

Supportive Treatment
- Treat underlying precipitating illnesses
- Monitor electrolytes (K⁺)
- Discontinue all protein intake and oral feedings until the diagnosis is confirmed
- Appropriate dietary adjustments

Malignant Hyperthermia

Laila Tutunji

Malignant hyperthermia (MH) is characterized by a sudden hypermetabolic reaction of skeletal muscle to certain inhaled anesthetics, mainly halothane, and the neuromuscular blocking agent, succinylcholine. There is usually an underlying familial susceptibility that leads to abnormal contraction coupling upon exposure to the offending agent.

(A) Risk factors: family history of malignant hyperthermia (especially when involving first degree relatives), Duchenne muscular dystrophy, scoliosis, heavy musculature

May manifest immediately during anesthesia induction, as masseter spasm, but more commonly, in the post-anesthesia care unit while recovering from general anesthesia.

Phases of Malignant Hyperthermia

1. Initial hypermetabolic phase that begins with an increase in O_2 consumption and CO_2 production, continuous muscle contractions, hyperthermia, rhabdomyolysis, myoglobinuria, acute tubular necrosis, hyperkalemia, tachycardia, hypertension, ventricular arrhythmias, acidosis, and DIC.

2. Eventually, hypermetabolism is replaced by shock, with hypotension, bradycardia and cardiac arrest.

(B) Acidosis in MH is secondary to increased oxygen consumption, anaerobic metabolism, and hypercarbia due to accumulation of large amounts of CO_2 that exceeds the lungs' capacity for clearance.

(C) Hyperthermia can be a late sign. **Do not wait for hyperthermia to develop** to initiate therapy if otherwise suspicious that a patient may be developing MH.

(D) **Dantrolene** is the drug of choice for aborting a hyperthermic reaction. It acts on excitation contraction coupling and decreases the release of calcium from the endoplasmic reticulum, and increases calcium re-uptake. Each mg of dantrolene is compounded with 150 mg of **mannitol**.

(E) Follow-up: after the first episode of MH, all immediate family members must be screened. For future anesthesia, halothane and succinylcholine must be avoided, using **nitrous oxide, curare and narcotic analgesics** instead. Premedication with oral **dantrolene** a few days prior to surgery should be considered.

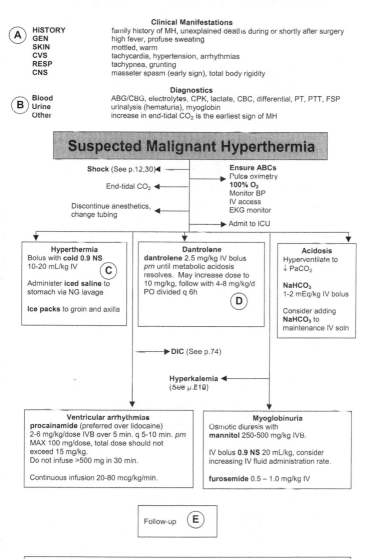

Clinical Manifestations

(A) **HISTORY** family history of MH, unexplained deaths during or shortly after surgery
GEN high fever, profuse sweating
SKIN mottled, warm
CVS tachycardia, hypertension, arrhythmias
RESP tachypnea, grunting
CNS masseter spasm (early sign), total body rigidity

Diagnostics

(B) **Blood** ABG/CBG, electrolytes, CPK, lactate, CBC, differential, PT, PTT, FSP
Urine urinalysis (hematuria), myoglobin
Other increase in end-tidal CO_2 is the earliest sign of MH

Suspected Malignant Hyperthermia

Shock (See p.12,30)

End-tidal CO_2

Discontinue anesthetics,
change tubing

Ensure ABCs
Pulse oximetry
100% O_2
Monitor BP
IV access
EKG monitor

Admit to ICU

Hyperthermia
Bolus with **cold 0.9 NS**
10-20 mL/kg IV (C)

Administer **iced saline** to
stomach via NG lavage

Ice packs to groin and axilla

Dantrolene
dantrolene 2.5 mg/kg IV bolus
prn until metabolic acidosis
resolves. May increase dose to
10 mg/kg, follow with 4-8 mg/kg/d
PO divided q 6h (D)

Acidosis
Hyperventilate to
↓ $PaCO_2$

NaHCO₃
1-2 mEq/kg IV bolus

Consider adding
NaHCO₃ to
maintenance IV soln

DIC (See p.74)

Hyperkalemia
(See p.210)

Ventricular arrhythmias
procainamide (preferred over lidocaine)
2-6 mg/kg/dose IVB over 5 min. q 5-10 min. *prn*
MAX 100 mg/dose, total dose should not
exceed 15 mg/kg.
Do not infuse >500 mg in 30 min.

Continuous infusion 20-80 mcg/kg/min.

Myoglobinuria
Osmotic diuresis with
mannitol 250-500 mg/kg IVB.

IV bolus **0.9 NS** 20 mL/kg, consider
increasing IV fluid administration rate.

furosemide 0.5 – 1.0 mg/kg IV

Follow-up (E)

Neuroleptic malignant syndrome: resembles MH, but occurs over days to months in patients
on neuroleptic agents such as haloperidol, thiothixene, and piperazine phenothiazine.
Manifestations include hyperthermia, hypermetabolism, tachycardia, muscle rigidity,
myoglobinuria, acute renal failure and multiorgan failure. Relieved by dantrolene or
bromocriptine. All patients with neuroleptic malignant syndrome should be treated as MH-
susceptible until proven otherwise.

Chapter 10 ♣ Neurologic Disorders

Coma
Katherine Ling-McGeorge

> Implies either
> - Bilateral hemispheric/cortical dysfunction, or
> - Brainstem/reticular activating system dysfunction

(A) Assess Glasgow Coma Scale/GCS (See p.305). Patients with GCS ≤ 8 should be admitted to the ICU.

(B) **Thiamine** 50 mg IV + 50 mg IM (prior to administering glucose)
Flumazenil (Romazicon®) 0.2 mg IV over 30 sec, MAX 2 mg total dose. Note - may cause seizure activity.

Neurologic Assessment
Lesion localization and differential diagnoses are imperative to therapy.

(C)

General appearance/level of consciousness	
lethargy	drowsiness
obtunded	blunted
stupor	barely arousable
coma	unresponsive
persistent vegetative state	brainstem function only

Vital signs	
fever	infection
↑ HR	shock, DKA, CHF
↓ BP	shock, adrenal failure
↓ HR, ↑BP	↑ ICP, poisoning

(D) Motor exam for cortical function
Observe spontaneous movements. Apply noxious stimuli (sternal rub, subungual pressure) to elicit posturing. Repeat stimuli to validate findings. To elicit voluntary movements, drop patient's arm on his/her face.

Motor exam/cortical function

Decorticate (arms flexed, abducted)	Cortical dysfunction
Decerebrate (extremities extended)	High brainstem dysfunction
Flaccid/hypotonic	Brainstem dysfunction, any level
Hypertonic	Corticospinal injury

(E) Brainstem evaluation
- Note that the **pupillary reflex** tends to remain intact with metabolic insults.

Pupillary reflex

bilateral	normal/small	reactive	toxic/metabolic
	midposition	fixed	midbrain dysfunction (parasympathetic, sympathetic)
	pinpoint	reactive	narcotics, barbiturates, organophosphates
		fixed	pontine lesion (sympathetic)
	large	reactive	anticholinergic agents, post-ictal, metabolic
		fixed	toxic/metabolic, anoxic
unilateral	small	minimal	ipsilateral sympathetic dysfunction
	large	fixed	midbrain or ipsilateral CN III injury, uncal herniation
hippus			midbrain

- **corneal reflex**: CN V sensory, CN VII motor
- **oculocephalic reflex/dolls eyes**
  Reflects absence of cortical influence on the brainstem. Indicates intact brainstem function.
  Rule out C-spine injury prior to performing maneuver.
  "Present" = eyes appear to gaze forward upon turning head laterally, i.e., eyes will deviate to the opposite side of head turning.
- **oculovestibular reflex/cold calorics**
  Determine that tympanic membranes are intact and ear canals free of cerumen prior to performing maneuver. Ascertain negative history for prior use of ototoxic drugs.

> Elevate head 30°. Place small catheter in the external canal near the tympanic membrane, and introduce ice water slowly from a syringe into the canal. Maximum volume per ear is approximately 120 mL. Allow 5 min for the oculovestibular system to stabilize before performing test in opposite ear.

In a normal, awake patient: will observe nystagmus, with the slow component toward the irrigated ear and fast component away.
In the comatose patient: will observe eyes tonically deviate toward the irrigated ear, with disappearance of the fast component. Severe brainstem injury obliterates the response entirely.

✱ Continued on p.170

Clinical Manifestations

HISTORY	onset, fever, preceding complaints, trauma, medications/toxins in household, substance abuse
Head	split sutures (hydrocephalus), intracranial bruits (AVM), VP shunt
Eyes	periorbital ecchymosis (blow-out orbital fx), retinal hemorrhages (child abuse), chemosis (cavernous sinus thrombosis)
Ears	Battle's sign (basilar skull fx), hemotympanum or CSF otorrhea (trauma)
Nose	CSF rhinorrhea (trauma)
Oropharynx	tongue lacerations (seizures), pigmentation (Addison's disease), gingival lines (plumbism)
Neck	rigidity (infection, intracranial hemorrhage), thyromegaly (thyrotoxicosis)
RESP (breath)	fruity (DKA), garlic (arsenic, paraldehyde, organophosphate), almonds (cyanide), alcohol (ethanol)
SKIN	erythema (CO, atropine, mercury), cyanosis (hypoxia, CNS emboli in R→L shunt with congenital heart disease), petechiae or splinter hemorrhages (infectious endocarditis, coagulopathy), icterus or spider hemangiomata (hepatic oncephalopathy), periungual fibroma (tuberous sclerosis), desquamation (vitamin A intoxication), rash (SLE, infection), pigmentation (Addison's disease), needle tracks (drugs)

Diagnostics

Blood	glucose, ABG/CBG, CBC, differential, electrolytes, BUN, creatinine, Ca^{++}, Mg^{++}, P, osmolality, culture, comprehensive toxicology screen. Consider COHb, LFTs, lactate, ammonia, metabolic screen, coagulation profile
Urine	urinalysis, drug screen
Imaging	head CT
Other	lumbar puncture (if not contraindicated), EKG, EEG

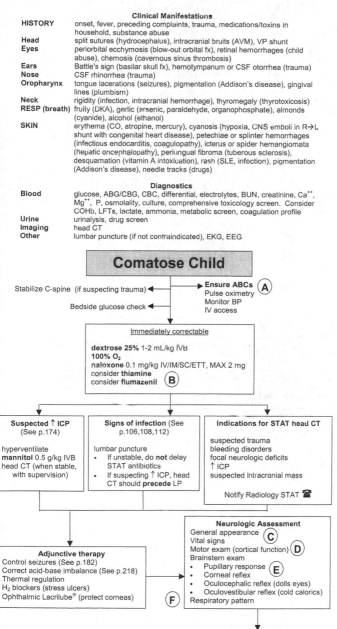

Comatose Child

Stabilize C-spine (if suspecting trauma) ←
→ **Ensure ABCs** (A)
Pulse oximetry
Monitor BP
IV access

Bedside glucose check ←

Immediately correctable

dextrose 25% 1-2 mL/kg IVB
100% O$_2$
naloxone 0.1 mg/kg IV/IM/SC/ETT, MAX 2 mg
consider **thiamine**
consider **flumazenil** (B)

Suspected ↑ ICP
(See p.174)

hyperventilate
mannitol 0.5 g/kg IVB
head CT (when stable, with supervision)

Signs of infection (See p.106,108,112)

lumbar puncture
- If unstable, do **not** delay STAT antibiotics
- If suspecting ↑ ICP, head CT should **precede** LP

Indications for STAT head CT

suspected trauma
bleeding disorders
focal neurologic deficits
↑ ICP
suspected intracranial mass

Notify Radiology STAT ☎

Adjunctive therapy
Control seizures (See p.182)
Correct acid-base imbalance (See p.218)
Thermal regulation
H$_2$ blockers (stress ulcers)
Ophthalmic Lacrilube® (protect corneas)

Neurologic Assessment
General appearance (C)
Vital signs
Motor exam (cortical function) (D)
Brainstem exam
- Pupillary response (E)
- Corneal reflex
- Oculocephalic reflex (dolls eyes)
- Oculovestibular reflex (cold calorics)
Respiratory pattern

(F)

✱ Continued on p.171

✳ Continued from p.168

(F) <u>Respiratory patterns</u>

- Cheyne-Stokes - bilateral hemispheric dysfunction, as seen with transtentorial herniation, DKA, CHF

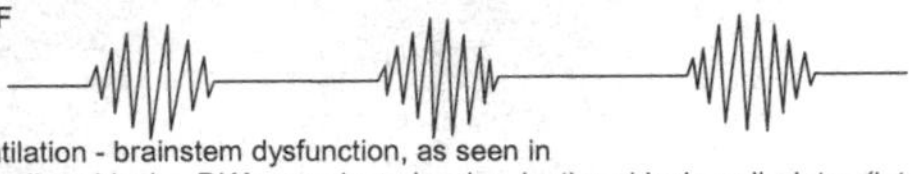

- Hyperventilation - brainstem dysfunction, as seen in
  o Metabolic acidosis - DKA, uremia, poisoning, lactic acidosis, salicylates (late)
  o Respiratory alkalosis - hepatic encephalopathy, salicylates (early)
  o Reye sydrome

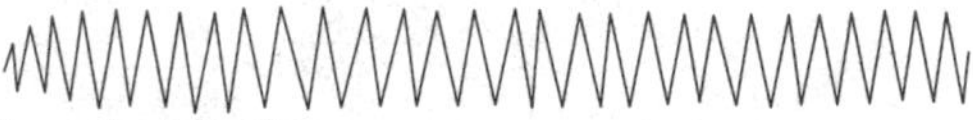

- Apneustic - pontine dysfunction

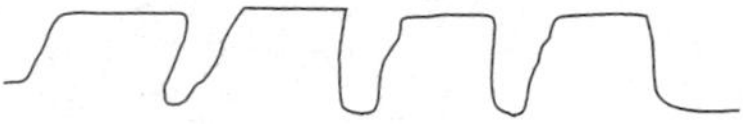

- Ataxic/agonal - medullary

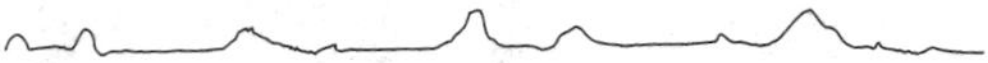

- Hypoventilation - drugs

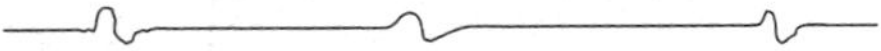

(G) Non-metabolic causes of coma: neoplasm, hemorrhage, CVA, vasculitis

(H) Toxins causing coma: barbiturates, phenytoin, narcotics, salicylates, lead, cyclic antidepressants, phenothiazines, amphetamines, iron, CO, alcohol, organophosphates, carbamates. Note - protect airway prior to performing GI decontamination

Other metabolic causes of coma: anoxia/post-CPR, hypoglycemia, DKA, adrenal insufficiency, porphyria, uremia, hepatic encephalopathy, hyperammonemia, Reye syndrome, inborn errors of metabolism, hyper/hypocalcemia, hyper/hyponatremia, hyper/hypomagnesemia, acidosis/alkalosis, CO_2 narcosis, hyperosmolar conditions, vitamin deficient/dependent states, HUS.

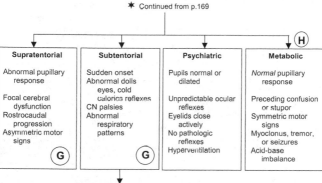

✱ Continued from p.169

Supratentorial	**Subtentorial**	**Psychiatric**	**Metabolic**
Abnormal pupillary response Focal cerebral dysfunction Rostrocaudal progression Asymmetric motor signs **G**	Sudden onset Abnormal dolls eyes, cold calorics reflexes CN palsies Abnormal respiratory patterns **G**	Pupils normal or dilated Unpredictable ocular reflexes Eyelids close actively No pathologic reflexes Hyperventilation	*Normal* pupillary response Preceding confusion or stupor Symmetric motor signs Myoclonus, tremor, or seizures Acid-base imbalance

Intubate early!

Guillain-Barré Syndrome

Ina Shamraj

An acute, inflammatory peripheral neuropathy, also known as acute inflammatory demyelinating polyneuropathy (AIDP), thought to be immune-mediated. Infrequently, it is the presenting syndrome of chronic inflammatory demyelinating polyneuropathy (CIDP).

(A) History of antecedent viral illness or surgical procedure, commonly URI, gastroenteritis, mononucleosis, or scarlet fever.

(B) Differential diagnoses: myopathy, transverse myelitis, botulism, myasthenia gravis, poliomyelitis, heavy metal poisoning, organophosphate poisoning, acute intermittent porphyria, and thiamine deficiency.

(C) GBS is frequently accompanied by autonomic dysfunction, which results in abnormal peripheral vasomotor tone and arrhythmias. This results in transient extremes of BP and arrhythmias. It is generally recommended to withhold treatment, as it can worsen the symptoms of autonomic dysfunction.

(D) The use of depolarizing agents in patients with GBS is associated with ventricular arrhythmias. Use of sedative and anesthetic agents can accentuate autonomic instability.

(E) Either **IV immunoglobulin** or **plasmapheresis/plasma exchange** is used as the primary treatment modality for acute GBS. Indications for treatment include: bulbar involvement, respiratory failure, and loss of ambulation. Plasmapheresis is usually only indicated within the first two weeks.

(F) Over the long term, these patients are prone to decubitus ulcers, deep vein thrombosis, and pulmonary embolism, due to immobility. In addition, urinary retention often leads to UTI's. Decreased respiratory effort can lead to pneumonia in patients with respiratory compromise. Continued management and supportive therapy should be directed toward the prevention of these complications.

(A) **Clinical Manifestations**

Patients in respiratory failure will not manifest signs of distress, because of muscle weakness (poor effort) and phrenic nerve involvement.

Vitals	autonomic instability, extremely high/low BP, arrhythmias
Motor	symmetric ascending distal weakness → paralysis, difficulty walking, floppy infant (progressive over days to weeks)
Sensory	loss of sensation or paresthesias in limbs, loss of vibratory/position sense (seen early, within a few days)
Other	**hyporeflexia/arreflexia**, altered mental status. Miller-Fischer variant: descending weakness, ataxia, ophthalmoplegia, facial palsy.

Diagnostics

FVC	(forced vital capacity) q 2-4 hours (See p.304)
ABG/CBG	monitor CO_2 retention
LP	cytoalbuminologic dissociation: elevated protein, minimal pleocytosis (1 wk after onset of symptoms)
EMG, NCV	acute denervation, greatly reduced motor conduction (1 week after onset of symptoms)

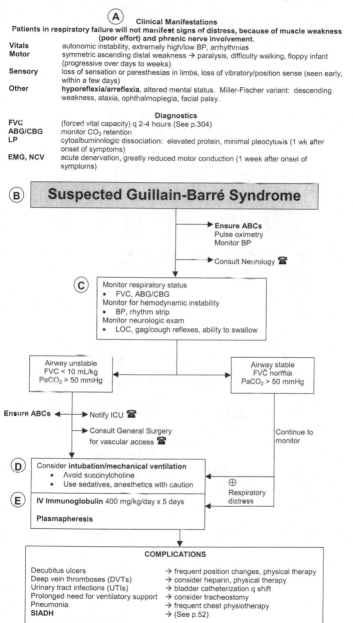

(B) # Suspected Guillain-Barré Syndrome

▶ **Ensure ABCs**
Pulse oximetry
Monitor BP

▶ Consult Neurology ☎

(C) Monitor respiratory status
• FVC, ABG/CBG
Monitor for hemodynamic instability
• BP, rhythm strip
Monitor neurologic exam
• LOC, gag/cough reflexes, ability to swallow

Airway unstable
FVC < 10 mL/kg
$PaCO_2 > 50$ mmHg

Airway stable
FVC normal
$PaCO_2 > 50$ mmHg

Ensure ABCs ◀ ▶ Notify ICU ☎

▶ Consult General Surgery
for vascular access ☎

Continue to
monitor

(D) Consider **intubation/mechanical ventilation**
• Avoid succinylcholine
• Use sedatives, anesthetics with caution

⊕
Respiratory
distress

(E) **IV Immunoglobulin** 400 mg/kg/day x 5 days

Plasmapheresis

COMPLICATIONS

Decubitus ulcers	→ frequent position changes, physical therapy
Deep vein thromboses (DVTs)	→ consider heparin, physical therapy
Urinary tract infections (UTIs)	→ bladder catheterization q shift
Prolonged need for ventilatory support	→ consider tracheostomy
Pneumonia	→ frequent chest physiotherapy
SIADH	→ (See p.52)

Increased Intracranial Pressure

Varsha Gharpure

> A rigid cranial vault encases the brain. Increased intracranial pressure (ICP) thus can result in brain herniation. Subsequent compression of the brainstem results in progressive deterioration in the level of consciousness, and if untreated, may lead to apnea and death.

(A) History suggestive of increased ICP: occipital headache, neck pain, vomiting, altered mental status, visual disturbances.
History suggestive of etiology: trauma, previous shunt surgery, ataxia, fever, otitis media, bleeding disorder, over judicious hydration in the treatment of diabetic ketoacidosis, predisposing factors for SIADH, dehydration.

(B) Avoid prolonged bag-mask ventilation to prevent gastric distention and emesis. Aim for a $PaCO_2$ of 30 mmHg. A lower $PaCO_2$ may be necessary for a short period of time if there is evidence of herniation. Utilize end-tidal CO_2 monitor if available.

(C) Rapid Sequence Intubation if impending herniation
- Lidocaine blunts the ICP spike, cough reflex, and cardiovascular effects of intubation.
- Midazolam should be injected 2-3 minutes prior to paralytic agent to avoid conscious paralysis.
- Thiopental, propofol, and etomidate decrease ICP by decreasing cerebral metabolism.
- Rocuronium is preferred due to rapid onset and shorter duration of action.

(D) **Maintain mean arterial pressure to preserve cerebral perfusion.** Sedative agents used for intubation can cause hypotension. Judicious use of fluids and inotropic support may be necessary.
- Thiopental and propofol cause peripheral vasodilatation and myocardial depression. *Reduce doses by half if severe multisystem trauma or hypovolemia is present.*
- Etomidate has minimal hemodynamic effects and is preferred in patients with hypovolemia. It may activate seizure foci. When used only for induction, etomidate causes insignificant adrenal suppression. Safety and efficacy have not been established for etomidate in children below 10 years of age.

(E) **Aspiration of reservoir**
Under sterile conditions, puncture reservoir with 25-gauge butterfly needle, and check column of CSF to assess pressure. Slowly aspirate aliquots of 5-10 mL CSF, until symptomatically improved. Send CSF for labs. Inability to draw back suggests proximal shunt obstruction. Neurosurgeon or other experienced personnel must be present. For ventricular tap, consult Neurosurgery. Subdural tap may be necessary in the apneic infant with suspected child abuse and subdural hematoma (**Subdural Tap**, see p.284 and **Child Abuse**, see p.42).

(F)

Etiology of Increased Intracranial Pressure		
Brain	Cerebral edema	
• Vasogenic edema	Secondary to abscess, meningitis, tumor	Disrupted blood-brain barrier, leaky inter-endothelial junctions
• Cytotoxic edema	Hypoxia, water intoxication	Intracellular fluid shift secondary to failure of ATP-dependent sodium pump or sudden decrease in extracellular volume
• Interstitial edema	Obstructive hydrocephalus, shunt malfunction	Increased CSF hydrostatic pressure causing CSF shift to interstitial space
Blood	AV malformation, dural sinus thrombosis, hemorrhage (trauma)	
CSF	Communicating and non-communicating hydrocephalus	
Other	Tumor, abscess, cyst, hemorrhage (trauma, AV malformation)	

(G) **Pentobarbital** 2 mg/kg IV, repeat every 20 minutes up to 10-15 mg/kg, followed by continuous infusion at 1-3 mg/kg/hour. Monitor blood pressure closely. May need inotropic support.

(A) Clinical Manifestations

VITALS	**Cushing's response - hypertension, bradycardia, bradypnea**
GENERAL	vomiting, check for presence of shunt/reservoir and/or evidence of trauma.
HEENT	headache, increased head circumference, bulging anterior fontanelle, meningeal signs, papilledema or retinal hemorrhage
CNS	altered mental status, posturing, seizures, diplopia, sunset eyes, extraocular muscle palsy, unequal pupils

Diagnostics

Blood	glucose, electrolytes, BUN, creatinine, osmolality, ABG/CBG, CBC, differential, drug screen, culture
Urine	electrolytes, UUN, creatinine, drug screen
Imaging	head CT, MRI, US (a) **if stable**, (b) if no immediate metabolic cause is evident

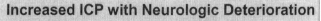

Increased ICP with Neurologic Deterioration

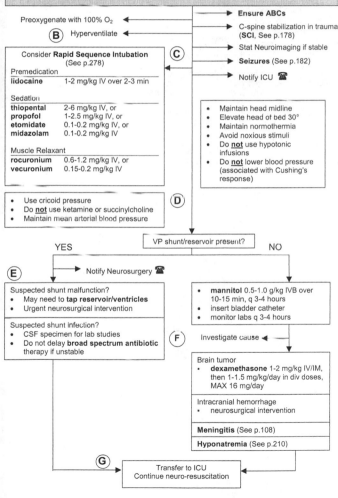

Ensure ABCs

Preoxygenate with 100% O_2 ←

(B) Hyperventilate ←

C-spine stabilization in trauma (**SCI**, See p.178)

Stat Neuroimaging if stable

(C)

Consider **Rapid Sequence Intubation**
(See p.278)

Seizures (See p.182)

Notify ICU ☎

Premedication

lidocaine 1-2 mg/kg IV over 2-3 min

Sedation

thiopental 2-6 mg/kg IV, or
propofol 1-2.5 mg/kg IV, or
etomidate 0.1-0.2 mg/kg IV, or
midazolam 0.1-0.2 mg/kg IV

Muscle Relaxant

rocuronium 0.6-1.2 mg/kg IV, or
vecuronium 0.15-0.2 mg/kg IV

- Maintain head midline
- Elevate head of bed 30°
- Maintain normothermia
- Avoid noxious stimuli
- Do **not** use hypotonic infusions
- Do **not** lower blood pressure (associated with Cushing's response)

- Use cricoid pressure
- Do **not** use ketamine or succinylcholine
- Maintain mean arterial blood pressure

(D)

VP shunt/reservoir present?

YES   NO

(E) Notify Neurosurgery ☎

Suspected shunt malfunction?
- May need to **tap reservoir/ventricles**
- Urgent neurosurgical intervention

Suspected shunt infection?
- CSF specimen for lab studies
- Do not delay **broad spectrum antibiotic** therapy if unstable

- **mannitol** 0.5-1.0 g/kg IVB over 10-15 min, q 3-4 hours
- insert bladder catheter
- monitor labs q 3-4 hours

(F) Investigate cause ←

Brain tumor
- **dexamethasone** 1-2 mg/kg IV/IM, then 1-1.5 mg/kg/day in div doses, MAX 16 mg/day

Intracranial hemorrhage
- neurosurgical intervention

Meningitis (See p.108)

Hyponatremia (See p.210)

(G) Transfer to ICU
Continue neuro-resuscitation

Myasthenia Gravis

Clarence Parks

(A) An autoimmune disorder of the neuromuscular junction. A decreased number of functional acetylcholine receptors results in muscle weakness. Affects all muscle groups, including respiratory apparatus, although most commonly the muscles for oculomotor movements and mastication.

- *Neonatal MG:* presents at birth, floppy infant, associated with transplacental antibody transmission, may involve an infant thymic factor.
- *Juvenile MG:* usually presents > 8 yrs age, waxes and wanes, associated with seizures
- *Congenital MG:* autosomal recessive. Mother is disease free. Antibody is absent. Acetylcholine receptor protein is defective. Often resistant to therapy.

Ach = acetylcholine
AChe = achetylcholinesterase

Differential diagnoses

Infectious	polio, echovirus, coxsackie, GBS, transverse myelitis, diphtheric neuropathy, tick paralysis
Congenital	vasculitis, vascular malformations in spinal cord, spinal cord masses
Metabolic/ environmental	hypokalemia, paralysis, porphyria, drug induced paralysis, heavy metals
Other	botulism, Guillain-Barré Syndrome

(B)

Drugs to avoid in patients with myasthenia gravis

Analgesics	meperidine, morphine
Anesthetics	lidocaine, procaine
Antiarrhythmics	procainamide, quinidine, quinine
Antibiotics	gentamicin, polymixins, streptomycin, tetracycline, tobramycin
Anticonvulsants	carbamazepine, phenytoin, valproic acid
Anxiolytics	benzodiazepines
Muscle relaxants	baclofen
Paralyzing agents	curare, succinylcholine

(A) **Clinical Manifestations**

Fluctuating weakness of ocular (prolonged upward gaze leads to ptosis), facial,
neck (infants: poor head control), oropharyngeal (infants: difficulty feeding), and limb muscles

Diagnostics

EMG: decremental response of muscle action potential (MAP) seen with 3/sec repetitive nerve
stimulation, until refractory to further stimulation (muscle fatigue).

	Clinical setting	Clinical manifestations	Treatment
Myasthenic crisis	Infections, menses, stress, under-medication, hazardous medication	Muscle weakness, tachycardia, mydriasis, respiratory distress	• AChe therapy • May need ventilatory support
Cholinergic crisis	AChe overdose	Diarrhea, cramps, miosis, bradycardia, fasciculations, salivation, diaphoresis	• Hold all AChe therapy • Consider atropine • May need ventilatory support

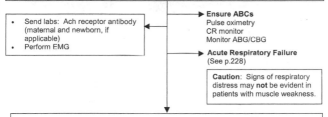

Patient with Suspected Myasthenia Gravis

• Send labs: Ach receptor antibody (maternal and newborn, if applicable)
• Perform EMG

➤ **Ensure ABCs**
Pulse oximetry
CR monitor
Monitor ABG/CBG

➤ **Acute Respiratory Failure**
(See p.228)

Caution: Signs of respiratory distress may **not** be evident in patients with muscle weakness.

Notify Neurology prior to performing the tests below. ☎
Monitor HR and BP. Double blind fashion with 0.9 NS placebo.

edrophonium (Tensilon®) test: 0.15 mg/kg/dose IV/IM/SC, MAX 10 mg
Assess strength and ocular movements, drug effects only last a few minutes.
or
neostigmine (Prostigmin®) test: 0.025-0.04 mg/kg IM
May be preferred in neonates, response noted within 10 minutes and peaks at 30 minutes

Have **atropine** available 0.01 mg/kg IM/SC, MIN 0.1 mg, MAX 2 mg, for potential side
effects of edrophonium (severe bradycardia, hypotension, cramps).

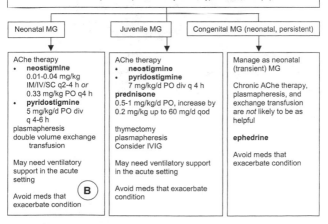

Neonatal MG	Juvenile MG	Congenital MG (neonatal, persistent)

AChe therapy
• **neostigmine**
  0.01-0.04 mg/kg
  IM/IV/SC q2-4 h *or*
  0.33 mg/kg PO q4 h
• **pyridostigmine**
  5 mg/kg/d PO div
  q 4-6 h
plasmapheresis
double volume exchange
transfusion

May need ventilatory
support in the acute
setting

Avoid meds that
exacerbate condition

(B)

AChe therapy
• **neostigmine**
• **pyridostigmine**
  7 mg/kg/d PO div q 4 h
prednisone
0.5-1 mg/kg/d PO, increase by
0.2 mg/kg up to 60 mg/d qod

thymectomy
plasmapheresis
Consider IVIG

May need ventilatory support
in the acute setting

Avoid meds that exacerbate
condition

Manage as neonatal
(transient) MG

Chronic AChe therapy,
plasmapheresis, and
exchange transfusion
are *not* likely to be as
helpful

ephedrine

Avoid meds that
exacerbate condition

Spinal Cord Injury (SCI)

Russell Clark

Causes: trauma (most common), vascular disorders, tumors, infections, and congenital disorders. Trauma includes: motor vehicle accidents (50%), auto vs. pedestrian, assault, falls, sports (diving, football, gymnastics, hockey), and child abuse. Higher incidence in older male children, due to associated high risk behaviors. Anatomic frequency distribution is cervical (61%), thoracolumbar (T11-L2, TLJ, 19%), thoracic (16%), and lumbosacral (4%). The atlanto-occipital complex is at greatest risk during the perinatal period. Prior to adolescence, dislocation and distraction injuries are more frequently seen than fractures, while traumatic fracture dislocation is more common after age 11 years. Following stabilization, a complete neurologic exam includes assessment of perianal sensation, voluntary rectal sphincter control, priapism, incontinence, and skin warmth or flushing (See p.181 for dermatomes). Serial neurologic exams will help distinguish between incomplete (*non*-progressive) SCI's from incomplete progressive SCI's, which benefit from surgical intervention.

(A)

Complete SCI - complete loss of sensorimotor and reflex activity below the level of the injury.
Incomplete SCI - preservation of some motor or sensory function below the level of injury.
Sacral sparing - the existence of motor/sensory activity at the anal mucocutaneous border. This distinguishes complete from incomplete SCI.

Spinal **C**ord **I**njury **W**ith**O**ut **R**adiographic **A**bnormality (SCIWORA)
Can be incomplete or complete. Almost only seen in children. Because of increased compliance of the developing bony skeleton and increased mobility of the pediatric spine, a child's vertebral column may sustain significant trauma without radiologic evidence.

Incomplete SCI Syndromes

Syndrome	Mechanism of injury	Site of injury	Neurologic deficit / Clinical presentation
Central cord	Anterior-posterior cord compression (congenital stenotic canals)	Cervical Centrally located neural fibers	• Motor weakness, distal > proximal, UE > LE • Possible urinary retention • Sacral sparing
Brown-Sequard		Lateral hemisection of the cord	• Ipsilateral motor weakness • Loss of proprioception and vibration • Loss of contralateral pain, pin prick, temperature sensation
Anterior cord	Disruption of anterior spinal artery flow to the anterior 2/3 of the cord	Anterior 2/3 of cord, including C1, T4, and L1 watersheds	• Complete paralysis • Bilaterally ↓ sensation to pain and touch • Intact proprioception/vibratory sense
Conus medularis		Distal cord	• Areflexic bladder, bowel, LE • Bilateral LE motor and sensory deficit • Preserved bulbocavernosus and micturition reflexes
Cauda equina		Lumbosacral nerve roots	• Varies, not necessarily bilateral • LE, bowel and bladder sensorimotor and reflex deficits • Possible radiculopathy

Medical conditions with increased risk for SCI

Trisomy 21	Rheumatoid arthritis	Congenital spinal stenosis
Spina bifida	Diastematomyelia	Tethered cord
Achondroplasia	Acquired osteoporosis	Forestier's disease
Paget's disease	Degenerative disk disease	Ankylosing spondylitis
Mucopolysaccharidosis	Klippel-Feil Syndrome	

(B) Spinal cord stabilization: restores the patient to an immobilized neutral supine position and allows access to maintain airway and circulation.
   • Use straight backboard: maintain neutral alignment of head/neck to the long axis of the body.
   • Apply cervical collar and towel rolls or sandbags on each side of the head.
   • Apply tape/Velcro straps to forehead, chest (nonrestrictive), pelvis, knees, and ankles.
   • Special consideration in infants: due to their disproportionately larger heads, their cervical spine flexes anteriorly when placed supine on flat surfaces. Ways to prevent this: modifying the backboard to provide a recess for the occiput, or using double mattress pads between the board and the patient to raise the trunk.
64% of SCI patients have concomitant injuries.

(C) Respiratory insufficiency can be immediate or delayed, due to muscle fatigue, soft tissue edema, or hematoma. Abdominal breathing may be observed. *Gentle* manual in-line axial traction may be needed to maintain the spine in a neutral position when considering endotracheal intubation.

(D) The goals of radiographic examination of a patient with suspected SCI are:
   • Detect and characterize the skeletal fracture, subluxation, and /or dislocation.
   • Differentiate intrinsic and extrinsic spinal lesions that may require surgical decompression in a patient with neurologic deficits.

✳ Continued on p.180

Clinical Manifestations

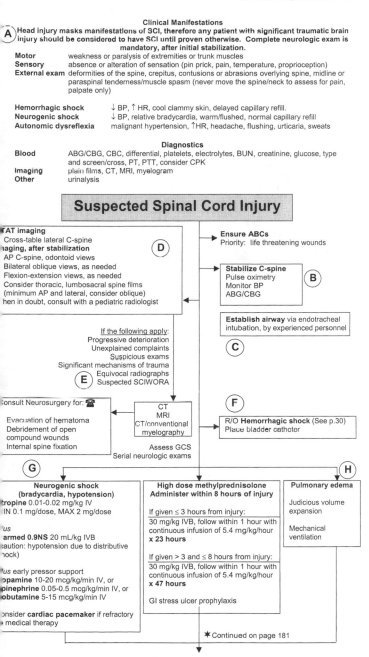

(A) Head injury masks manifestations of SCI, therefore any patient with significant traumatic brain injury should be considered to have SCI until proven otherwise. Complete neurologic exam is mandatory, after initial stabilization.

Motor	weakness or paralysis of extremities or trunk muscles
Sensory	absence or alteration of sensation (pin prick, pain, temperature, proprioception)
External exam	deformities of the spine, crepitus, contusions or abrasions overlying spine, midline or paraspinal tenderness/muscle spasm (never move the spine/neck to assess for pain, palpate only)

Hemorrhagic shock	↓ BP, ↑ HR, cool clammy skin, delayed capillary refill.
Neurogenic shock	↓ BP, relative bradycardia, warm/flushed, normal capillary refill
Autonomic dysreflexia	malignant hypertension, ↑HR, headache, flushing, urticaria, sweats

Diagnostics

Blood	ABG/CBG, CBC, differential, platelets, electrolytes, BUN, creatinine, glucose, type and screen/cross, PT, PTT, consider CPK
Imaging	plain films, CT, MRI, myelogram
Other	urinalysis

Suspected Spinal Cord Injury

STAT imaging
Cross-table lateral C-spine
Imaging, after stabilization **(D)**
AP C-spine, odontoid views
Bilateral oblique views, as needed
Flexion-extension views, as needed
Consider thoracic, lumbosacral spine films
(minimum AP and lateral, consider oblique)
When in doubt, consult with a pediatric radiologist

→ **Ensure ABCs**
Priority: life threatening wounds

Stabilize C-spine
Pulse oximetry
Monitor BP
ABG/CBG **(B)**

Establish airway via endotracheal intubation, by experienced personnel **(C)**

If the following apply:
Progressive deterioration
Unexplained complaints
Suspicious exams
Significant mechanisms of trauma
Equivocal radiographs **(E)**
Suspected SCIWORA

(F)

Consult Neurosurgery for: ☎
Evacuation of hematoma
Debridement of open compound wounds
Internal spine fixation

CT
MRI
CT/conventional myelography
Assess GCS
Serial neurologic exams

R/O **Hemorrhagic shock** (See p.30)
Place bladder catheter

(G)

Neurogenic shock
(bradycardia, hypotension)
atropine 0.01-0.02 mg/kg IV
MIN 0.1 mg/dose, MAX 2 mg/dose

Plus
warmed 0.9NS 20 mL/kg IVB
(caution: hypotension due to distributive shock)

Plus early pressor support
dopamine 10-20 mcg/kg/min IV, or
epinephrine 0.05-0.5 mcg/kg/min IV, or
dobutamine 5-15 mcg/kg/min IV

Consider **cardiac pacemaker** if refractory to medical therapy

High dose methylprednisolone
Administer within 8 hours of injury

If given ≤ 3 hours from injury:
30 mg/kg IVB, follow within 1 hour with continuous infusion of 5.4 mg/kg/hour x 23 hours

If given > 3 and ≤ 8 hours from injury:
30 mg/kg IVB, follow within 1 hour with continuous infusion of 5.4 mg/kg/hour x 47 hours

GI stress ulcer prophylaxis

(H)

Pulmonary edema
Judicious volume expansion
Mechanical ventilation

✱Continued on page 181

✴ Continued from p.178

Cross-table lateral C-spine taken with patient immobilized on the trauma board can identify 80-90% of significant abnormalities. Imaging must include the C7-T1 articulation and the top of T1. Pulling down on the patient's hands during imaging may help the patient relax the shoulder girdle muscles to better visualize the cervical spine. A *swimmer's view* also images the cervico-thoracic junction when the above efforts fail.

- Additional plain films (after patient stabilization): *AP C-spine and odontoid* (open mouth) views are mandatory to identify the remaining 10% of significant abnormalities. *Bilateral oblique views* and *flexion-extension views* as needed.
- Consider imaging the *thoracic and lumbosacral spine* in all patients with severe trauma and those with altered mental status.
- Atlanto-occipital dislocation is a difficult radiographic diagnosis!
- For cervical spine, any subluxation greater than 4 mm or angulation greater than 11° indicates major ligamentous injury. Pre-dental space should be < 5 mm in children. The anterior margin of the foramen magnum should lie within 5 mm directly above the tip of the odontoid. Pediatric patients often exhibit a 2-3 mm C2-C3 and C3-C4 pseudosubluxation. Special criteria apply to the occiput through C2 levels and also for different age ranges in pediatrics. When in doubt, consult with pediatric radiologist.

(E) Additional neuroimaging
- CT best defines skeletal anatomy
- CT or conventional myelography - can define impingement on the spinal cord.
- MR imaging - best for soft tissue definition, cord compression, vascular anatomy, foreign bodies, bony fragments, cord edema, spinal canal stenosis or impingement, hematomas, tumors, ligamentous injury, disc herniation, and Chiari malformations. Ligamentous injury results in chronic instability without fracture. MR is particularly valuable in the diagnosis of SCIWORA.

(F) Always rule out concomitant *hemorrhagic shock* in the trauma victim. Hemorrhagic shock presents classically with **hypotension, tachycardia, cool clammy skin, delayed capillary refill**.

(G) *Neurogenic shock* results from temporary disruption of efferent sympathetic tracts in SCI at or above the injured level, due to edema, compression, relative ischemia, or inflammation. There is a loss of sympathetic vasomotor tone, with peripheral vasodilatation and hypotension; paradoxical bradycardia or asystole occurs from unopposed parasympathetic vagal tone. The patient will appear **warm, flushed**, dry, and **hypotensive** with relative **bradycardia** and **normal capillary refill**. Use caution in administering fluids, since intravascular volume is actually mal-distributed and may require early pressor support. If bradycardia persists despite medical intervention, the patient may require a cardiac pacemaker.

(H) *Pulmonary edema* may result from massive sympathetic discharge, leading to a disruption of pulmonary capillary endothelium. It may also be due to over-aggressive fluid resuscitation in a patient in neurogenic shock and manifests after pressor support is initiated.

(I) Supportive care:
- Temperature control: limited ability to shiver, ↓ cutaneous vasomotor control
- Respiratory support: unopposed vagal tone results in copious secretions.
- Nasogastric tube placement.
- GI stress ulcer prophylaxis.
- DVT prophylaxis (DVT seen in 72%; death due to PE 37%).
- Nutritional support.
- Prevention of decubitus ulcer.
- Bowel and bladder care.
- Physical medicine/rehabilitation, prevention of contractures, and control of spasticity.

(J) *Autonomic dysreflexia* occasionally occurs with SCI at or higher than the midthoracic level. Unopposed nociceptive afferents from below the injury level can cause malignant hypertension, tachycardia, headache, flushing, urticaria, and diaphoresis. Treat hypertension, until able to identify and eliminate the nociceptive stimulus.

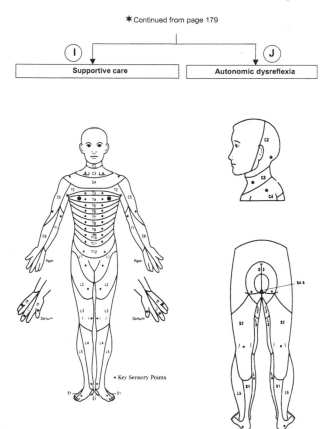

✳ Continued from page 179

I → Supportive care
J → Autonomic dysreflexia

• Key Sensory Points

ASIA IMPAIRMENT SCALE
(modified from Frankel)

A = Complete. No sensory or motor function is preserved in the sacral segments S4-S5.

B = Incomplete. Sensory but not motor function is preserved below the neurological level and extends through sacral segments S4-S5.

C = Incomplete. Motor function is preserved below the neurological level; the majority of key muscle groups below the neurological level have a power grade less than 3.

D = Incomplete. Motor function is preserved below the neurological level; the majority of key muscle groups below the neurological level have a power grade greater than or equal to 3.

E = Normal. Sensory and motor function is normal.

*From International Standards for Neurological Classification of Spinal Cord Injury,
Atlanta: American Spinal Injury Association, 2000, p10-11. With permission.*

Status Epilepticus

Jeff A. Clark

> Single seizure or repeated seizure lasting at least 15-30 min during which the patient does not regain consciousness.

(A) Seizure types
1. febrile
2. idiopathic - absence of underlying brain pathology, commonly from withdrawal or subtherapeutic levels of antiepileptic drugs (AED)
3. symptomatic - occurs in association with ongoing neurologic or metabolic abnormality

Treatment goals
- maintain normal cardiorespiratory function and cerebral oxygenation (ABCs)
- stop clinical and electrical seizure activity
- identify and treat precipitating factors
- correct metabolic disturbances and systemic complications

(B) Etiology
- fever
- antiepileptic medication change or withdrawal
- metabolic - electrolyte disturbances, ↓ glucose, hepatic failure, uremia
- hypoxia/ischemia
- hemolytic uremic syndrome
- ↑ ICP, including shunt malfunction
- infection - CNS and non-CNS
- trauma
- toxic ingestion/exposure - alcohol, cyclic antidepressants, hypoglycemic agents, organophosphates, theophylline, cyclosporine, lead, etc.
- intracranial tumor

(C) **Paraldehyde** is no longer approved for human use, with the exception of use through an investigational protocol. Dose 0.3 mL/kg PR mixed 1:1 with mineral oil, MAX 5 mL, dispense via glass syringe.

Fosphenytoin takes 15-20 min to take effect.

(D) For the child who is currently on **phenobarbital**, it is reasonable to give 5 mg/kg IVB pending the phenobarbital level. Phenytoin has a narrow therapeutic range, therefore in the child who was previously taking phenytoin, await result of level prior to determining and administering phenytoin IV bolus dose.

(E) Complications of status epilepticus
- hyper/hypotension
- arrhythmias/conduction abnormalities
- congestive heart failure
- cardiac arrest
- pulmonary edema
- aspiration pneumonia
- hyper/hypoglycemia
- SIADH
- diabetes insipidus
- ↑ cortisol, ↑ prolactin
- rhabdomyolysis
- acute tubular necrosis
- fever
- dehydration
- DIC

(A) **Clinical Manifestations**

Typically generalized tonic-clonic movements or focal activity lasting > 15-30 min with ⊕ LOC
In neonates, may only see eye deviation, chewing/sucking motions, apnea
↑ BP, ↑ HR, altered RR

Diagnostics

Blood ABG/CBG, electrolytes, BUN, creatinine, Ca^{++}, Mg^{++}, P, glucose, CBC, differential, AED (anti-epileptic drug) levels. Consider drug screen, metabolic screen, ammonia

Urine urinalysis, consider drug screen

Imaging consider head CT if indicated ☆

Other consider lumbar puncture (if not contraindicated) ☆

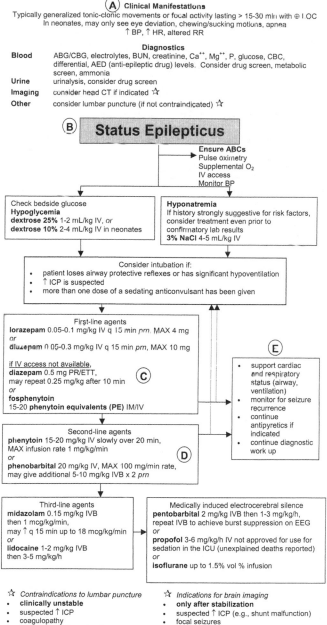

(B) **Status Epilepticus**

Ensure ABCs
Pulse oximetry
Supplemental O_2
IV access
Monitor BP

Check bedside glucose
Hypoglycemia
dextrose 25% 1-2 mL/kg IV, *or*
dextrose 10% 2-4 mL/kg IV in neonates

Hyponatremia
If history strongly suggestive for risk factors, consider treatment even prior to confirmatory lab results
3% NaCl 4-5 mL/kg IV

Consider intubation if:
- patient loses airway protective reflexes or has significant hypoventilation
- ↑ ICP is suspected
- more than one dose of a sedating anticonvulsant has been given

First-line agents
lorazepam 0.05-0.1 mg/kg IV q 15 min *prn*, MAX 4 mg
or
diazepam 0.05-0.3 mg/kg IV q 15 min *prn*, MAX 10 mg

if IV access not available,
diazepam 0.5 mg PR/ETT, (C)
may repeat 0.25 mg/kg after 10 min
or
fosphenytoin
15-20 **phenytoin equivalents (PE)** IM/IV

Second-line agents
phenytoin 15-20 mg/kg IV slowly over 20 min,
MAX infusion rate 1 mg/kg/min
or (D)
phenobarbital 20 mg/kg IV, MAX 100 mg/min rate,
may give additional 5-10 mg/kg IVB x 2 *prn*

(E)
- support cardiac and respiratory status (airway, ventilation)
- monitor for seizure recurrence
- continue antipyretics if indicated
- continue diagnostic work up

Third-line agents
midazolam 0.15 mg/kg IVB
then 1 mcg/kg/min,
may ↑ q 15 min up to 18 mcg/kg/min
or
lidocaine 1-2 mg/kg IVB
then 3-5 mg/kg/h

Medically induced electrocerebral silence
pentobarbital 2 mg/kg IVB then 1-3 mg/kg/h,
repeat IVB to achieve burst suppression on EEG
or
propofol 3-6 mg/kg/h IV not approved for use for sedation in the ICU (unexplained deaths reported)
or
isoflurane up to 1.5% vol % infusion

☆ *Contraindications to lumbar puncture*
- **clinically unstable**
- suspected ↑ ICP
- coagulopathy
- infection over the entry site

☆ *Indications for brain imaging*
- **only after stabilization**
- suspected ↑ ICP (e.g., shunt malfunction)
- focal seizures
- trauma

Seizures

Girija Natarajan

A paroxysmal involuntary disturbance of brain function that may manifest as an impairment or loss of consciousness, abnormal motor activity, behavior abnormalities, sensory disturbances, or autonomic dysfunction.

(A) International Seizure Classification

Generalized seizures

1. typical absence - sudden cessation of motor activity or speech or awareness, no aura or post-ictal impairment, < 30 sec duration, EEG 2 per sec spike and generalized wave activity
2. atypical absence - associated motor or myoclonic movements or atonia
3. generalized tonic clonic - typical aura and post-ictal state
4. tonic - sustained muscle contractions
5. clonic - flexor spasm of extremities
6. myoclonic - brief, repetitive, symmetric muscle contractions with loss of tone
7. atonic - abrupt loss of muscle tone
8. infantile spasms

Partial seizures (focal onset)

1. simple - motor, sensory, autonomic, psychic; duration 10-20 sec, no automatisms; EEG unilateral or multifocal spike or sharp wave activity
2. complex - aura present in 30%, automatisms in 50-75%, duration 1-2 min, impaired consciousness; EEG anterior, temporal, multifocal spikes or sharp waves, normal in 20%
3. partial evolving into secondarily generalized seizures

Unclassified seizures

Special syndromes

1. febrile convulsions
2. isolated seizures
3. seizures related to acute metabolic or toxic event

Causes of *symptomatic* seizures: association with ongoing neurologic or metabolic abnormality

- electrolyte abnormalities (especially Na^+), hyper/hypoglycemia
- inborn errors of metabolism (seizures recurrent)
- hepatic, renal, or multi-organ failure
- ischemic, hypertensive encephalopathy (seizures recurrent)
- meningitis, encephalitis
- systemic diseases - SLE, AIDS
- drug-related - cocaine, cyclosporine, chemotherapy, alcohol, cyclic antidepressants, hypoglycemic agents, organophosphates, theophylline, lead
- intracranial tumor
- head injury
- neurodegenerative disease
- congenital malformations - neurocutaneous syndromes, Aicardi syndrome (seizures recurrent)
- structural CNS lesions - schizencephaly, lissencephaly (seizures recurrent)

Differential diagnoses for seizure activity

- syncope (routine, cardiogenic, cough)
- breath-holding spells in toddlers
- pseudoseizure (hysteria)
- narcolepsy/sleep apnea
- benign paroxysmal vertigo
- complicated migraine
- Sandifer's syndrome (opisthotonic posturing associated with gastroesophageal reflux)

(B) Indications for anti-epileptic drug (AED) levels

- initiation of AED treatment to confirm therapeutic levels
- in the noncompliant patient
- patients presenting with status epilepticus
- during accelerated growth spurts
- on polytherapy - particularly with valproate, phenobarbital, lamotrigine
- uncontrolled or changing type of seizure
- signs of drug toxicity
- hepatic or renal disease
- suspected drug interactions
- in the child with cognitive or physical disabilities in whom toxicity is difficult to assess

(C) Routine interictal EEGs are abnormal in only 60% of patients.

Prolonged video EEG - conducted in a hospital setting with AEDs withheld, sphenoidal and possibly subdural electrodes; tested under conditions of hyperventilation, photic stimulation, and sleep deprivation

✱ Continued on p.186

(A) **Clinical Manifestations**

History	fever, duration/frequency of seizures, post-ictal state, precipitating factors, h/o drug ingestion or head injury; family h/o epilepsy, febrile convulsions or metabolic diseases; toxin or medication exposure
GEN	other medical problems such as cardiovascular disease, failure to thrive, unilateral growth arrest of limb, vomiting
HEENT	chorioretinitis, coloboma, retinal hemorrhages, phakomas, abnormal facies
CNS	mood swings, headache (early AM or sudden), preceding aura, focal motor activity or neurological deficit, altered consciousness, loss of milestones
SKIN	neurocutaneous stigmata, evidence of trauma

Diagnostics

Blood	ABG/CBG, glucose, electrolytes, BUN, creatinine, Ca^{++}, Mg^{++}, P, CBC, differential; consider cultures, LFTs, ammonia, drug screen, HIV, ANA, AED levels if applicable (B)
Urine	urinalysis
Imaging	head CT/MRI if indicated ☆
Other	EEG, lumbar puncture if indicated ☆ (C)

For refractory seizure disorders: prolonged video EEG, SPECT/PET scan, intra-carotid amyl barbital injection

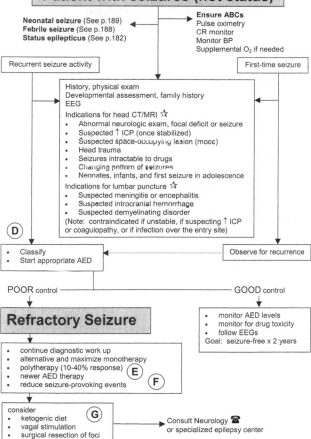

Patient with seizures (not status)

Neonatal seizure (See p.189)
Febrile seizure (See p.188)
Status epilepticus (See p.182)

Ensure ABCs
Pulse oximetry
CR monitor
Monitor BP
Supplemental O$_2$ if needed

Recurrent seizure activity

First-time seizure

History, physical exam
Developmental assessment, family history
EEG

Indications for head CT/MRI ☆
- Abnormal neurologic exam, focal deficit or seizure
- Suspected ↑ ICP (once stabilized)
- Suspected space-occupying lesion (mass)
- Head trauma
- Seizures intractable to drugs
- Changing pattern of seizures
- Neonates, infants, and first seizure in adolescence

Indications for lumbar puncture ☆
- Suspected meningitis or encephalitis
- Suspected intracranial hemorrhage
- Suspected demyelinating disorder
(Note: contraindicated if unstable, if suspecting ↑ ICP or coagulopathy, or if infection over the entry site)

(D)
- Classify
- Start appropriate AED

Observe for recurrence

POOR control

GOOD control

Refractory Seizure

- monitor AED levels
- monitor for drug toxicity
- follow EEGs
Goal: seizure-free x 2 years

- continue diagnostic work up
- alternative and maximize monotherapy
- polytherapy (10-40% response)
- newer AED therapy
- reduce seizure-provoking events
(E) (F)

consider (G)
- ketogenic diet
- vagal stimulation
- surgical resection of foci

→ Consult Neurology ☎
or specialized epilepsy center

✳ Continued from p. 184

SPECT/PET scan - for localizing hypometabolic or hypoperfused regions
WADA intra-carotid amyl barbital injection prior to surgery to identify dominant hemisphere and
risk to language function by planned surgical resection of seizure foci

(D)
Anti-Epileptic Drugs (AED) Preferences

AED	Generalized	Absence	Partial seizure	Myoclonic
First-line	carbamazepine valproate phenytoin	valproate ethosuximide	carbamazepine valproate phenytoin	valproate
Alternatives	phenobarbital primidone felbamate gabapentin lamotrigine	clonazepam lamotrigine nitrazepam	phenobarbital, primidone, felbamate, gabapentin, lamotrigine, tiagabine, topiramate, clonazepam	clonazepam lamotrigine nitrazepam

Infantile spasms
- First-line: **ACTH/adrenocorticotropic hormone** 150 units/m^2/d IM div q 12 h x 2-11 wk, taper
- Alternatives: valproate, nitrazepam, vigabatrin, lamotrigine, topiramate, surgery, ketogenic diet

Anti-Epileptic Drug (AED) Profiles

AED	Dose range (mg/kg)	Therapeutic level (mcg/mL)	Side effects
carbamazepine (CBZ)	10-30	8-12	dizziness, diplopia, liver dysfunction, anemia, neutropenia, SIADH
clonazepam	< 30 kg: 0.05-0.2 > 30 kg: 1.5 MAX 20 mg	> 0.013	drowsiness, irritability, behavioral problems, depression, salivation
ethosuximide	20-40	40-100	liver dysfunction, rash, leukopenia
phenobarbital (PB)	3-5	15-40	hyperactivity, attention deficit, temper tantrums, impaired cognition, Stevens Johnson syndrome
phenytoin (PHT)	3-9	10-20	hirsutism, acne, gum hypertrophy, rash, Stevens Johnson, ataxia, blood dyscrasias
valproic acid (VPA)	10-30	50-100	vomiting, sedation, tremor, weight gain, hepatotoxicity, amenorrhea, marrow suppression

Refractory Seizures

Seizures that occur while the patient has an AED concentration, of at least 1 standard
medication appropriate for the seizure type, in the usual effective therapeutic range at the time,
within 1 year of the onset of epilepsy. Associated with Lennox Gastaut syndrome, symptomatic
epilepsy due to CNS structural malformations, mental or motor handicap, abnormal neurologic
exam, delay in start of treatment, interictal activity, slow background activity on EEG, seizures
of multiple types. 35% of complex partial and 20% of GTC seizures are refractory.

(E)
New Anti-Epileptic Drugs
Not considered first-line therapy, to be co-managed with a pediatric neurologist

AED	Indications	Mechanism	Dose (mg/kg)	Toxicity	Drug interactions
gabapentin (Neurontin®)	partial seizure	induces GABA synthesis, acts on Ca^{++} and Na^{++} channel, ↓'s monoamine release	30-90 in children > 12 y	behavioral changes, ataxia, tremor, ↑ weight	no interaction
lamotrigine	Lennox Gastaut, partial seizures, generalized, atonic, infantile spasms, juvenile myoclonic epilepsy (JME)	acts on voltage dependent sodium channel	1-15	rash (more with VPA), ataxia, diplopia, ↑ alertness and attention	T ½ ↓'d by CBZ, PHT, PB; synergistic with VPA
tiagabine	partial seizure	selective inhibition of GABA reuptake	0.1-1.5	headache, drowsiness, ataxia, tremor, poor attention	

✳ Continued on p. 187

✳ Continued from p.186

topiramate	partial seizure, infantile spasm, Lennox Gastaut	blocks voltage dependent sodium channel, GABA effect, glutamate receptor antagonist	1-10	drowsiness, speech difficulties, ↓weight, diplopia, psychomotor slowing, ataxia, paresthesias	PHT < CBZ < VPA decrease levels
vigabatrin	infantile spasms, associated with tuberous sclerosis, partial and generalized seizures, Lennox Gastaut	irreversible GABA transferase inhibitor	50-150	hyperactivity, ↑ weight, ataxia, optic atrophy, visual field constriction, drowsiness	levels of PHT, PB ↓

(F) Reduce seizure-provoking events: fever, sleep deprivation, metabolic derangement, drugs

(G) Ketogenic diet - useful in complex partial, myoclonic, atonic seizures, and Lennox Gastaut syndrome. Best result in 2-5 years. A high fat, low carbohydrate and protein diet raises plasma ketone levels, which potentiate GABA activity.

Vagal stimulation - in refractory partial seizures in children > 12 years old.

Surgical resection - anterior temporal resection and limited mesial temporal resection is 70% successful in controlling seizure activity. Extratemporal neocortex resection - 45% successful. Corpus callosum resection - palliative only.

Febrile Seizures

Girija Natarajan

A seizure accompanied by fever without CNS infection in infants and children between 6 months and 5 years of age. Seen in 2-5% of children. Risk of recurrence is 50% in children < 12 mos age and 30% in children > 12 mos age. Genetic predisposition noted.

Subsequent *risk of developing epilepsy* in simple febrile seizures is slightly higher than that of the general population. A higher risk is associated in those with complex febrile seizures, infants < 6 mos, family history of non-febrile seizures, and abnormal neurological development before the onset of seizures.

The *likelihood of meningitis* is higher in children with febrile seizures who had a focal seizure, signs such as rash, petechiae, cyanosis, hypotension, grunting respirations, meningeal signs, hyper/hypotonia, ataxia, bulging fontanelles, nystagmus, or an inability to track or respond to painful stimuli.

Clinical Manifestations

Simple febrile seizure	age 6 mos - 5 y, *and*
	⊕ fever, *and*
	generalized seizure < 15 min, *and*
	normal neurological examination, *and*
	no history of previous neurologic or CNS abnormality
Complex febrile seizure	focal seizure > 15 min, multiple episodes within 24 h
Symptomatic febrile seizure	known CNS malformations, neurodegenerative disease, or history of prior afebrile seizure

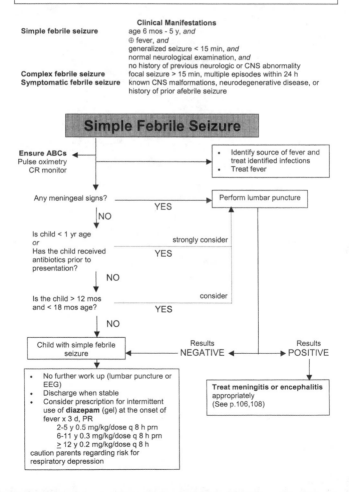

Simple Febrile Seizure

Ensure ABCs
Pulse oximetry
CR monitor

- Identify source of fever and treat identified infections
- Treat fever

Any meningeal signs? —— **YES** —→ Perform lumbar puncture

NO

Is child < 1 yr age
or
Has the child received antibiotics prior to presentation?

strongly consider **YES**

NO

Is the child > 12 mos and < 18 mos age?

consider **YES**

NO

Child with simple febrile seizure ←—— Results **NEGATIVE** ←—— Results **POSITIVE**

- No further work up (lumbar puncture or EEG)
- Discharge when stable
- Consider prescription for intermittent use of **diazepam** (gel) at the onset of fever x 3 d, PR
    2-5 y 0.5 mg/kg/dose q 8 h prn
    6-11 y 0.3 mg/kg/dose q 8 h prn
    ≥ 12 y 0.2 mg/kg/dose q 8 h
caution parents regarding risk for respiratory depression

Treat meningitis or encephalitis appropriately
(See p.106,108)

Clinical Manifestations

Perinatal history	maternal diabetes or PIH, fetal distress, hypoxia, birth injury, birth weight, type of formula (phosphate content),
GEN	any stereotypic movement or autonomic disturbance, blinking, chewing, bicycling
HEENT	abnormal facies, microcephaly, chorioretinitis
RESP	apnea
GI	vomiting, poor feeding
CNS	lethargy, hypotonia, bradycardia
SKIN	neurocutaneous stigmata

Diagnostics

Blood	ABG/CBG, glucose, electrolytes, BUN, creatinine, Ca^{++}, Mg^{++}, ammonia; consider amino acids, lactate, pyruvate, long chain fatty acid assay, serum level of local anesthetic if indicated, TORCH titers, cultures, karyotype
Urine	drug screen, organic acids, 2,4-dinitrophenylhydrazine
Imaging	head US/CT/MRI
Other	meconium drug screen, lumbar puncture (infection, hemorrhage, glycine, lactate), EEG (prolonged or repeated due to common clinical electrical dissociation)

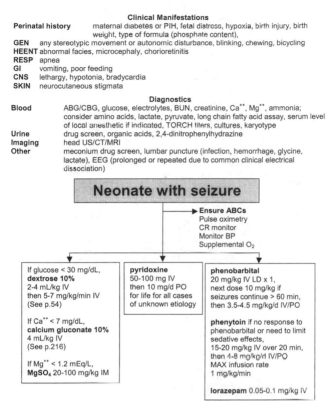

Neonate with seizure

→ **Ensure ABCs**
Pulse oximetry
CR monitor
Monitor BP
Supplemental O$_2$

If glucose < 30 mg/dL,
dextrose 10%
2-4 mL/kg IV
then 5-7 mg/kg/min IV
(See p.54)

If Ca^{++} < 7 mg/dL,
calcium gluconate 10%
4 mL/kg IV
(See p.216)

If Mg^{++} < 1.2 mEq/L,
MgSO$_4$ 20-100 mg/kg IM

pyridoxine
50-100 mg IV
then 10 mg/d PO
for life for all cases
of unknown etiology

phenobarbital
20 mg/kg IV LD x 1,
next dose 10 mg/kg if
seizures continue > 60 min,
then 3.5-4.5 mg/kg/d IV/PO

phenytoin if no response to
phenobarbital or need to limit
sedative effects,
15-20 mg/kg IV over 20 min,
then 4-8 mg/kg/d IV/PO
MAX infusion rate
1 mg/kg/min

lorazepam 0.05-0.1 mg/kg IV

Clinical Classification of Neonatal Seizures

Type	Presentation	EEG	Associated conditions	Prog
Focal	rhythmic jerking of face, trunk, limbs	unifocal, abnormal	metabolic causes, SAH, focal injury, infarct	good
Multifocal clonic	involves multiple muscle groups	multifocal, abnormal	neonatal or hypoxic ischemic encephalopathy (HIE)	poor
Tonic	generalized rigidity +/- eye deviation	burst suppression/low amplitude	prematurity, IVH, diffuse cerebral disease, drug withdrawal	poor
Myoclonic	involves distal muscles, rapid jerks	burst suppression or hypsarrhythmia	diffuse cerebral disease	poor
Subtle	buccal and oculomotor movements, pedaling, color change, autonomic dysfunction	normal	neonatal or hypoxic ischemic encephalopathy (HIE)	

Possible etiologies based on onset of clinical presentation

Day 1-2:	intracranial hemorrhage, HIE, ↓ glucose, ↓ Ca^{++}, injection of local anesthetic, cerebral dysgenesis
Day 3-7:	intracranial hemorrhage, inborn errors of metabolism, infections, drug withdrawal, epilepsy syndromes, dysgenesis
Day 7-10:	↓ Ca^{++}, infection, drug withdrawal

Etiologies based on incidence: hypoxic ischemic encephalopathy (35-42%), intracranial hemorrhage/infarction (15-20%), CNS infection (12-17%), CNS malformation (5%), metabolic (3-5%), other (5-20%).

Acute Hemiparesis

Cheryl Ackley Bagenstose

A sudden onset of ipsilateral weakness of the upper and lower extremities.

(A) Differential diagnosis of acute hemiparesis
- **cerebrovascular accident (CVA), ischemic/embolic/hemorrhagic**
- meningitis, encephalitis
- cerebral neoplasm
- post-ictal Todd paralysis
- insulin-dependent diabetes mellitus (associated with URI, headache, facial/arm involvement > legs)
- hypoglycemia
- subdural/epidural hemorrhage

- complicated migraine
- familial hemiplegic migraine
- hemiparetic seizures
- alternating hemiplegia of childhood
- OTC deficiency
- homocystinuria
- pyruvate dehydrogenase deficiency
- MELAS (*m*itochondrial encephalopathy, *l*actic *a*cidosis, *s*troke-like episodes)

(B) Imaging
Head CT without contrast - readily accessible, fast, may have normal findings in the first 12-24 h post-ischemic stroke
Contrast-enhanced CT - defines abscesses and tumors
Head MRI - less accessible, longer imaging time, usually requires sedation, may show infarct within 6 h of event, better visualization of brain parenchyma and ability to date intracranial hemorrhages, may fail to identify small aneurysms and other vascular abnormalities
Positron emission tomography (PET) and single photon emission computed tomography (SPECT) are not useful in acute diagnostic phase

(C) **Causes of ischemic/embolic CVA**
Vascular - moyamoya, fibromuscular dysplasia, dissecting aneurysm
Infectious - viral encephalitis, meningitis (bacterial, fungal, viral, TB - causing thrombophlebitis and arterial occlusion), retropharyngeal abscess, bacterial endocarditis, septic emboli, cerebral abscess, cavernous venous sinus thrombosis 2° to otitis/mastoiditis, retrograde orbital infection, cat-scratch disease or *Mycoplasma pneumoniae* (carotid artery arteritis adjacent to infected nodes)
Trauma to the head, neck (carotid artery injury). Birth trauma.
Drugs - cocaine, marijuana, glue sniffing, OCP, head/neck radiation therapy
Metabolic -diabetes, homocystinuria, Fabry disease, mitochondrial disorders, urea cycle defects, hyperlipidemia
Hematologic/oncologic - sickle cell disease, polycythemia, protein C or S deficiency, antithrombin III deficiency, antiphospholipid antibodies, DIC, leukemia, lymphoma
Cardiac - arrhythmia (most commonly atrial fibrillation), atrial myxoma, paradoxical emboli via PFO in cyanotic heart defects, post-cardiac surgery or catheterization, hyperlipidemia
Autoimmune - SLE, polyarteritis nodosum, Takayasu arteritis, vasculitides
Neurocutaneous - neurofibromatosis, Sturge-Weber syndrome, tuberous sclerosis
Other - severe dehydration, air emboli, fat emboli, pregnancy or post-partum, idiopathic (30% with negative work-ups)

(D) **Causes of hemorrhagic CVA**
Vascular - arteriovenous malformation, cerebral aneurysm
Hematologic - hemophilia, thrombocytopenia
Trauma - subdural/epidural hematoma

(A) Clinical Manifestations

SKIN   cyanosis, jaundice, petechiae, malar rash, café-au-lait, neurofibromas, hemangiomas
NECK   bruits, stiffness, swelling, ecchymosis
CVS   murmurs, clicks, ↑ BP, unequal pulses, assess hydration status
GI   nausea, vomiting
CNS   headache, seizures, ↓ level of consciousness, asymmetric UE/LE weakness, ataxia, altered gait, vertigo, asymmetric or decreased reflexes, CN palsies, intracranial bruits, hemianopsia, dysphasia, nystagmus, changes in vision, paresthesias

Diagnostics

Blood   CBC, differential, PT, PTT, BUN, creatinine, glucose, cholesterol, triglycerides, LFTs, toxicology screen, ESR, ANA. Consider: fibrinogen, serum amino acids, lactate, pyruvate, hemoglobin electrophoresis, protein C and S, antithrombin III, lupus anticoagulant, anticardiolipin antibody, C3, C4, rheumatoid factor, HIV, RPR/VDRL, cultures
Urine   urinalysis (RBC, protein). Consider: organic acids, homocystine levels, culture
Imaging   head CT, MRI/MRA, cerebral angiography (B)
Other   lumbar puncture, EKG, echocardiogram

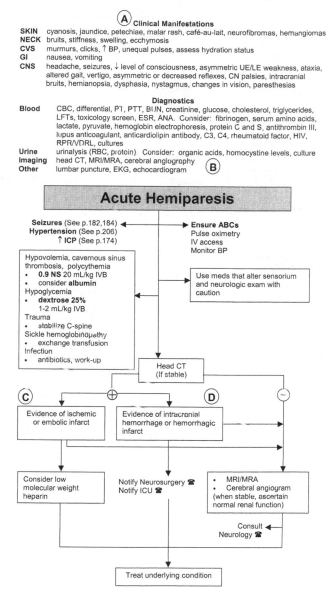

Acute Psychosis

Ina Shamraj

> A state of disorganized thought, involving delusions and/or hallucinations, and occasionally disorganized speech or behavior. Gross impairment in reality testing. May be classified as primary (functional) psychotic disorders and secondary (organic) psychosis.

(A) Mental status exam for patients with psychotic disorders should always include direct questions about types of hallucinations: "Do you hear things that other people don't hear?", delusions, and negative symptoms.

Must rule out secondary (organic) causes of psychosis first.

(B) Primary Psychotic Disorders	**(B)** Secondary (Organic) Psychosis	**(C)** Ingestions
Schizophrenia Schizophreniform disorder Schizoaffective disorder Delusional disorder Psychotic disorder NOS* Bipolar disorder Post-traumatic stress disorder Obsessive-compulsive disorder Autism Tourette's	Hypoxia Hepatic encephalopathy Uremia Adrenal dysfunction Hyperthyroidism Diabetic ketoacidosis Thiamine deficiency B12 deficiency Lupus Head trauma Intracranial mass Vasculitis Acute intermittent porphyria Meningitis/encephalitis Sepsis Multiple sclerosis	PCP Cocaine Peyote Amphetamines LSD Alcohol/delirium tremens Mushrooms Mescaline Heavy metals (lead) Iron Carbon monoxide Steroids Antipsychotics Sympathomimetics Antihistamines Anticholinergics Antibiotics Anticonvulsants Antidepressants Antihypertensives NSAIDS Theophylline

*NOS = Not otherwise specified

(D) **Haloperidol** administration
- Side effects: dry mouth, blurred vision, tachycardia, constipation.
- Postural hypotension → **IV fluids** or **vasopressors**.
- Acute dystonic reaction → **diphenhydramine** 1-2 mg/kg IV.
- Neuroleptic malignant syndrome → supportive care, monitor renal function.

(E) **Diphenhydramine** and **lorazepam** may be used as adjuncts, with awareness that they may cause paradoxical agitation.

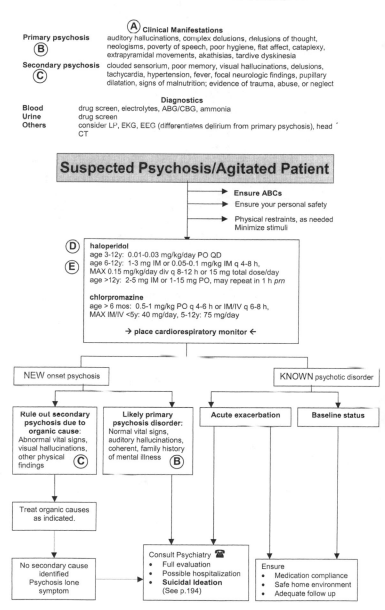

Ⓐ Clinical Manifestations

Primary psychosis
Ⓑ
auditory hallucinations, complex delusions, delusions of thought, neologisms, poverty of speech, poor hygiene, flat affect, cataplexy, extrapyramidal movements, akathisias, tardive dyskinesia

Secondary psychosis
Ⓒ
clouded sensorium, poor memory, visual hallucinations, delusions, tachycardia, hypertension, fever, focal neurologic findings, pupillary dilatation, signs of malnutrition; evidence of trauma, abuse, or neglect

Diagnostics

Blood   drug screen, electrolytes, ABG/CBG, ammonia
Urine   drug screen
Others   consider LP, EKG, EEG (differentiates delirium from primary psychosis), head CT

Suspected Psychosis/Agitated Patient

➤ **Ensure ABCs**
➤ Ensure your personal safety

➤ Physical restraints, as needed
  Minimize stimuli

Ⓓ **haloperidol**
Ⓔ age 3-12y: 0.01-0.03 mg/kg/day PO QD
age 6-12y: 1-3 mg IM or 0.05-0.1 mg/kg IM q 4-8 h,
MAX 0.15 mg/kg/day div q 8-12 h or 15 mg total dose/day
age >12y: 2-5 mg IM or 1-15 mg PO, may repeat in 1 h *prn*

chlorpromazine
age > 6 mos: 0.5-1 mg/kg PO q 4-6 h or IM/IV q 6-8 h,
MAX IM/IV <5y: 40 mg/day, 5-12y: 75 mg/day

→ place cardiorespiratory monitor ←

| NEW onset psychosis | | KNOWN psychotic disorder | |

Rule out secondary psychosis due to organic cause: Abnormal vital signs, visual hallucinations, other physical findings Ⓒ

Likely primary psychosis disorder: Normal vital signs, auditory hallucinations, coherent, family history of mental illness Ⓑ

Acute exacerbation

Baseline status

Treat organic causes as indicated.

No secondary cause identified
Psychosis lone symptom

Consult Psychiatry ☎
• Full evaluation
• Possible hospitalization
• **Suicidal Ideation**
(See p.194)

Ensure
• Medication compliance
• Safe home environment
• Adequate follow up

Suicide

Ina Shamraj

> Threat or attempt to end one's life. Even children who do not understand the finality
> of death can attempt or commit suicide.

(A) Take all threats of suicide seriously. In the United States, suicide is the fourth leading cause of
death in children ages 10-14 years and the third leading cause of death in children ages 15-19
years.

(B) More than 1/3 of suicide cases involve substance abuse. Even if trauma is the method of suicide,
always consider intoxication.

(C) Lethality of attempt: obtain a detailed description from the patient of reasons for the attempt,
plans and methods, availability of rescue.

(D) Treat associated conditions accordingly.
- 90% of successful adolescents who attempt or commit suicides have a **diagnosable
  psychiatric illness**, especially major depression, other mood disorder, schizophrenia, or
  substance abuse.
- **Medical conditions** associated with increased frequency of suicidal thoughts include
  pregnancy, cancer, diabetes, neurodegenerative disorders, facial injuries.

(E) *Risks for attempted suicide*: substance abuse, family suicide, problems/changes in the family,
problems at school, sexual abuse.

Risks for successful suicide: mood disorders, previous attempts, violent means, male sex.
Reassure your patient that thoughts of killing oneself in times of stress are not unusual.

Other risk factors: adolescent age, precipitating event, school failure, access to weapons,
planned attempt, impulsivity, feelings of hopelessness and helplessness, high parental stress.

(F) If seen in the Emergency Department, a patient needs evaluation by a mental health professional
and may need hospitalization.

If seen in clinic, a 'no-suicide' contract can be established with arrangements for psychiatric
follow-up within 1-2 days. The patient should have immediate access to telephone or other
support to diffuse potentially volatile situations. Note that only 50% of patients will comply with
follow up.

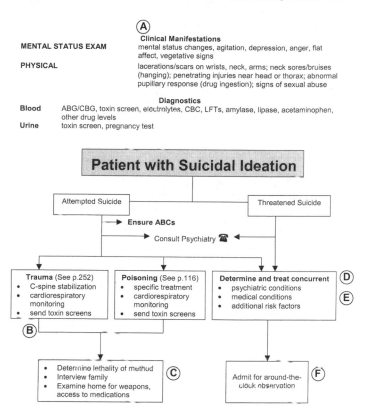

(A)

Clinical Manifestations

MENTAL STATUS EXAM mental status changes, agitation, depression, anger, flat affect, vegetative signs

PHYSICAL lacerations/scars on wrists, neck, arms; neck sores/bruises (hanging); penetrating injuries near head or thorax; abnormal pupillary response (drug ingestion); signs of sexual abuse

Diagnostics

Blood ABG/CBG, toxin screen, electrolytes, CBC, LFTs, amylase, lipase, acetaminophen, other drug levels

Urine toxin screen, pregnancy test

Patient with Suicidal Ideation

Attempted Suicide

Threatened Suicide

→ **Ensure ABCs**

→ Consult Psychiatry ☎ ◄

Trauma (See p.252)
- C-spine stabilization
- cardiorespiratory monitoring
- send toxin screens

(B)

Poisoning (See p.116)
- specific treatment
- cardiorespiratory monitoring
- send toxin screens

Determine and treat concurrent
- psychiatric conditions
- medical conditions
- additional risk factors

(D)

(E)

- Determine lethality of method
- Interview family
- Examine home for weapons, access to medications

(C)

Admit for around-the-clock observation

(F)

Chapter 11 ♣ Ophthalmologic Emergencies

Aditi Sharangpani

(A)

Clinical Symptom	Suspected Disease Process
acute unilateral vision loss, transient	TIA involving retina (consider central retinal artery occlusion if lasting), migraine, optic neuritis
acute bilateral vision loss	TIA involving occipital brain
floaters	vitreous opacities, retinal detachment
flashing lights	migraine, retinal detachment
"curtain" drawn down	TIA, retinal detachment
diplopia	CN palsy or extraocular muscle weakness
halos around lights	glaucoma (from corneal edema), cataracts
pruritis	allergic conjunctivitis
acute onset superficial pain	trauma, foreign body or secondary corneal abrasion
burning	conjunctivitis, corneal irritation, dry eye, allergy
deep intense pain	uveitis, glaucoma, optic neuritis, referred vascular pain (migraine, aneurysm), sinusitis, associated ↑IOP
pain upon pressing globe	Lid/orbital inflammation, scleritis/episcleritis, uveitis, glaucoma
photophobia	conjunctivitis, keratitis, uveitis, migraine

Clinical Sign	Suspected Disease Process
CN III, IV, VI palsies	↑ intracranial pressure, meningitis, trauma
impaired extraocular muscle (EOM) movement	orbital cellulitis, orbital fracture + trapped EOM
ptosis, ophthalmoplegia	myasthenia gravis
anisocoria	CN III palsy pre-herniation, Aide's tonic pupil (benign), note: normal variant in 25%
absent pupillary reaction to light	abnormality of the retina or optic nerve
pupillary irregularity	prolapsed iris, ruptured globe
Marcus-Gunn/afferent pupillary defect (APD): dilation of contralateral pupil upon light stimulation of the injured eye	visual defect
iridodonesis: "trembling of the iris"	lens dislocation
subcutaneous emphysema, crepitis	nasal or facial bone fracture
↓/↑ sensation of infraorbital nerve distribution	orbital floor fracture
blepharospasm	glaucoma, corneal inflammation, blepharitis

Fluorescein Staining

Preferentially use fluorescein-impregnated sterile strips. Solutions often become contaminated with Pseudomonas. Instill drops of anesthetic. Drip sterile saline along paper strip into inner canthus or conjunctiva. Direct Wood's lamp or fluorescent light to detect staining due to foreign body (or entry point for foreign body into the globe), corneal abrasion, or diffuse staining due to viral infections. Seidel test: non-stained 'streaming' seen with globe content leakage, considered positive.

Topical antibiotics: administer QID

gentamicin 0.3% oint, drops	**tobramycin** 0.3% oint, drops	**erythromycin** 0.5% oint
sulfacetamide 10% oint, drops	**ciprofloxacin** 0.35% drops	**bacitracin** oint

Cycloplegic agents to ↓ ciliary spasm and minimize posterior synechiae formation

cyclopentolate 0.5, 1.0% drops	1 drop TID (mydriasis 1-2d)
tropicamide 0.5, 1.0% drops	1 drop (mydriasis 6h)
atropine 0.5, 1.0%	1-2 drops qD-TID

Agents reducing intraocular pressure

carbonic anhydrase inhibitor	**acetazolamide** 20-40 mg/kg/d IV div. q6h *or* 8-30 mg/kg/d PO div. q6-8h, MAX 1 g/d
β-blockers	**timolol** 0.25-0.5% 1 drop BID; **betaxolol** 0.5% 1 drop BID
hyperosmotic drugs	**mannitol** 0.5-1.0 g/kg IV; **glycerol** 1-1.8 g/kg PO
cholinergic drugs	**pilocarpine** 2% 1 drop up to 6X/d, adjust as needed for IOP

Topical anesthetic: **proparacaine** 0.5% 1 drop
Use of ophthalmologic steroid drops should <u>only</u> be used on consultation with Ophthalmology.

(B) Corneal burns
S/S: severe pain, tearing, photophobia, foreign-body sensation, conjunctival injection, corneal edema or opacification, ↓visual acuity
Alkali chemical injuries are more severe than acid ones, because alkali are highly lipid-soluble, penetrating the cornea more rapidly. Acids coagulate proteins of the corneal epithelium, producing a barrier to deep penetration (exception: hydrofluoric acid).

(C) Globe rupture
S/S: Marked ↓visual acuity, abnormally deep anterior chamber, limited EOM, may be associated with hyphema, full thickness scleral or corneal laceration, irregular pupil, subluxed lens.

(D) Hyphema
S/S: photophobia, blurred or ↓visual acuity, ocular pain, blood in the anterior chamber.
Due to ruptured blood vessels of the iris or ciliary body into the anterior chamber; either traumatic (71-94% blunt), surgical, or spontaneous causes, including tumors, blood dyscrasias, vascular

✱ (Continued on p.198)

Clinical Manifestations

GEN fever, associated HEENT infections (sinusitis, dental abscess), history of blunt or projectile trauma (include "forbidden activities", i.e., BB guns, fireworks)

PMH prior eye injury; medications, contact lenses; intrauterine drug exposure/infection, prematurity, sickle cell disease, diabetes, malignancy, hypertension, migraines

See Associated Ophthalmologic Signs/Symptoms on p.196. 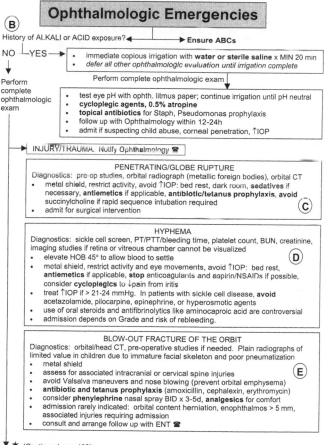(A)

Complete Ophthalmologic Exam

- Visual acuity by levels: by chart per age (fix/follow for > 6 wk olds, Allen pic card for > 2 yo, E chart for > 4 yo, Snellen chart for > 5-6 yo) → by ability to count fingers → by recognition of faces (parents) → to hand movements → to light
- External inspection: globe (size, position), pupils (size, equality, light reflex), lids (edema, lacrimal duct, undersurface for foreign bodies), palpate orbital rims (for tumor, step off or crepitus in fracture), conjunctiva, facial asymmetry, ecchymosis, excessive tearing
- Slit lamp exam: conjunctiva and cornea (abrasions, foreign bodies), anterior chamber (particulate matter, uveitis, foreign bodies, hyphema or blood, hypopyon or pus)
- Tonometry (IOP measurement): **defer** if suspecting infection, globe rupture or laceration
- Funduscopic exam: for retinal hemorrhages, papilledema
- Visual fields: if defect respects the meridian, it is at the level of the chiasm, tract, or brain
- Fluorescein staining: for corneal defects

Diagnostics: Consideration given below as per suspected diagnosis.

Ophthalmologic Emergencies

(B) History of ALKALI or ACID exposure? ◄──────────► **Ensure ABCs**

NO └─YES──►

- immediate copious irrigation with **water or sterile saline** x MIN 20 min
- *defer all other ophthalmologic evaluation until irrigation complete*

↓

Perform complete ophthalmologic exam

Perform complete ophthalmologic exam

- test eye pH with ophth. litmus paper; continue irrigation until pH neutral
- **cycloplegic agents, 0.5% atropine**
- **topical antibiotics** for Staph, Pseudomonas prophylaxis
- follow up with Ophthalmology within 12-24h
- admit if suspecting child abuse, corneal penetration, ↑IOP

────► INJURY/TRAUMA. Notify Ophthalmology ☎

PENETRATING/GLOBE RUPTURE

Diagnostics: pre-op studies, orbital radiograph (metallic foreign bodies), orbital CT

- metal shield, restrict activity, avoid ↑IOP: bed rest, dark room, **sedatives** if necessary, **antiemetics** if applicable, **antibiotic/tetanus prophylaxis, avoid succinylcholine** if rapid sequence intubation required (C)
- admit for surgical intervention

HYPHEMA

Diagnostics: sickle cell screen, PT/PTT/bleeding time, platelet count, BUN, creatinine, imaging studies if retina or vitreous chamber cannot be visualized

- elevate HOB 45° to allow blood to settle (D)
- metal shield, restrict activity and eye movements, avoid ↑IOP: bed rest, **antiemetics** if applicable, **stop** anticoagulants and aspirin/NSAIDs if possible, consider **cycloplegics** to ↓pain from iritis
- treat ↑IOP if > 21-24 mmHg. In patients with sickle cell disease, **avoid** acetazolamide, pilocarpine, epinephrine, or hyperosmotic agents
- use of oral steroids and antifibrinolytics like aminocaproic acid are controversial
- admission depends on Grade and risk of rebleeding.

BLOW-OUT FRACTURE OF THE ORBIT

Diagnostics: orbital/head CT, pre-operative studies if needed. Plain radiographs of limited value in children due to immature facial skeleton and poor pneumatization

- metal shield
- assess for associated intracranial or cervical spine injuries (E)
- avoid Valsalva maneuvers and nose blowing (prevent orbital emphysema)
- **antibiotic and tetanus prophylaxis** (amoxicillin, cephalexin, erythromycin)
- consider **phenylephrine** nasal spray BID x 3-5d, **analgesics** for comfort
- admission rarely indicated: orbital content herniation, enophthalmos > 5 mm, associated injuries requiring admission
- consult and arrange follow up with ENT ☎

▼ ✱ (Continued on p.199)

✱ (Continued from p.196)

anomalies, drugs (aspirin, anticoagulants). Grade I: < 1/3 anterior chamber, 25% rebleed; II: 1/3-½ anterior chamber; III: > ½ anterior chamber, 67% rebleed; IV: total ("eight ball hyphema")
Complications: rebleed, ↑IOP leading to glaucoma, corneal blood staining, synechiae.

(E) Blow-out fracture of the orbit (orbital floor, medial wall - weakest structural points)
S/S: diplopia upon ↑/↓ gaze due to trapped inferior rectus or oblique muscles, ↓/↑ sensation over inferior nerve distribution (medial 1/3 lower lid, maxilla, upper gingiva), enophthalmos (herniation of orbital fat through fracture), crepitus, ecchymosis, epistaxis, normal acuity.
Less likely in children < 7 yo due to lack of pneumatization. Orbital roof fractures with associated CNS injuries are more common in children.
Disposition: 85% resolve without surgical intervention; indications include persistent diplopia, restricted EOM, enophthalmos > 5 mm. Late complications include sinusitis, orbital infection.

(F) Corneal abrasions, foreign bodies
S/S: severe pain, photophobia, conjunctival/scleral injection, tearing, blurred vision, foreign body sensation, headache, blepharospasm.
Assess with fluorescein staining and lid eversion. Contact lenses cause bilateral defects.
Vertical abrasions suggest foreign body beneath lid. Can have intraocular foreign body without apparent ocular damage. Corneal uptake in dendritic pattern suggestive of HSV keratitis.

Others: Lens dislocation - blurred vision, pain, ↑IOP, cloudy cornea, iridodonesis, "floating shadow". Transient cortical blindness due to blunt head trauma. Lid laceration - repair by ophthalmologist if involves avulsion, lid margin, or canalicular apparatus.

(G) Orbital/Septal Cellulitis
S/S: painful/indurated superficial + deep orbital tissue involvement, fever 75%, unilateral 95%, proptosis, impaired visual acuity, afferent pupillary defect, restricted painful EOM
2° to extension from adjacent structures: periorbital cellulitis, sinusitis, dental abscess, retained orbital foreign body, orbital fracture. Most commonly *S. pneumonia, S. aureus, S. pyogenes, H. influenzae* type B in unimmunized children (violaceous hue)
Complications: ophthalmoplegia, periosteal or brain abscess, meningitis, septic cavernous sinus thrombosis, optic neuritis, septicemia

(H) Periorbital/Preseptal Cellulitis
S/S: no evidence of orbital involvement, i.e., no proptosis, normal visual acuity, EOMI.
Preceding URI, fever if bacteremic, otherwise due to trauma, bites, allergies, tumor. Unilateral.

(I) Conjunctivitis
S/S: red eye, discharge, sticky eyelids, chemosis, normal visual acuity, normal anterior chamber and IOP, foreign body sensation, pruritis if allergic
Ophthalmia neonatorum by age: at 6-12h, due to silver nitrate drops, resolves; at 2-5d with mucopurulent discharge due to *N. gonorrhoeae*; at 5-14d, consider *C. trachomatis*. Beyond neonatal period, due to adenovirus, Staph, Strep, *H. influenza* nontypable (conjunctivitis-otitis syndrome may need PO antibiotics)

(J) Endophthalmitis: hypopyon or pus (WBC cells) seen in anterior chamber, plus infected vitreous.

(K) Central retinal artery occlusion (CRAO)
S/S: sudden painless monocular loss of vision, "count fingers" or "light perception" acuity in 90%, partial field defects, APD. In affected retina: edema within 20 min, unilateral diffuse pallor, empty or dark red stationary "boxcaring" rouleaux within arteries, cherry-red fovea, pale optic disc.
Due to emboli (hypertension, valvular disease, diabetes, vasculitis), thrombosis (SLE, sickle cell).

(L) Vitreous hemorrhage
S/S: sudden painless loss of vision, dark spots or floaters in visual axis, loss of red light reflex, inability to visual the fundus, mild afferent pupillary defect.
2° diagnosis requiring identification of specific cause for treatment. Etiologies include tearing of blood vessels due to trauma or spontaneous bleed due to neovascularization; associated diseases include proliferative retinopathy, diabetes mellitus, sickle cell disease, retinal telangiectasia, SAH/SDH, leukemia or intraocular tumors.

(M) Retinal detachment (RD): most commonly due to trauma in children
S/S: "curtain" or shadow over visual field, floaters, flashes of light, peripheral or central vision loss, normal visual acuity, may be asymptomatic or delayed in presentation
Due to retinal breaks (structural, developmental, trauma), vitreous bands (diabetes, vasculopathy, perforating injury, severe chorioretinitis, ROP, sickle cell, toxocariasis), or abnormal retinal fluid collections (choroid tumors, retinoblastoma, inflammatory disorders).

(N) Acute closed-angle glaucoma
S/S: tearing, photophobia, blepharospasm, irritability 2° to corneal edema/irritation. Cornea hazy, enlarged due to elasticity in children, Haab's striae (breaks in Descemet's membrane → linear ridging). Buphthalmos or "ox eye". ↓Acuity, nausea, vomiting, mid-dilated pupils.
Consider developmental glaucoma (1:10,000 live births) in an irritable photophobic child or when "big eyes" are noted. Children may require sedation or general anesthesia for proper exam.

✱ (Continued from p.197)

CORNEAL ABRASIONS, FOREIGN BODIES

Diagnostics: when suspecting penetrating intraocular foreign body, consider orbital radiographs (high-velocity injury) or ocular CT/MRI/US (nonmetallic).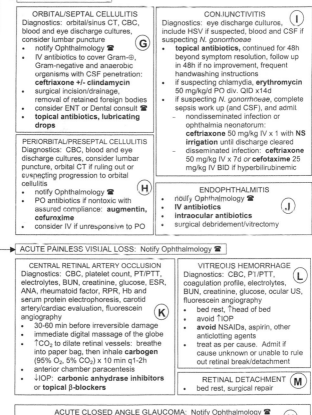

- perform **fluorescein** staining
- remove superficial (nonembedded) foreign bodies by: irrigate with **0.9NS** at oblique angle, *or* moist cotton tipped applicator, *or* 25-gauge needle with slitlamp
- **antibiotic prophylaxis,** cover Pseudomonas in contact lens wearers
- **tetanus prophylaxis,** if contaminants include dirt, fecal material, or saliva
- patching is controversial, poorly tolerated in children. Contraindications: contact lens-related injuries, infection-prone injuries (fingernail, vegetable matter, wood).
- analgesics, discontinue contact lenses use.
- follow up in 24-48h with Ophthalmologist

EYE INFECTIONS

ORBITAL/SEPTAL CELLULITIS

Diagnostics: orbital/sinus CT, CBC, blood and eye discharge cultures, consider lumbar puncture

- notify Ophthalmology ☎
- IV antibiotics to cover Gram-⊕, Gram-negative and anaerobic organisms with CSF penetration: **ceftriaxone +/- clindamycin**
- surgical incision/drainage, removal of retained foreign bodies
- consider ENT or Dental consult ☎
- **topical antibiotics, lubricating drops**

PERIORBITAL/PRESEPTAL CELLULITIS

Diagnostics: CBC, blood and eye discharge cultures, consider lumbar puncture, orbital CT if ruling out or suspecting progression to orbital cellulitis

- notify Ophthalmology ☎
- PO antibiotics if nontoxic with assured compliance: **augmentin, cefuroxime**
- consider IV if unresponsive to PO

CONJUNCTIVITIS

Diagnostics: eye discharge cultures, include HSV if suspected, blood and CSF if suspecting *N. gonorrhoeae*

- **topical antibiotics,** continued for 48h beyond symptom resolution, follow up in 48h if no improvement, frequent handwashing instructions
- if suspecting chlamydia, **erythromycin** 50 mg/kg/d PO div. QID x14d
- if suspecting *N. gonorrhoeae,* complete sepsis work up (and CSF), and admit
  - nondisseminated infection or ophthalmia neonatorum: **ceftriaxone** 50 mg/kg IV x 1 with **NS irrigation** until discharge cleared
  - disseminated infection: **ceftriaxone** 50 mg/kg IV x 7d *or* **cefotaxime** 25 mg/kg IV BID if hyperbilirubinemic

ENDOPHTHALMITIS

- notify Ophthalmology ☎
- **IV antibiotics**
- **intraocular antibiotics**
- surgical debridement/vitrectomy

ACUTE PAINLESS VISUAL LOSS: Notify Ophthalmology ☎

CENTRAL RETINAL ARTERY OCCLUSION

Diagnostics: CBC, platelet count, PT/PTT, electrolytes, BUN, creatinine, glucose, ESR, ANA, rheumatoid factor, RPR, Hb and serum protein electrophoresis, carotid artery/cardiac evaluation, fluorescein angiography

- 30-60 min before irreversible damage
- immediate digital massage of the globe
- ↑CO_2 to dilate retinal vessels: breathe into paper bag, then inhale **carbogen** (95% O_2, 5% CO_2) x 10 min q1-2h
- anterior chamber paracentesis
- ↓IOP: **carbonic anhydrase inhibitors** or **topical β-blockers**

VITREOUS HEMORRHAGE

Diagnostics: CBC, PT/PTT, coagulation profile, electrolytes, BUN, creatinine, glucose, ocular US, fluorescein angiography

- bed rest, ↑head of bed
- avoid ↑IOP
- **avoid** NSAIDs, aspirin, other anticlotting agents
- treat as per cause. Admit if cause unknown or unable to rule out retinal break/detachment

RETINAL DETACHMENT

- bed rest, surgical repair

ACUTE CLOSED ANGLE GLAUCOMA: Notify Ophthalmology ☎

Diagnostics: tonometry IOP > 20mmHg suspicious (normal 10-20mmHg).

- ↓aqueous humor production:
  carbonic anhydrase inhibitor, acetazolamide 20-40 mg/kg/d IV div. q6h or 8-30 mg/kg/d PO div. q6-8h, MAX 1 g/d (contraindicated in sickle cell disease)
  β-blocker, timolol 0.25-0.5% 1 drop BID or **betaxolol** 0.5% 1 drop BID
- ↓intraocular volume: **mannitol** 0.5-1 g/kg IV or **glycerol** 1-1.8 g/kg PO
- ↓pupil size: **cholinergic agent, pilocarpine** 2% 1 drop q15min x 5 then 1 drop q2-3h in affected eye, 1 drop q6h in unaffected eye
- move lens posteriorly: by supine positioning

Chapter 12 ♠ Renal, Fluids, and Electrolytes

Acute Renal Failure
Amit Sarnaik

Acute renal failure is the sudden reduction or cessation of renal function to the point where body fluid homeostasis is compromised, leading to accumulation of nitrogenous waste products, with or without reduction of urine output.

Etiology

	Type	Mechanism	Clinical Situations
(A)	Prerenal	Hypovolemia	Severe dehydration, excessive GI losses, burns, acute blood loss, adrenal insufficiency
		Hypotension/ ↓ cardiac output	Sepsis, myocardial failure, third spacing, anaphylaxis, ischemia
		Glomerulonephritis	Post-infectious, lupus, Henoch-Schönlein purpura
	Renal	Acute tubular necrosis	Shock, drugs, heavy metals, hemoglobinuria, myoglobinuria, hypoxia, ischemia, post-renal transplant
		Renovascular coagulation and thrombosis	Hemolytic uremic syndrome (most common cause of acute renal failure in children), renal vein thrombosis, TTP, DIC
		Acute interstitial nephritis	Drugs, infections
		Anatomic abnormalities	Renal polycystic disease, hypoplasia, agenesis
		Tumors and tumor-related therapy	Infiltration by malignancy, tumor lysis syndrome, bilateral nephrectomy for tumor removal
		Immunologic	Renal transplant rejection
	Post-renal	Obstruction	Ureteropelvic junction (most common), posterior urethral valves, ureterocele, calculi, tumor
		Vesicoureteral reflux	Multicystic kidney disease, bladder abnormalities

(B)

Partial list of exogenous nephrotoxic agents			
acetaminophen	captopril	heavy metals	prednisone
acyclovir	carbamazepine	methanol	rifampin
aminoglycoside	carbon monoxide	NSAIDs	sulfonamides
amoxicillin	cocaine	opioids	tetracycline
amphotericin B	ethylene glycol	penicillin	vancomycin
ascorbic acid	furosemide	phosphates	radiographic contrast

(C) Replace fluid losses/restore fluid volume **despite** anuric phase. If the only cause of anuria or oliguria is fluid depletion, fluid resuscitation should restore urine flow within 6 hours or less. Always assess for ongoing losses if acute renal failure persists in spite of adequate volume expansion. Consider CVP monitoring to more accurately reflect intravascular volume status.

(D)

Causes of post-renal oliguria: obstruction
Urethral: posterior urethral valves, phimosis, strictures
Bladder: neurogenic, clots, malignancies, calculi
Ureteral: *intrinsic* – clot, calculi, stenosis, hydronephrosis
            extrinsic – malignancy, ligation, radiation therapy

(E) The goal of therapy is to maintain a stable serum sodium and a decrease in total body weight by 0.5-1% per day

(F) Myoglobinuria may be seen following rhabdomyolysis or crush injuries. Urinalysis is usually *positive* by reagent strips for blood (myoglobin), but *negative* for RBC microscopically. Administer **mannitol** 0.25 g/kg IV q 6h, alkalinize urine with **NaHCO$_3$** IV, and ensure adequate hydration and urine output (> 2 mL/kg/h)

(G) Consider oral phosphate binders or Ca^{++} supplements. **CaCO$_3$** 25 mEq elemental Ca^{++}/kg PO q 6 h

(H) Administer **NaHCO$_3$** 1 mEq/kg IV over 1 h, correcting remaining deficit over 8-24 h
NaHCO$_3$ tablet 650 mg = 8 mEq HCO$_3$

Clinical Manifestations

HISTORY	preceding throat infection, gastroenteritis, exposure to drugs or toxins
GEN	pallor, edema, weakness, fatigue
SKIN	rash, petechiae, purpura
CVS	hypertension, congestive heart failure, signs of pericarditis
RESP	tachypnea, cough, hemoptysis, rales
GI	nausea, vomiting, anorexia, bleeding, flank mass, ascites
CNS	headache, seizures, confusion, lethargy, coma

Diagnostics

Blood	ABG/CBG, CBC, differential, peripheral smear, BUN, creatinine, electrolytes, osmolality, Ca^{++}, Mg^{++}, P, glucose, uric acid, alkaline phosphatase
Urine	urinalysis, UUN, creatinine, electrolytes, osmolality, specific gravity, hemoglobin and myoglobin if indicated
Imaging	chest radiograph, abdominal radiograph, abdominal and renal ultrasound with doppler, radionuclide scan
Others	Consider C3, C4, ANA, ASO titers, hepatitis profile, ANCA

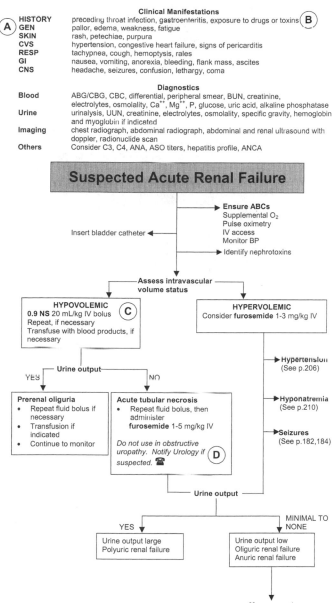

Suspected Acute Renal Failure

Ensure ABCs
Supplemental O_2
Pulse oximetry
IV access
Monitor BP

Insert bladder catheter

Identify nephrotoxins

Assess intravascular volume status

HYPOVOLEMIC (C)
0.9 NS 20 mL/kg IV bolus
Repeat, if necessary
Transfuse with blood products, if necessary

HYPERVOLEMIC
Consider **furosemide** 1-3 mg/kg IV

Urine output

YES — NO

Prenal oliguria
- Repeat fluid bolus if necessary
- Transfusion if indicated
- Continue to monitor

Acute tubular necrosis
- Repeat fluid bolus, then administer **furosemide** 1-5 mg/kg IV

Do not use in obstructive uropathy. Notify Urology if suspected. ☎ (D)

Hypertension
(See p.206)

Hyponatremia
(See p.210)

Seizures
(See p.182,184)

Urine output

YES

MINIMAL TO NONE

Urine output large
Polyuric renal failure

Urine output low
Oliguric renal failure
Anuric renal failure

Management
*Continued on p.203

NOTES

✳ Continued from p.201

Management of Acute Renal Failure

Monitor lab values
q 4-6 h

☎ Notify Nephrology
Monitor central venous
pressure and BP

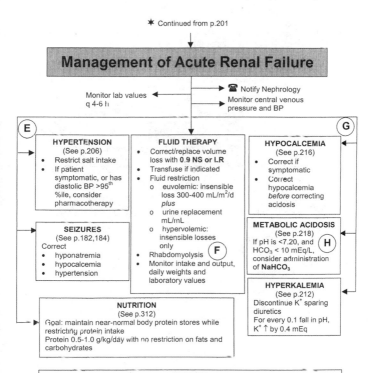

E

HYPERTENSION
(See p.206)
- Restrict salt intake
- If patient symptomatic, or has diastolic BP >95th %ile, consider pharmacotherapy

SEIZURES
(See p.182,184)
Correct
- hyponatremia
- hypocalcemia
- hypertension

FLUID THERAPY
- Correct/replace volume loss with **0.9 NS or LR**
- Transfuse if indicated
- Fluid restriction
  - euvolemic: insensible loss 300-400 mL/m²/d *plus*
  - urine replacement mL/mL
  - hypervolemic: insensible losses only
- Rhabdomyolysis **F**
- Monitor intake and output, daily weights and laboratory values

NUTRITION
(See p.312)
Goal: maintain near-normal body protein stores while restricting protein intake
Protein 0.5-1.0 g/kg/day with no restriction on fats and carbohydrates

G

HYPOCALCEMIA
(See p.216)
- Correct if symptomatic
- Correct hypocalcemia *before* correcting acidosis

METABOLIC ACIDOSIS
(See p.218)
If pH is <7.20, and HCO₃ < 10 mEq/L, consider administration of **NaHCO₃** **H**

HYPERKALEMIA
(See p.212)
Discontinue K⁺ sparing diuretics
For every 0.1 fall in pH, K⁺ ↑ by 0.4 mEq

DIALYSIS
Venous access (See p.268,282)
Early initiation has significantly improved the survival of children with acute renal failure
Indications
- Fluid overload not amenable to pharmacologic therapy leading to severe hypertension, congestive heart failure, pulmonary edema
- Severe metabolic acidosis
- Hyperkalemia > 6.5 mEq/L not responsive to pharmacologic measures
- Severe azotemia: BUN > 100-120 mg/dL and rising, or at lower levels but rising very quickly
- Symptomatic uremia: encephalopathy, pericarditis, GI bleeding
- Persistent hypocalcemia and secondary seizures

Hemolytic Uremic Syndrome
Hrishikesh Dingankar

A triad of acute microangiopathic hemolytic anemia, thrombocytopenia and impaired renal function. The most common cause of acute renal failure in children.

Etiology:

1.   Typical or classic form: caused by verocytotoxin producing organisms like *E. coli* (especially O157:H7), and *Shigella dysenteriae*. After ingestion of contaminated food, about 40% of individuals will develop bloody diarrhea within 24 hours; of those, 2-4% will develop hemolytic uremic syndrome (HUS). Other etiologic factors include viral infections, oral contraceptives, and cyclosporine A.
2.   Atypical or non-classic form: rarely, HUS may be familial (variable inheritance) or recurrent.

(A) Clinical features:

1.   90% of cases occur in children less than 5 y. Typically preceded by bloody or non-bloody diarrhea.
2.   Diarrhea → hemolysis in 5-7 days → renal insufficiency in 3-5 days with oliguria, fluid overload, and hypertension (seen in 50% of children).
3.   Platelet count of <100,000/mm^3 in 50% of patients at time of presentation.
4.   Neurologic involvement (most frequently seizures) is evident in 20-30% of children.
5.   Abdominal pain, elevation of liver enzymes.

(B) Investigations:

1.   CBC with differential and peripheral smear:
     *   Anemia: intravascular hemolysis (schistocytes, ↑ reticulocyte count, ↑ LDH, ↓ haptoglobin, negative Coomb's test, negative osmotic fragility test)
     *   Thrombocytopenia: median platelet count of 50,000/mm^3
     *   Leucocytosis: > 20,000/mm^3 indicates severe disease and poor prognosis
2.   Renal function: ↑ BUN and creatinine, proteinuria and microscopic hematuria with cellular casts
3.   Hypoalbuminemia resulting from capillary leak secondary to endothelial damage.
4.   Coagulopathy: PT, aPTT, D-dimers, and FSP are rarely abnormal
5.   Bacteriology: *E. coli* is usually only present in the stools for a few days, therefore, *E. coli* O157:H7 is more likely to be detected if IgM and IgG antibodies are tested for in addition to stool cultures.

(C) Differential diagnosis includes DIC, thrombotic thrombocytopenic purpura (TTP), vasculitides, and cavernous hemangiomas. TTP is more common in adults, and neurological symptoms are more pronounced.

(D) **Synsorb-Pk®**: developed from Chromosorb, a silicon dioxide covalently coupled to synthetic Pk receptors. Verotoxin has high affinity to Synsorb-Pk®. Synsorb-Pk® given within 4 days of the onset of diarrhea due to verotoxin-producing *E. coli* has been shown to decrease the risk of developing HUS by 54%. Further trials are in progress. Early use of Synsorb-Pk® is limited by the current lack of a rapid diagnostic test to diagnose an infection with verotoxin-producing *E. coli*.

Treatment methods found to be ineffective in HUS: heparin, fibrinolytics, anti-platelet agents, FFP, plasmapheresis and IVIG.

Prognosis

Classic form:

*   Mortality is 3-5%,
*   Residual and persistent renal changes in 3-5%
     o   chronic renal failure
     o   persistent hematuria/proteinuria, and hypertension
*   90% recover completely

Non-classic form: higher incidence of residual and persistent changes.

Clinical Manifestations

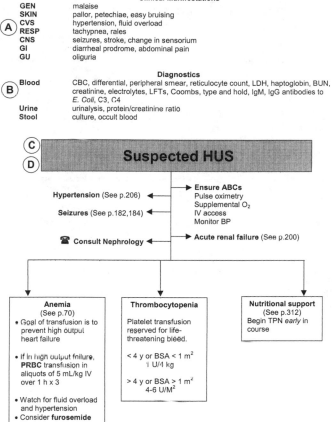

	GEN	malaise
	SKIN	pallor, petechiae, easy bruising
A	CVS	hypertension, fluid overload
	RESP	tachypnea, rales
	CNS	seizures, stroke, change in sensorium
	GI	diarrheal prodrome, abdominal pain
	GU	oliguria

Diagnostics

B	Blood	CBC, differential, peripheral smear, reticulocyte count, LDH, haptoglobin, BUN, creatinine, electrolytes, LFTs, Coombs, type and hold, IgM, IgG antibodies to *E. Coli*, C3, C4
	Urine	urinalysis, protein/creatinine ratio
	Stool	culture, occult blood

C
D
Suspected HUS

Hypertension (See p.206) ◄———

Seizures (See p.182,184) ◄———

———► **Ensure ABCs**
Pulse oximetry
Supplemental O_2
IV access
Monitor BP

☎ **Consult Nephrology** ◄——— ———► **Acute renal failure** (See p.200)

Anemia
(See p.70)
- Goal of transfusion is to prevent high output heart failure

- If in high output failure, **PRBC** transfusion in aliquots of 5 mL/kg IV over 1 h x 3

- Watch for fluid overload and hypertension
- Consider **furosemide**

Thrombocytopenia

Platelet transfusion reserved for life-threatening bleed.

< 4 y or BSA < 1 m^2
1 U/4 kg

> 4 y or BSA > 1 m^2
4-6 U/M^2

Nutritional support
(See p.312)
Begin TPN *early* in course

Hypertensive Crisis, Encephalopathy

K. Jane Lee

> Hypertensive crisis includes hypertensive emergency and hypertensive urgency.
>
> **Hypertensive emergency** - markedly increased blood pressure associated with hypertension-related end organ damage, most often affecting CNS (CVA, seizures, encephalopathy), the cardiovascular system (CHF, MI, aortic dissection), and the kidneys (acute renal insufficiency).
>
> **Hypertensive urgency** - markedly increased blood pressure without end organ damage.
>
> **Hypertensive encephalopathy** is seen when the systemic blood pressure exceeds the limits of cerebral blood flow autoregulation, resulting in vasodilatation, breakdown of the blood-brain barrier, and cerebral edema and ischemia.

(A) Diagnostic evaluation should include history of:
- Prescription, over the counter, and illicit drug use
- Use of umbilical catheters in the neonatal period
- Symptoms of weight loss, FTT, pallor, flushing, sweating, palpitations (neuroblastoma, pheochromocytoma)
- Family history of cardiovascular disease, renal disease, and tumors

Additional clinical manifestations suggestive of etiology include: thyromegaly, abdominal bruits or masses, periorbital or sacral edema, findings consistent with Cushing, Turners, and Williams syndrome.

Consider the following additional laboratory studies: renin, aldosterone, C3, C4, ASO titers, T4, TSH, ESR, ANA, cortisol, abdominal ultrasound, echocardiogram, renal scan, VCUG.

In a patient presenting with signs and symptoms of cerebral dysfunction, other causes (increased intracranial pressure, trauma, tumor, infarction, infection, ingestion) must be considered. Evidence of other end-organ damage is supportive of hypertension as the etiology.

(B) Although there are age dependent values for severe hypertension, hypertensive crisis is **not** based strictly on these values and is instead a clinical diagnosis.

An appropriate sized cuff is one in which the width of the bladder (short edge) is 1.25 – 1.5 times the diameter of the upper arm. This takes into account weight differences in people with the same length arm.

(C) There is no specific blood pressure value at which encephalopathy is seen, since cerebral blood flow autoregulation curve will shift in response to chronic hypertension. The upper limit of autoregulation is usually 30-40% above the basal mean arterial pressure. Blood pressure should be lowered by 20-25% of the mean arterial pressure or to a diastolic pressure of 100-110 mmHg, whichever is higher, over 1-3 hours. Lowering the blood pressure is diagnostic as well as therapeutic. If cerebral dysfunction does not resolve within hours of lowering blood pressure to an appropriate level, other causes must be investigated. Avoid hypotension which will result in cerebral hypoperfusion.

(D) In a hypertensive emergency, blood pressure should be lowered by 20-25% of the mean arterial pressure or to a diastolic pressure of 100-110 mmHg, whichever is higher, within 1-3h. Abruptly lowering the blood pressure to normal values can result in cerebral hypoperfusion and dysautoregulation.

(E) In hypertensive urgency, blood pressure should be lowered slowly to the levels described above over a 24 hour period. This can be done in a non-ICU setting using oral medication.

(F) **Sodium nitroprusside**
Toxicity is usually not seen in first 72 hours of use. Follow thiocyanate and methemoglobin levels.
- cyanide toxicity - metabolic acidosis, confusion, hemodynamic deterioration
- thiocyanate toxicity - abdominal pain, delirium, headache, nausea, muscle spasms, restlessness

Labetalol
Contraindicated in patients with bronchospasm, sinus bradycardia < 50 bpm, heart block, or CHF.

(G) **Diazoxide**
Pure arterial vasodilator with resultant increase in heart rate and cardiac output. Contraindicated in patients with left heart failure or aortic dissection. May cause hyperglycemia and fluid retention.

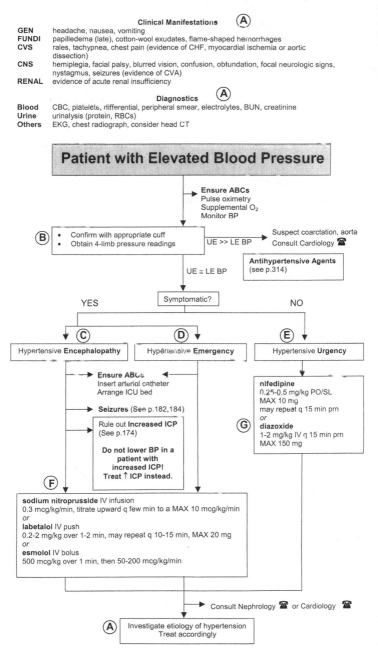

Clinical Manifestations (A)

GEN	headache, nausea, vomiting
FUNDI	papilledema (late), cotton-wool exudates, flame-shaped hemorrhages
CVS	rales, tachypnea, chest pain (evidence of CHF, myocardial ischemia or aortic dissection)
CNS	hemiplegia, facial palsy, blurred vision, confusion, obtundation, focal neurologic signs, nystagmus, seizures (evidence of CVA)
RENAL	evidence of acute renal insufficiency

Diagnostics (A)

Blood	CBC, platelets, differential, peripheral smear, electrolytes, BUN, creatinine
Urine	urinalysis (protein, RBCs)
Others	EKG, chest radiograph, consider head CT

Patient with Elevated Blood Pressure

Ensure ABCs
Pulse oximetry
Supplemental O₂
Monitor BP

(B)
- Confirm with appropriate cuff
- Obtain 4-limb pressure readings

UE >> LE BP → Suspect coarctation, aorta
Consult Cardiology ☎

Antihypertensive Agents
(see p.314)

UE ≅ LE BP

Symptomatic?

YES   NO

(C) Hypertensive **Encephalopathy**
(D) Hypertensive **Emergency**
(E) Hypertensive **Urgency**

Ensure ABCs
Insert arterial catheter
Arrange ICU bed

Seizures (See p.182,184)

Rule out **Increased ICP**
(See p.174)

**Do not lower BP in a patient with increased ICP!
Treat ↑ ICP instead.**

(E)
nifedipine
0.25-0.5 mg/kg PO/SL
MAX 10 mg
may repeat q 15 min prn
or
(G) **diazoxide**
1-2 mg/kg IV q 15 min prn
MAX 150 mg

(F)
sodium nitroprusside IV infusion
0.3 mcg/kg/min, titrate upward q few min to a MAX 10 mcg/kg/min
or
labetalol IV push
0.2-2 mg/kg over 1-2 min, may repeat q 10-15 min, MAX 20 mg
or
esmolol IV bolus
500 mcg/kg over 1 min, then 50-200 mcg/kg/min

Consult Nephrology ☎ or Cardiology ☎

(A) Investigate etiology of hypertension
Treat accordingly

Hypernatremic Dehydration

Girija Natarajan

> Hypernatremic dehydration is usually seen in infants who are fed boiled skim milk or improperly mixed electrolyte solutions with high salt content. Infants are at a greater risk for this type of dehydration because of greater water loss secondary to higher body surface area:weight ratio.

(A) Etiology:

A. High total body sodium
1. Administration of hypertonic saline: 3% sodium, sodium bicarbonate, hypernatremic enemas
2. Improper feeding with boiled skim milk, rehydrating solutions
3. High breast milk sodium
4. Hyperaldosteronism

B. Normal total body sodium (pure water loss)
1. Neurogenic hypernatremia
2. Diabetes insipidus: central, nephrogenic (congenital or acquired)
3. Extrarenal: sweating
4. Inadequate access to free water due to impaired mental status
5. Primary hypodipsia

C. Low total body sodium
1. Renal: osmotic diuresis, diabetes mellitus, tubulointerstitial or obstructive nephropathy
2. Extrarenal: diarrhea, burns, ileus, pancreatitis

(B) Change in vital signs or evidence of poor perfusion may not appear until 12-18% weight loss. If degree of dehydration by history is greater than by physical examination, consider hypernatremic dehydration.

(C) Common accompanying electrolyte abnormalities are hypocalcemia and hypoglycemia.

(D) If U/P osmolality is < 2, DI should be considered as a cause. Polyuria will be present, and urinalysis will show normal parameters except for a specific gravity < 1.006 or urine osmolality < 200 mOsm/L despite dehydration.

Treatment for nephrogenic DI
- **chlorothiazide** 20-40 mg/kg/day PO
- low salt diet
- **indomethacin**

(E) Sample calculation:

| Weight | 7.0 kg | measured serum sodium | 165 mEq/L |
| % dehydration | 10% | desired serum sodium | 145 mEq/L |

	Maintenance (for 48 hours)	Replacement	Maintenance+ Replacement = Total[b]
Water	100 mL/kg/day x 7 kg x 2 days = 1400 mL	10% x 7.0 kg = 700 mL [a]free water deficit 580 mL Remainder as NS 120 mL	1400 + 700 mL = 2100 mL over 48 h
Na$^+$	3 mEq/100 mL x 700 mL/1 x 2 d = 42 mEq	(120 mL) x (154 mEq/L) (1L/1000 mL) = 18 mEq	42 mEq + 18 mEq = 60 mEq

[a]free water deficit

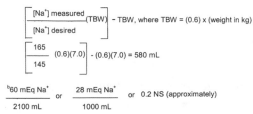

$$\left[\frac{[Na^+]\ measured}{[Na^+]\ desired}(TBW) \right] - TBW, \text{ where } TBW = (0.6) \times (\text{weight in kg})$$

$$\left[\frac{165}{145}(0.6)(7.0) \right] - (0.6)(7.0) = 580 \text{ mL}$$

$$[b]\frac{60 \text{ mEq Na}^+}{2100 \text{ mL}} \quad \text{or} \quad \frac{28 \text{ mEq Na}^+}{1000 \text{ mL}} \quad \text{or} \quad 0.2 \text{ NS (approximately)}$$

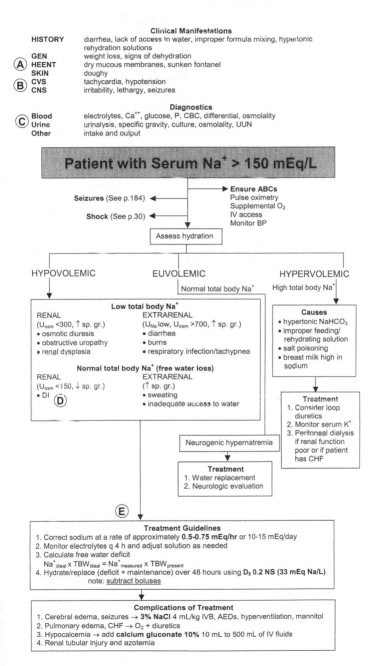

Clinical Manifestations

HISTORY	diarrhea, lack of access to water, improper formula mixing, hypertonic rehydration solutions
GEN	weight loss, signs of dehydration
(A) HEENT	dry mucous membranes, sunken fontanel
SKIN	doughy
(B) CVS	tachycardia, hypotension
CNS	irritability, lethargy, seizures

Diagnostics

(C) Blood	electrolytes, Ca^{++}, glucose, P, CBC, differential, osmolality
Urine	urinalysis, specific gravity, culture, osmolality, UUN
Other	intake and output

Patient with Serum Na$^+$ > 150 mEq/L

→ **Ensure ABCs**
Pulse oximetry
Supplemental O$_2$
IV access
Monitor BP

Seizures (See p.184) ◄

Shock (See p.30) ◄

Assess hydration

HYPOVOLEMIC

EUVOLEMIC
Normal total body Na$^+$

HYPERVOLEMIC
High total body Na$^+$

Low total body Na$^+$

RENAL
(U$_{osm}$ <300, ↑ sp. gr.)
• osmotic diuresis
• obstructive uropathy
• renal dysplasia

EXTRARENAL
(U$_{Na}$ low, U$_{osm}$ >700, ↑ sp. gr.)
• diarrhea
• burns
• respiratory infection/tachypnea

Normal total body Na$^+$ (free water loss)

RENAL
(U$_{osm}$ <150, ↓ sp. gr.)
• DI **(D)**

EXTRARENAL
(↑ sp. gr.)
• sweating
• inadequate access to water

Causes
• hypertonic NaHCO$_3$
• improper feeding/rehydrating solution
• salt poisoning
• breast milk high in sodium

Treatment
1. Consider loop diuretics
2. Monitor serum K$^+$
3. Peritoneal dialysis if renal function poor or if patient has CHF

Neurogenic hypernatremia

Treatment
1. Water replacement
2. Neurologic evaluation

(E)

Treatment Guidelines
1. Correct sodium at a rate of approximately **0.5-0.75 mEq/hr** or 10-15 mEq/day
2. Monitor electrolytes q 4 h and adjust solution as needed
3. Calculate free water deficit
   Na$^+_{ideal}$ X TBW$_{ideal}$ = Na$^+_{measured}$ X TBW$_{present}$
4. Hydrate/replace (deficit + maintenance) over 48 hours using **D$_5$ 0.2 NS (33 mEq Na/L)**
   note: <u>subtract boluses</u>

Complications of Treatment
1. Cerebral edema, seizures → **3% NaCl** 4 mL/kg IVB, AEDs, hyperventilation, mannitol
2. Pulmonary edema, CHF → O$_2$ + diuretics
3. Hypocalcemia → add **calcium gluconate 10%** 10 mL to 500 mL of IV fluids
4. Renal tubular injury and azotemia

Hyponatremia

Aditi Sharangpani

> Hyponatremia is defined as a serum sodium of < 130 mEq/L
> True hyponatremia: due to redistribution of intracellular sodium into the extracellular space
> False hyponatremia (pseudohyponatremia) may be due to:
> - Hyperglycemia – for every 100 mg/dL increase in glucose over 150 mg/dL, sodium level is falsely decreased by 1.6 mEq/L
> - Hyperlipidemia – falsely low sodium is produced by limitations of flame photometry measurement of sodium. Serum osmolality is normal.

(A) Clinical manifestations of hyponatremia depend on several factors:
- Rate of drop
- Plasma volume status
- Duration of hyponatremia
- Degree of hyponatremia

(B) CNS manifestations are generally the result of cerebral edema. Slowly developing hyponatremia is better tolerated than an acute drop in serum sodium. Most patients with hyponatremia who present with coma have a serum sodium < 120 mEq/L.

(C) Suspect adrenal insufficiency in states of hyponatremia accompanied by hyperkalemia (in the absence of renal failure).

(D) Consider WIC syndrome: Women Infants and Children (WIC) is a program that provides free formula and nutritional support to infants and children. Occasionally, mothers on the program dilute the infant formula to make it last over a longer period of time. Children who are given this diluted formula may develop hyponatremia.

(E) With SIADH, patients are euvolemic, or even hypervolemic.

(F) To determine the fluid correction for 24 hours:
1. Calculate sodium requirement
   Na^+ requirement = Na^+ deficit + Na^+ maintenance
   Na^+ deficit = (135 - measured Na^+) x weight in kg x 0.6
   Na^+ maintenance = 2-4 mEq Na^+ x weight in kg (per 24 h period)
2. Determine the fluid requirement
   Fluid requirement = fluid deficit + fluid maintenance
   Fluid deficit (liters) = % dehydration x ideal body weight in kg
   Fluid maintenance   0-10 kg → 100 mL/kg/day
                           plus 11-20 kg → 50 mL/kg/day
                           plus > 20 kg → 20 mL/kg/day
3. Calculate the sodium concentration of the replacement fluid
   Divide Na^+ requirement by fluid requirement (in liters)
   0.2 NS contains approximately 34 mEq sodium/liter
   0.3 NS contains approximately 50 mEq sodium/liter
   0.45 NS contains approximately 75 mEq sodium/liter

Note:
Hyponatremia associated with hyperglycemia generally resolves as hyperglycemia is corrected
Use ideal body weight if patient is overweight

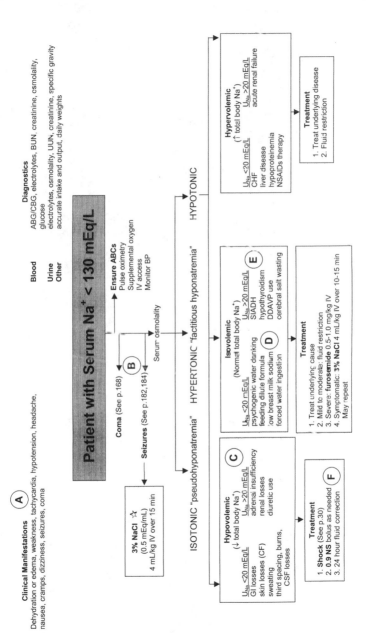

Clinical Manifestations Ⓐ

Dehydration or edema, weakness, tachycardia, hypotension, headache, nausea, cramps, dizziness, seizures, coma

Diagnostics

Blood ABG/CBG, electrolytes, BUN, creatinine, osmolality, glucose

Urine electrolytes, osmolality, UUN, creatinine, specific gravity

Other accurate intake and output, daily weights

Patient with Serum Na⁺ < 130 mEq/L

Ensure ABCs
Pulse oximetry
Supplemental oxygen
IV access
Monitor BP

Coma (See p.168)

Seizures (See p.182,184)

Ⓑ Serum osmolality

3% NaCl ☆
(0.5 mEq/mL)
4 mL/kg IV over 15 min

ISOTONIC "pseudohyponatremia"   HYPERTONIC "factitious hyponatremia"   HYPOTONIC

Hypovolemic Ⓒ
(↓ total body Na⁺)

U_{Na} <20 mEq/L
GI losses
skin losses (CF)
sweating
third spacing, burns,
CSF losses

U_{Na} >20 mEq/L
adrenal insufficiency
renal losses
diuretic use

Treatment Ⓕ
(See p.30)
1. Shock
2. 0.9 NS bolus as needed
3. 24 hour fluid correction

Isovolemic Ⓓ
(Normal total body Na⁺)

U_{Na} <20 mEq/L
psychogenic water drinking
feeding dilute formula
low breast milk sodium
forced water ingestion

U_{Na} >20 mEq/L Ⓔ
SIADH
hypothyroidism
DDAVP use
cerebral salt wasting

Treatment
1. Treat underlying cause
2. Mild to moderate: fluid restriction
3. Severe: furosemide 0.5-1.0 mg/kg IV
4. Symptomatic: 3% NaCl 4 mL/kg IV over 10-15 min
   May repeat

Hypervolemic
(↑ total body Na⁺)

U_{Na} <20 mEq/L
CHF
liver disease
hypoproteinemia
NSAIDs therapy

U_{Na} >20 mEq/L
acute renal failure

Treatment
1. Treat underlying disease
2. Fluid restriction

Hyperkalemia

Susan E. Gunderson

Hyperkalemia is defined as a serum K^+ level of > 5.5 mEq/L in a non-hemolyzed sample.

(A) Etiology of hyperkalemia

Potassium overload	↓ Intracellular Uptake	Pseudohyperkalemia

• PO/IV supplements
• Transfusion of "old" blood
• Cell lysis (tumor lysis)
• Poisoning
 	
↓ Renal excretion
• Renal failure
• Dehydration/shock
• Congenital adrenal hyperplasia (21 hydroxylase deficiency)
• Hypoaldosteronism
	• Acidosis
	• Shock
	• DKA
	• Digitalis toxicity
	• β-Adrenergic blockade
	• Succinylcholine
	• Familial periodic paralysis
		• Hemolyzed specimen
		• Clotted specimen if:
		  WBC > 1,000,000/mm^3
		  Platelets > 10,000,000/mm^3

EKG Changes: **(B)**

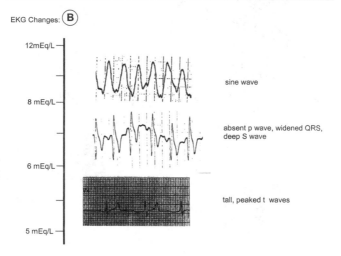

12mEq/L —

sine wave

8 mEq/L —

absent p wave, widened QRS, deep S wave

6 mEq/L —

tall, peaked t waves

5 mEq/L —

(C) Calcium chloride/gluconate 10% protects the myocardium from cardiac toxicity by membrane stabilization. Calcium chloride is the preferred preparation because it contains a higher amount of ionized calcium as compared to calcium gluconate. Extravasation of calcium into soft tissues can cause necrosis.

NaHCO$_3$ increases intracellular potassium uptake. To avoid precipitation, it should not be infused with calcium.

Insulin with glucose solution increases intracellular potassium uptake.

β-adrenergic agents increase intracellular potassium uptake and induce kaliuresis – controversial.

Kayexalate® binds potassium (ion exchange), in exchange for sodium, therefore decreasing total body K^+.

Clinical Manifestations

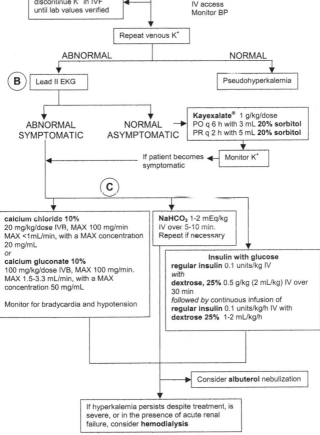

A HISTORY renal failure, drug ingestion, family history of hyperkalemic periodic paralysis
CVS arrhythmias, hypotension
CNS paresthesias, weakness, paralysis

Diagnostics

Blood electrolytes, BUN, creatinine
Others EKG

Hyperkalemia

Ensure ABCs
▶ Pulse oximetry
Supplemental O₂
EKG monitor
IV access
Monitor BP

If patient is on IV fluids, discontinue K⁺ in IVF until lab values verified

Repeat venous K⁺

ABNORMAL — NORMAL

B Lead II EKG — Pseudohyperkalemia

ABNORMAL SYMPTOMATIC — NORMAL ASYMPTOMATIC — **Kayexalate®** 1 g/kg/dose PO q 6 h with 3 mL **20% sorbitol** PR q 2 h with 5 mL **20% sorbitol**

If patient becomes symptomatic ◀— Monitor K⁺

C

calcium chloride 10%
20 mg/kg/dose IVB, MAX 100 mg/min
MAX <1mL/min, with a MAX concentration
20 mg/mL
or
calcium gluconate 10%
100 mg/kg/dose IVB, MAX 100 mg/min.
MAX 1.5-3.3 mL/min, with a MAX
concentration 50 mg/mL

Monitor for bradycardia and hypotension

NaHCO₃ 1-2 mEq/kg
IV over 5-10 min.
Repeat if necessary

Insulin with glucose
regular insulin 0.1 units/kg IV
with
dextrose, 25% 0.5 g/kg (2 mL/kg) IV over 30 min
followed by continuous infusion of
regular insulin 0.1 units/kg/h IV with
dextrose 25% 1-2 mL/kg/h

Consider **albuterol** nebulization

If hyperkalemia persists despite treatment, is severe, or in the presence of acute renal failure, consider **hemodialysis**

Hypermagnesemia

Susan E. Gunderson

Defined as a serum magnesium of > 2 mEq/L

Etiology

Increased Intake	Renal Insufficiency	Other
• antacids • laxatives • enemas • lithium intoxication • accidental Mg^{++} overdose	• renal failure • hyperparathyroidism • adrenal insufficiency	• massive hemolysis • infants of mothers with pre-eclampsia treated with $MgSO_4$

RBCs contain a high amount of magnesium, about 3X that in serum. With massive hemolysis, hypermagnesemia may occur.

Pathophysiology
Magnesium is a physiologic calcium blocker. The most serious consequence of hypermagnesemia is a result of calcium antagonism in the conduction system of the cardiovascular system.

Consequences of hypermagnesemia at different levels

Serum Magnesium	Clinical Manifestations
4.0 mEq/L	Hyporeflexia
>5.0 mEq/L	Prolonged AV conduction
>10 mEq/L	Complete heart block
>13 mEq/L	Asystole

Management
The treatment of choice for severe hypermagnesemia, especially in the presence of renal insufficiency, is hemodialysis. If the patient develops asystole and cardiac arrest from an overdose, intravenous **calcium chloride** or **calcium gluconate** may antagonize the effects of magnesium on conduction, and can be used as a temporizing measure until hemodialysis can be instituted. The administration of **furosemide** and intravascular volume expansion may also help in excretion of magnesium.

Clinical Manifestations

(A) HISTORY increased intake, possible sources of intoxication, renal failure, mother with pre-eclampsia receiving MgSO₄, patients on chemotherapy or other IV therapy receiving supplemental magnesium

GEN poor feeding
CVS bradycardia, hypotension, asystole, cardiac arrest **(B)**
RESP hypoventilation, respiratory arrest
CNS irritability, lethargy, hyporeflexia, coma

Diagnostics

(C) Blood Mg^{++}, Ca^{++}, electrolytes, ABG/CBG, BUN, creatinine
Other EKG: prolongation of P-R interval, 3° block

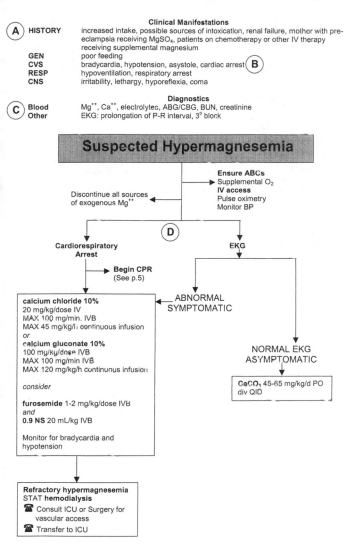

Suspected Hypermagnesemia

Ensure ABCs
Supplemental O_2
IV access
Pulse oximetry
Monitor BP

Discontinue all sources of exogenous Mg^{++}

(D)

Cardiorespiratory Arrest

Begin CPR
(See p.5)

EKG

calcium chloride 10%
20 mg/kg/dose IV
MAX 100 mg/min. IVB
MAX 45 mg/h continuous infusion
or
calcium gluconate 10%
100 mg/kg/dose IVB
MAX 100 mg/min IVB
MAX 120 mg/kg/h continuous infusion

consider

furosemide 1-2 mg/kg/dose IVB
and
0.9 NS 20 mL/kg IVB

Monitor for bradycardia and hypotension

ABNORMAL SYMPTOMATIC

NORMAL EKG ASYMPTOMATIC

CaCO₃ 45-65 mg/kg/d PO div QID

Refractory hypermagnesemia
STAT **hemodialysis**
☎ Consult ICU or Surgery for vascular access
☎ Transfer to ICU

Hypocalcemia

Susan E. Gunderson

Definition of hypocalcemia
neonate   total serum calcium < 7 mg/dL, ionized calcium < 1 mmol/L
infant/child   total serum calcium < 8 mg/dL, ionized calcium < 1-1.3 mmol/L

Calcium circulates in 3 forms
- protein bound (50%)
- ionized or free (40%)
- complexed to anions (10%)

(A) Albumin is responsible for 80% of the protein that binds to calcium, therefore hypoalbuminemia may result in a decrease in the amount of total calcium but does not affect ionized calcium levels. However, because ionized calcium is the physiologically active form, clinical manifestations occur predominantly with low ionized calcium.

Etiology of hypocalcemia related to PTH

(B)

Decreased PTH	Normal or Increased PTH
• Transient/physiologic (neonatal) • Hypoparathyroidism • Hypomagnesemia • Pancreatitis	• Pseudohypoparathyroidism • Renal failure • Liver disease/malabsorption • Vitamin D deficiency • Drugs: furosemide, aminoglycoside, cimetidine • Heparin, theophylline • Alkalosis • Cardiopulmonary bypass • Fat embolism • Sepsis • Blood transfusion

Etiology of hypocalcemia in the neonatal period

Prenatal (maternal factors)	Perinatal	Postnatal
• Vitamin D deficiency • Hyperparathyroidism • Physiologic ↑ PTH (diabetes)	• Perinatal stress • Hypoxia/anoxia • Prematurity, IUGR	• Postnatal stress • RDS • Sepsis/shock • $NAHCO_3$ infusion • Post-transfusion

Transient or late onset neonatal (3-10 d age)
- physiologically underactive PTH glands are unable to respond to high phosphate diet
- high phosphate decreases serum calcium through calcium phosphate deposits

Etiology of hypocalcemia related to other factors

Hypomagnesemia	Hyperphosphatemia	Vitamin D deficiency
• Decreased intake • Increased intracellular uptake • Renal and/or GI loss	• Increased intake • Cell lysis • Renal failure and/or ↓ PTH	• Decreased intake • Liver disease/ malabsorption • Rickets (type I and II)

Clinical Manifestations

HISTORY	renal disease, dietary deficiency, use of diuretics or other drugs, liver disease pancreatitis, maternal factors
GEN	poor feeding, failure to thrive
CVS	hypotension, arrhythmias which can be refractory
CNS	hyperreflexia, irritability, tremors, tetany, seizures, Chvostek's and Trousseau's signs are helpful if positive, but are nonspecific and insensitive indicators of hypocalcemia

Diagnostics

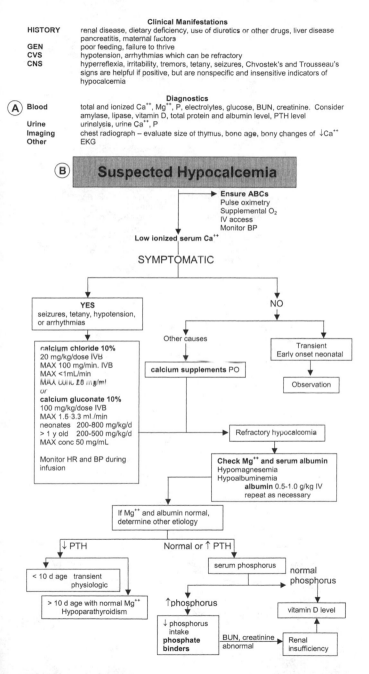

(A) Blood	total and ionized Ca^{++}, Mg^{++}, P, electrolytes, glucose, BUN, creatinine. Consider amylase, lipase, vitamin D, total protein and albumin level, PTH level
Urine	urinalysis, urine Ca^{++}, P
Imaging	chest radiograph – evaluate size of thymus, bone age, bony changes of ↓Ca^{++}
Other	EKG

(B) **Suspected Hypocalcemia**

→ **Ensure ABCs**
Pulse oximetry
Supplemental O_2
IV access
Monitor BP

Low ionized serum Ca^{++}

SYMPTOMATIC

YES
seizures, tetany, hypotension, or arrhythmias

NO

calcium chloride 10%
20 mg/kg/dose IVB
MAX 100 mg/min. IVB
MAX <1mL/min
MAX conc 20 mg/ml
or
calcium gluconate 10%
100 mg/kg/dose IVB
MAX 1.5-3.3 mL/min
neonates 200-800 mg/kg/d
> 1 y old 200-500 mg/kg/d
MAX conc 50 mg/mL

Monitor HR and BP during infusion

Other causes

calcium supplements PO

Transient
Early onset neonatal

Observation

Refractory hypocalcemia

Check Mg^{++} and serum albumin
Hypomagnesemia
Hypoalbuminemia
albumin 0.5-1.0 g/kg IV
repeat as necessary

If Mg^{++} and albumin normal, determine other etiology

↓ PTH

Normal or ↑ PTH

< 10 d age transient physiologic

> 10 d age with normal Mg^{++}
Hypoparathyroidism

serum phosphorus

normal phosphorus

↑phosphorus

↓ phosphorus intake
phosphate binders

BUN, creatinine abnormal

Renal insufficiency

vitamin D level

Metabolic Acidosis

Hrishikesh Dingankar

A decrease in blood pH resulting from a primary reduction in plasma bicarbonate.
Pathophysiology

HCO_3^- loss or ↓ H^+ load → ↓ HCO_3^- → metabolic acidosis

Compensation decreases the magnitude of the pH change but does not completely normalize the pH

- Lungs ↑ elimination of CO_2, full effect achieved by 12-24 h
- Kidneys ↑ production and secretion of NH_3 and excretion of titratable acids; full effect achieved by 5-7 days

(A) Serum anion gap represents the amount of *unmeasured* anions (phosphate, sulfates, negatively-charged proteins) in blood. Normally accounts for 8-16 mEq/L.

Anion gap = Na^+ - (HCO_3^- + Cl^-)

Urine anion gap – major urinary cations are Na^+, K^+, NH_4^+; anions are Cl^- and HCO_3^-

If urine Cl^- > urine Na^+ + K^+ → indicates NH_4^+ secretion by kidney

If urine Cl^- < urine Na^+ + K^+ → indicates ↑ HCO_3^- loss in urine

Classification and etiology:

Normal Anion Gap Acidosis		
Pathophysiology	GI or renal HCO_3^- loss with compensatory hyperchloremia and maintenance of normal anion gap	
Etiology	Urine Cl^- > urine Na^++K^+ urine pH < 5.5 GI losses: diarrhea, small bowel/pancreatic drainage, bowel augmentation, cystoplasty/urinary diversion Renal losses: proximal RTA Misc: adrenal insufficiency, carbonic anhydrase inhibitor use	Urine Cl^- < urine Na^++K^+ urine pH > 5.5 Distal RTA
Increased Anion Gap Acidosis		
Pathophysiology	Accumulation of acidic anions in blood which cause ↓ HCO_3^- (buffering) and ↓ Cl^- resulting in an anion gap	
Etiology	Endogenous: ketoacidosis (DKA, starvation), lactic acidosis (primary or secondary), inborn errors of metabolism, renal failure	Exogenous: toxins and drugs (salicylates, alcohols)

Mnemonics **USEDCARP** and **MUDPILES**

Normal anion gap acidosis	Increased anion gap acidosis
Ureteroenterostomy	**M**ethanol
Small bowel fistula	**U**remia
Extra chloride	**D**iabetic ketoacidosis
Diarrhea	**P**araldehyde
Carbonic anhydrase inhibitor use	**I**ron/INH/Inhalants (CO, CN)
Adrenal Insufficiency	**L**actic acidosis
Renal tubular acidosis	**E**thanol/Ethylene glycol
Pancreatic fistula	**S**alicylates/Starvation/Solvents (toluene)

Metabolic acidosis most commonly results from decreased tissue perfusion:

Pyruvate + NADH + H^+ → lactate + NAD^+ (reduction of pyruvate)

With tissue anoxia: ↓ oxidation of pyruvate → ↑ pyruvate

↓ oxidation of NADH to NAD^+

The reduction of pyruvate produces more lactate during episodes of tissue anoxia, which is converted by the liver to glucose with release of HCO_3^-. With ↑ production of lactate or with hepatic insufficiency, the ability of the liver for gluconeogenesis is impaired, therefore lactate accumulates.

(B) Osmolar gap = measured osmolality – calculated osmolality, normal < 10

Calculated osmolality = 2[Na^+ mEq/L] + [BUN mg/dL]/2.8 + [glucose mg/dL]/18

✱ Continued on p.219

✳ Continued from p.218

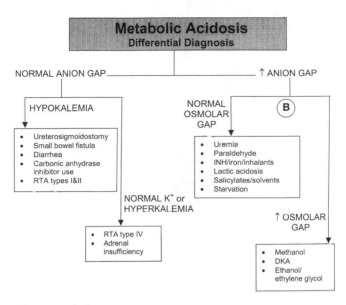

Metabolic Acidosis
Differential Diagnosis

NORMAL ANION GAP ——————————————— ↑ ANION GAP

HYPOKALEMIA

- Ureterosigmoidostomy
- Small bowel fistula
- Diarrhea
- Carbonic anhydrase inhibitor use
- RTA types I&II

NORMAL OSMOLAR GAP   (**B**)

- Uremia
- Paraldehyde
- INH/iron/inhalants
- Lactic acidosis
- Salicylates/solvents
- Starvation

NORMAL K⁺ or HYPERKALEMIA

- RTA type IV
- Adrenal insufficiency

↑ OSMOLAR GAP

- Methanol
- DKA
- Ethanol/ethylene glycol

(**C**) Management principles:

HCO_3^- deficit (mEq) = [desired HCO_3^- - measured HCO_3^-] x weight (kg) x 0.6 (V_d of HCO_3^-)

Metabolic acidosis is a biochemical derangement that results from an underlying disease process, therefore, treatment should be aimed at correction of the disease.

Severe metabolic acidosis with pH < 7.1 and/or HCO_3^- < 6-8 mEq/L can have deleterious effects on the myocardium and other organ systems. Correction of acidosis and low HCO_3^- is therefore recommended.

Disadvantages of **NaHCO₃** administration:
1. ↑ sodium load - hypernatremia/hyperosmolality can cause intracranial bleed in premature infants
2. Hypercarbia: $NaHCO_3 \leftrightarrows Na^+ + H_2O + CO_2$
3. May aggravate pre-existing hypocalcemia and hypokalemia by inducing cellular shifts

Other therapeutic options for correction of metabolic acidosis:
THAM (tris-hydroxy-methyl-amino-methane)
$\qquad$ THAM + $H_2CO_3 \rightarrow 2\ HCO_3^- + 2\ Na^+$

Carbicarb an equimolar solution of $NaHCO_3 + Na_2CO_3$
$\qquad Na_2CO_3 + CO_2 + H_2O \rightarrow 2H_2CO_3 + 2Na^+$

DCA (dichloroacetate)
$\qquad$ activates pyruvate dehydrogenase kinase and decreases lactate production

Dialysis for severe intractable metabolic acidosis

Clinical Manifestations

Symptoms due to acidosis hyperventilation, Kussmaul respirations, altered sensorium, hypotension, poor peripheral perfusion
other symptoms are disease-specific

Diagnostics

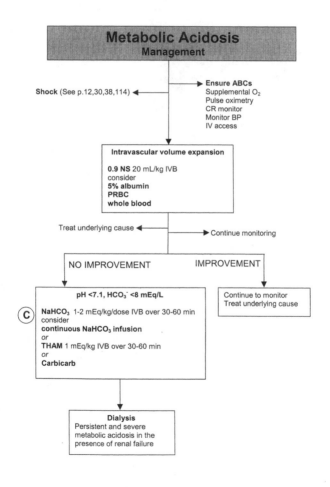

A **Blood** ABG/CBG, electrolytes, BUN, creatinine, osmolality, ketones, glucose, drug screen (include alcohol panel)
culture, Ca^{++}, Mg^{++}, CBC, differential

B **Urine** urinalysis, pH, electrolytes, drug screen, culture

Other consider imaging, echocardiogram, EKG depending on the suspected underlying disease.

Metabolic Acidosis
Management

Shock (See p.12,30,38,114) ◄

► **Ensure ABCs**
Supplemental O_2
Pulse oximetry
CR monitor
Monitor BP
IV access

Intravascular volume expansion

0.9 NS 20 mL/kg IVB
consider
5% albumin
PRBC
whole blood

Treat underlying cause ◄

► Continue monitoring

NO IMPROVEMENT

IMPROVEMENT

pH <7.1, HCO_3^- <8 mEq/L

C **$NaHCO_3$** 1-2 mEq/kg/dose IVB over 30-60 min
consider
continuous $NaHCO_3$ infusion
or
THAM 1 mEq/kg IVB over 30-60 min
or
Carbicarb

Continue to monitor
Treat underlying cause

Dialysis
Persistent and severe metabolic acidosis in the presence of renal failure

NOTES

Dehydration

Susan E. Gunderson

A The most common cause of dehydration in children is acute infectious gastroenteritis, usually viral. Infants can lose significant amounts of water and electrolytes within a brief period of time. In the management of these children, it is important to replace their deficit and provide maintenance IV fluids. However, it is equally important to continually reassess these children, to ascertain that there is a good response to therapy, as well as to determine ongoing losses in order to provide adequate replacement of those losses.

B If weight loss is unknown, estimate severity from signs and symptoms of extracellular fluid (ECF) loss

Signs and Symptoms	Mild Dehydration	Moderate Dehydration	Severe Dehydration
Heart rate (pulse)	normal	rapid	rapid and weak
Respirations	normal	deep	rapid and deep
Blood pressure	normal	orthostatic hypotension	decreased or absent
Urine output	normal	decreased	absent
Capillary refill time	normal	delayed	
Fontanel/eyes	normal	sunken	
Tears	normal	absent	
Mucous membranes	normal	dry	

☆ **HYPOTENSION IS A LATE SIGN OF DEHYDRATION**

C The purpose of IV boluses is to rapidly re-expand intravascular volume or circulating volume. **NEVER USE HYPOTONIC SOLUTIONS FOR IV BOLUSES.**

D **Isonatremic dehydration** (Na^+ 130-150 mEq/L) – proportionate loss of water and Na^+ from ECF; no water shift between ECF and ICF. Severity is determined from % weight loss (in kg)

Hyponatremic dehydration (Na^+ < 130 mEq/L) – ECF sodium loss greater than water loss. *Signs and symptoms appear earlier* as water shifts intracellularly.

Hypernatremic dehydration (Na^+ > 150 mEq/L) – ECF water loss greater than sodium loss. *Signs and symptoms delayed* as water shifts into ECF, maintaining ECF volume. Occasionally, fluid shifts may lead to cerebral hemorrhage, especially in infants. In addition to signs and symptoms of dehydration, patients may also have warm, doughy skin, hypertonia, hyperreflexia, and irritability.
Avoid rapid correction of acute hypernatremic dehydration as a sudden fall in intracellular fluid osmolality may lead to cerebral edema (see p.174).

E

	Mild Dehydration		Moderate Dehydration		Severe Dehydration	
	Infants	Older children	Infants	Older children	Infants	Older children
% body weight loss	5	3	10	6	15	9
Fluid deficit (mL/kg)	50	30	100	60	150	90

In hyponatremic or hypernatremic dehydration, estimation of degree of dehydration based on signs and symptoms of ECF loss may be misleading.

F Maintenance + replacement (of deficit and ongoing losses) restores ECF volume. Maintenance fluids replace physiologic losses (sweat, stools, insensible, urine); most commonly estimated from caloric expenditure (not applicable in infants < 14 days of age)

Body Weight	Caloric Expenditure (water requirement/day)	Holliday-Segar method: every
2.5 – 10 kg	100 kcal (mL)/kg	100 calories expended
11 – 20 kg	1,000 kcal (mL) + 50 kcal (mL)/kg over 10 kg	requires 100 mL water, 3 mEq
> 20 kg	1,500 kcal (mL) + 20 kcal (mL)/kg over 20 kg	of Na^+ and 2 mEq K^+

✳ Continued on p.224

Diagnostics

Blood	ABG/CBG, electrolytes, BUN, creatinine, glucose, osmolality, Ca^{++}, Mg^{++}, P, CBC, differential
Urine	urine output and specific gravity
Other	stool culture, stool for occult blood, Rotazyme®

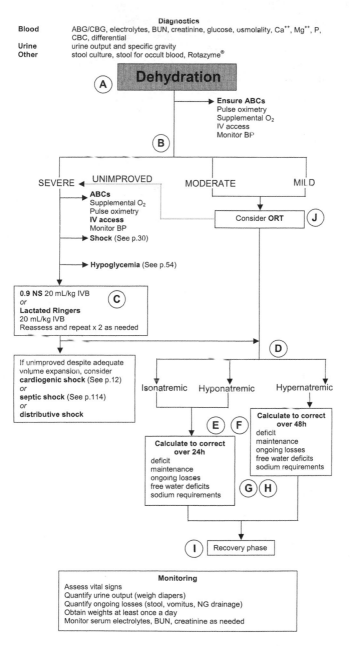

✳ Continued from p.222

Dehydration worksheet (G)

Fluids (for 1st 24 hours)	Water (mL)	Sodium (mEq/L)
Maintenance	B	B
Deficit	C	C
Na$^+$ deficit (hyponatremic)	--	D
Free water deficit (hypernatremic dehydration)	E	--
SUBTOTAL		
Subtract bolus(es)	F	F
TOTAL	G	G

Sample calculation:
A. Weight = 4.5 kg infant with 10% dehydration, pre-illness weight = 4.5 kg + [0.10 x 4.5 kg] ≅ 5kg
   Total body water (TBW) = 0.6 x pre-illness weight = 0.6 x 5 kg = 3 kg = 3L = 3000 mL

B. Maintenance estimated from Holliday and Segar method using pre-illness weight
   Water   100 mL x 5 kg = <u>500 mL/d water</u>
   Na$^+$ 3 mEq/100 mL x 500 mL = <u>15 mEq Na$^+$/day</u>

C. Water deficit   5 kg – 4.5 kg = 0.5 kg = 0.5 L = <u>500 mL</u>
   Na$^+$ deficit   0.5 L x [% from ECF] x [conc of Na$^+$ in ECF]
                      0.5 L x 60% x 140 mEq/L = <u>42 mEq Na$^+$</u>

D. Hyponatremic dehydration **only**
   Na$^+$ deficit   = [135 mEq/L – measured Na$^+$] x TBW
   If Na$^+$ = 120 mEq/L   = [135 mEq/L – 120 mEq/L] x 0.6 x 5 kg = <u>45 mEq Na$^+$</u>

E. Hypernatremic dehydration **only**
   Free water deficit (L) = [Measured Na$^+$ x TBW/145 mEq/L] – TBW
   If Na$^+$ = 150 mEq/L   = [150 mEq/L x 0.6 x 5 kg/145 mEq/L] – [0.6 x 5 kg] = 0.1 L = <u>100 mL</u>

F. 0.9 NS (154 mEq/L Na$^+$)
   20 mL/kg bolus   20 mL x 4.5 kg = <u>90 mL</u>; 154 mEq/L x 0.09 L ≅ <u>14 mEq Na$^+$</u>

G. IV fluid rate for 24 h correction: isonatremic and hyponatremic dehydration
      Total water (G) ÷ 24 h = IV rate in mL/h (24 h)

   IV fluid rate for 48 h correction: hypernatremic dehydration
   [Total water (G) + additional 24 h maintenance fluid (B)] ÷ 48 h = mL/h (48 h)

   Approximate Na$^+$ solution to deliver total Na$^+$ over 24 or 48 h
      Total Na$^+$ ÷ total water (L) = Na$^+$ mEq/L
      Select fluid based on calculated Na$^+$ needs
         0.45 NS = 77 mEq/L
         0.3 NS = 51 mEq/L
         0.2 NS = 34 mEq/L

(H) Add glucose to IV fluids to minimize protein catabolism and provide energy source for the brain
    Add K$^+$ to IV fluids once urine output is established and adequate renal function ascertained

(I) Resume age-appropriate diet, avoiding foods high in fat and/or simple carbohydrates. Lactose-free formula does not shorten the duration of illness. There is no physiologic basis for bowel rest or the use of diluted formula.

(J) In mild to moderate dehydration, consider **oral rehydration therapy (ORT)** – as effective as IV therapy for replacement of deficit and ongoing losses
   o Contraindications to use of ORT
      ▪ severe dehydration with or without shock
      ▪ intractable vomiting
      ▪ ileus
      ▪ altered mental status
   o administer 5 mL ORT solution every 5 minutes, increasing amount as tolerated
   o mild dehydration → 12.5 mL/kg/h + 10 mL/kg/stool + estimated volume of emesis
   o moderate dehydration → 25 mL/kg/h + 10 mL/kg/stool + estimated volume of emesis

NOTES

Chapter 13 ♣ Respiratory Disorders

Acute Bronchiolitis

Adiaha Spinks

> Acute bronchiolitis is the most common lower respiratory tract infection in children < 2 years of age. Peak admission occurs in infants < 6 months of age. It is commonly caused by RSV (Respiratory Syncytial Virus) during the months of October through April and in the early spring by Parainfluenza Virus type 3.

(A) Apneic episodes may be the presenting symptom, especially in premature infants.

(B)

RSV Nasal Wash

Bulb Syringe Technique

Materials:	Sterile ear bulb syringe, medicine cup, 3-5 mL sterile saline, sterile specimen tube
Procedure:	Dispense 3-5 mL of sterile saline into medicine cup. Draw saline into bulb syringe. Incline patient's head at about 70° angle. Occlude one nostril with a gloved finger. Insert bulb syringe into other nostril, squirt saline, and immediately reaspirate. Remove syringe from nostril and empty contents into sterile tube. Submit to laboratory.

Butterfly® Tubing Technique

Materials:	23 or 24 gauge Butterfly® tubing infusion set with needle cut off, 5-8 mL sterile saline in a syringe, specimen tube
Procedure:	Attach syringe with saline into butterfly tubing. Insert tip of tubing into patient's nostril. Instill saline through the tubing. Reaspirate. Transfer washing into specimen tube or container. Submit to laboratory.

Pending RSV results, continue respiratory precautions.

(C) Inhaled bronchodilators have been used to afford symptomatic relief of symptoms. However, there is no evidence that it decreases admission rates or improves oxygen saturation. Primary treatment continues to be supportive management with adequate hydration and oxygen supplementation.

(D) Children with underlying chronic lung disease (e.g., BPD), reactive airway disease, tend to have severe symptoms. These children may benefit from systemic corticosteroids. If unable to obtain IV access, consider **dexamethasone** 1.5 mg/kg **aerosol**.

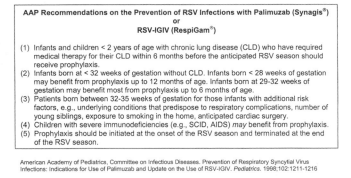

AAP Recommendations on the Prevention of RSV Infections with Palimuzab (Synagis®)
or
RSV-IGIV (RespiGam®)

(1) Infants and children < 2 years of age with chronic lung disease (CLD) who have required medical therapy for their CLD within 6 months before the anticipated RSV season should receive prophylaxis.
(2) Infants born at < 32 weeks of gestation without CLD. Infants born < 28 weeks of gestation may benefit from prophylaxis up to 12 months of age. Infants born at 29-32 weeks of gestation may benefit most from prophylaxis up to 6 months of age.
(3) Patients born between 32-35 weeks of gestation for those infants with additional risk factors, e.g., underlying conditions that predispose to respiratory complications, number of young siblings, exposure to smoking in the home, anticipated cardiac surgery.
(4) Children with severe immunodeficiencies (e.g., SCID, AIDS) *may* benefit from prophylaxis.
(5) Prophylaxis should be initiated at the onset of the RSV season and terminated at the end of the RSV season.

American Academy of Pediatrics, Committee on Infectious Diseases. Prevention of Respiratory Syncytial Virus Infections: Indications for Use of Palimuzab and Update on the Use of RSV-IGIV. *Pediatrics*. 1998;102:1211-1216

(A) **Clinical Manifestations**
Apnea, rhinorrhea, nasal flaring, cough, tachypnea, dyspnea, retractions, wheezing, irritability,
poor feeding, lethargy

Diagnostics
(B) ABG/CBG, CBC, differential, RSV-ELISA nasal washing, electrolytes, BUN, creatinine,
glucose, chest radiograph

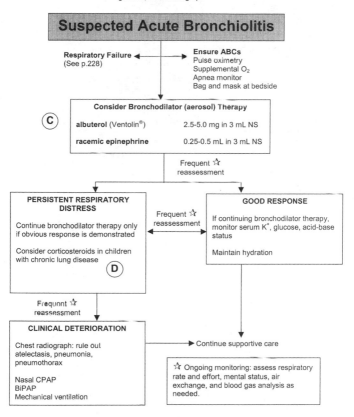

Suspected Acute Bronchiolitis

Respiratory Failure ◄──────► **Ensure ABCs**
(See p.228)   Pulse oximetry
                                   Supplemental O_2
                                   Apnea monitor
                                   Bag and mask at bedside

Consider Bronchodilator (aerosol) Therapy

(C)

albuterol (Ventolin®)	2.5-5.0 mg in 3 mL NS
racemic epinephrine	0.25-0.5 mL in 3 mL NS

Frequent ☆
reassessment

PERSISTENT RESPIRATORY DISTRESS

Continue bronchodilator therapy only
if obvious response is demonstrated

Consider corticosteroids in children
with chronic lung disease

(D)

Frequent ☆
reassessment

GOOD RESPONSE

If continuing bronchodilator therapy,
monitor serum K^+, glucose, acid-base
status

Maintain hydration

Frequent ☆
reassessment

CLINICAL DETERIORATION

Chest radiograph: rule out
atelectasis, pneumonia,
pneumothorax

Nasal CPAP
BiPAP
Mechanical ventilation

──────► Continue supportive care

☆ Ongoing monitoring: assess respiratory
rate and effort, mental status, air
exchange, and blood gas analysis as
needed.

Acute Respiratory Failure

Michael Fiore

(A) Respiratory failure: inability to maintain alveolocapillary gas exchange to meet the metabolic demands of the body

Respiratory distress: increased work in breathing as characterized by tachypnea, retractions, stridor, wheezing, nasal flaring, and/or grunting

There is a significant amount of interaction between the respiratory system and other organ systems. A certain degree of respiratory insufficiency can be tolerated by itself, but with additional stresses such as fluid overload, infections, myocardial dysfunction and metabolic abnormalities, decompensation readily occurs.

Overt respiratory failure may occur without manifesting signs of respiratory distress (e.g., neuromuscular disease), while a patient may display signs of severe respiratory distress with no pulmonary disease (severe metabolic acidosis with Kussmaul respirations, salicylic acid ingestion).

(B) Causes of Acute Respiratory Failure in Children

Inadequate respiratory drive	Increased ICP: obstructed shunt, tumor, trauma
	Infectious: meningitis, encephalitis
	Depressant drugs: opiates, benzodiazepines, barbiturates
	Others: central apnea, status epilepticus
Neuromuscular	Guillain-Barré Syndrome, myasthenia gravis, botulism, SMA
Chest wall abnormalities	Flail chest, kyphoscoliosis
Airway	Extrathoracic: tonsillar/adenoidal hypertrophy, laryngomalacia, croup, foreign body, subglottic stenosis, epiglottitis
	Intrathoracic, extrapulmonary: vascular rings, mediastinal tumors
	Intrathoracic, intrapulmonary: bronchiolitis, asthma
	Note: foreign bodies can lodge anywhere in the airway, symptoms vary according to location.
Pulmonary parenchyma	Pneumonia, ARDS, pulmonary edema, pneumothorax
Excess metabolic demands	Shock, sepsis, toxins

- **When examining a child in respiratory distress, the physician should never interfere with the child's own compensatory mechanisms**

(C) Signs and Symptoms of Respiratory Distress

Symptoms	Extrathoracic	Intrathoracic Extrapulmonary	Intrapulmonary	Parenchymal
Tachypnea	—	+	+	++++
Stridor	++++	—	—	—
Grunting	—	—	—	++++
Retractions	++++	++	++	++
Wheezing	—	++	++++	—

Table courtesy of Dr. A.P. Sarnaik.

- Lab investigations, imaging, and blood gas analysis all require time. **Do not delay emergent, life-saving treatment to obtain these studies**.
- ABG/CBG, pulse oximetry may show hypoxemia and/or hypercarbia

Pitfalls of Pulse Oximetry (D)

There may be inherent inaccuracy of up to 4%.
1. Based on the oxyhemoglobin dissociation curve. The curve flattens with $PaO_2 > 70$ mmHg, therefore, large changes in PaO_2 will result in only small changes in pulse oximeter recording.
2. Presence of abnormal hemoglobin, such as COHb or metHb, will lead to over estimations of O_2 saturation, because the pulse oximeter only detects saturated and unsaturated Hb, not what the Hb is saturated with.
3. Conditions with peripheral vasoconstriction and decreased pulsatile flow, such as shock, can lead to inaccurate readings.
4. If the pulse oximeter alarms frequently, determine the cause instead of turning the machine off.

(E) Children with respiratory insufficiency should be given the maximum amount of oxygen possible, even with normal pulse oximetry or in the absence of cyanosis and other signs of hypoxia.

(F) A nasal canula does not reliably deliver a consistent amount of oxygen. Delivery of ≥ 4 L/min is drying to the nasal mucosa and is uncomfortable. If > 2 L/min O_2 is needed, consider O_2 by mask.

✳ Continued on p.230

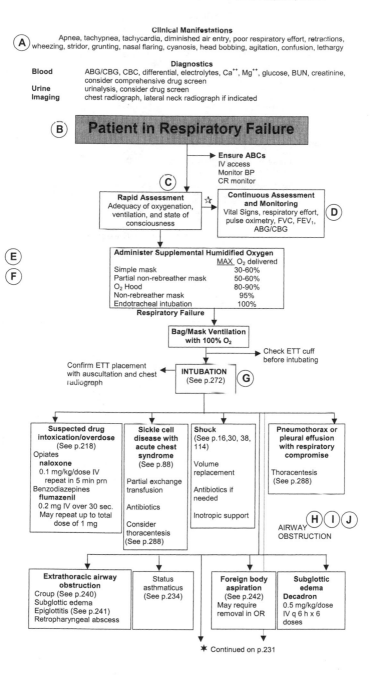

Clinical Manifestations

(A) Apnea, tachypnea, tachycardia, diminished air entry, poor respiratory effort, retractions, wheezing, stridor, grunting, nasal flaring, cyanosis, head bobbing, agitation, confusion, lethargy

Diagnostics

Blood	ABG/CBG, CBC, differential, electrolytes, Ca^{++}, Mg^{++}, glucose, BUN, creatinine, consider comprehensive drug screen
Urine	urinalysis, consider drug screen
Imaging	chest radiograph, lateral neck radiograph if indicated

(B) **Patient in Respiratory Failure**

Ensure ABCs
IV access
Monitor BP
CR monitor

(C) **Rapid Assessment**
Adequacy of oxygenation, ventilation, and state of consciousness

(D) **Continuous Assessment and Monitoring**
Vital Signs, respiratory effort, pulse oximetry, FVC, FEV$_1$, ABG/CBG

(E)
(F)

Administer Supplemental Humidified Oxygen

	MAX O$_2$ delivered
Simple mask	30-60%
Partial non-rebreather mask	50-60%
O$_2$ Hood	80-90%
Non-rebreather mask	95%
Endotracheal intubation	100%

Respiratory Failure

Bag/Mask Ventilation with 100% O$_2$

Check ETT cuff before intubating

Confirm ETT placement with auscultation and chest radiograph

(G) **INTUBATION** (See p.272)

Suspected drug intoxication/overdose (See p.218)
Opiates
naloxone
0.1 mg/kg/dose IV repeat in 5 min prn
Benzodiazepines
flumazenil
0.2 mg IV over 30 sec.
May repeat up to total dose of 1 mg

Sickle cell disease with acute chest syndrome (See p.88)
Partial exchange transfusion
Antibiotics
Consider thoracentesis (See p.288)

Shock (See p.16,30, 38, 114)
Volume replacement
Antibiotics if needed
Inotropic support

Pneumothorax or pleural effusion with respiratory compromise
Thoracentesis (See p.288)

(H)(I)(J)
AIRWAY OBSTRUCTION

Extrathoracic airway obstruction
Croup (See p.240)
Subglottic edema
Epiglottitis (See p.241)
Retropharyngeal abscess

Status asthmaticus (See p.234)

Foreign body aspiration (See p.242)
May require removal in OR

Subglottic edema
Decadron
0.5 mg/kg/dose IV q 6 h x 6 doses

✻ Continued on p.231

✳ Continued from p.228

A simple mask delivers 30-60% oxygen at a flow rate of 10-12 L/min. A partial rebreathing mask can deliver up to 60% O_2 at a flow of 10-12 L/min. A non-rebreather mask has one-way valves between the exhalation port and the exterior and between the bag and reservoir and is able to deliver up to 95% O_2 and prevents CO_2 rebreathing.

(G) Indications for endotracheal intubation:
- to maintain airway patency
- to institute mechanical ventilation
- to protect the patient from aspiration lung injury
- to facilitate pulmonary toilet

(H) Nebulization:
Racemic epinephrine acts by decreasing airway edema and congestion, thereby improving airflow
Albuterol is a β-2 agonist with potent bronchodilator properties. It can be administered intermittently or continuously.

(I) **Helium-oxygen** mixture: airflow becomes turbulent rather than laminar in the presence of airway obstruction. In this situation, resistance depends on gas density instead of viscosity. Replacing nitrogen with helium reduces resistance in the obstructed airway. **HeliOx** may be administered by mask or the endotracheal tube. Administration through an oxygen hood is not recommended, as the helium remains on the top of the hood, making it relatively inaccessible to the supine child.

(J) **Corticosteroids** have been found to be of benefit in the treatment of croup. **Decadron** IV or inhaled **budesonide** may be used.

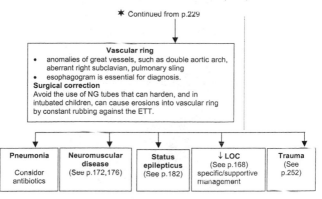

✳ Continued from p.229

Vascular ring
- anomalies of great vessels, such as double aortic arch, aberrant right subclavian, pulmonary sling
- esophagogram is essential for diagnosis.

Surgical correction
Avoid the use of NG tubes that can harden, and in intubated children, can cause erosions into vascular ring by constant rubbing against the ETT.

Pneumonia	Neuromuscular disease	Status epilepticus	↓LOC	Trauma
Consider antibiotics	(See p.172,176)	(See p.182)	(See p.168) specific/supportive management	(See p.252)

Mechanical Ventilation

Components of mechanical ventilatory strategy:
- initiation of inspiration (mode): intermittent mandatory ventilation (IMV), synchronized IMV (SIMV), assist/control
- inspiratory flow characteristics: sine wave or square wave flow
- termination of inspiration (cycle): time-cycled or volume-cycled
- expiratory flow maneuvers: positive end expiratory pressure (PEEP)

High frequency ventilation (oscillatory or jet): ventilation at high rates (1-15 Hertz) and low tidal volumes provide effective ventilation without using high airway pressures. This technique has been found to be especially useful in children with ARDS, pulmonary hemorrhage or interstitial pneumonia.

Unproven modalities for the management of respiratory failure include ECMO, surfactant administration, inhaled nitric oxide, partial liquid ventilation.

☆ Do not administer sedative agents to unintubated children with respiratory insufficiency who develop agitation or irritability, as this may reflect hypoxia/air hunger.

Apnea

Thomas Brousseau

Apnea is defined as the cessation of breathing for > 15 seconds, or less, if accompanied by pallor, cyanosis, and/or bradycardia. The two subtypes are central and obstructive apnea.

Must be distinguished from periodic breathing, which is a normal breathing pattern seen in infants, consisting of > 2-second respiratory pauses interspersed with regular respirations. This is **not** accompanied by color change or bradycardia.

(A) **Apparent life-threatening event (ALTE):** an episode that is frightening to the observer and is characterized by a combination of apnea, color change, change in muscle tone (usually hypotonic or limp), choking or gagging.

Check bedside glucose, maintain thermoneutral environment, avoid neck flexion or hyperextension.

(B) If historical events are inconsistent with physical findings, suspect **child abuse** (See p.42). Ensure proper documentation.

(C) **Obstructive apnea:** characterized by airway obstruction, which impairs or prevents ventilation despite sufficient respiratory effort. Causes include laryngospasm, croup, hypertrophy of tonsils and adenoids, tumors, tracheomalacia, craniofacial abnormalities, epiglottitis, foreign body aspiration, gastroesophageal reflux (may have a central mechanism) and vascular rings.

(D) **Central apnea:** characterized by a lack of respiratory effort. Causes include: infection (RSV, sepsis, encephalitis, meningitis, pertussis), seizures, IVH, ↑ ICP, prematurity, toxic ingestion, head injury, central hypoventilation syndrome, and metabolic disorders (hypocalcemia, hypoglycemia, hyponatremia, hypermagnesemia, acidosis).

Clinical Manifestations

GEN	pallor, cyanosis
CVS	tachycardia, bradycardia, cardiac arrest
RESP	may be associated with stridor, wheezing, rhinorrhoa, cough, respiratory arrest
CNS	macrocephaly, signs of ↑ ICP, hypotonia, seizures, lethargy

Diagnostics

Blood	ABG/CBG, CBC, differential, electrolytes, BUN, creatinine, glucose, Ca^{++}, Mg^{++}, drug screen
Urine	urinalysis, drug screen
Imaging	chest radiograph, head CT scan, lateral neck radiograph
Others	sepsis work-up to include lumbar puncture, RSV nasal wash
Consider	EEG, EKG, esophagogram, sleep pneumogram, metabolic screen

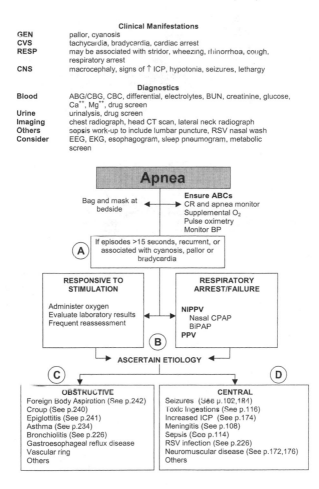

Apnea

Bag and mask at bedside ← → **Ensure ABCs**
CR and apnea monitor
Supplemental O_2
Pulse oximetry
Monitor BP

(A) If episodes >15 seconds, recurrent, or associated with cyanosis, pallor or bradycardia

RESPONSIVE TO STIMULATION	**RESPIRATORY ARREST/FAILURE**
Administer oxygen Evaluate laboratory results Frequent reassessment	**NIPPV** Nasal CPAP BiPAP **PPV**

(B)

→ ASCERTAIN ETIOLOGY ←

(C) (D)

OBSTRUCTIVE	**CENTRAL**
Foreign Body Aspiration (See p.242) Croup (See p.240) Epiglottitis (See p.241) Asthma (See p.234) Bronchiolitis (See p.226) Gastroesophageal reflux disease Vascular ring Others	Seizures (See p.102,184) Toxic Ingestions (See p.116) Increased ICP (See p.174) Meningitis (See p.108) Sepsis (See p.114) RSV infection (See p.226) Neuromuscular disease (See p.172,176) Others

Status Asthmaticus

Clarence Parks

- Asthma is a chronic inflammatory disorder of the airways involving mast cells, eosinophils and T lymphocytes. The inflammation results in recurrent episodes of wheezing, dyspnea and cough. Episodes are associated with widespread airflow obstruction that reverses spontaneously or with treatment. In addition, asthma is associated with increased airway responsiveness to a variety of stimuli.
- Status asthmaticus is an acute exacerbation of asthma that is unresponsive to routine treatment with inhaled bronchodilators. It can vary from mild to severe, with bronchospasm, airway inflammation and mucous plugging that can result in difficulty in breathing, CO_2 retention, hypoxemia, and respiratory failure.

Two phases of asthma:
Early asthma reaction (EAR): within minutes of exposure to an allergen, mast cells degranulate, and release histamine, prostaglandin D_2 and leukotrienes. These substances result in airway smooth muscle contraction increased capillary permeability, mucous secretion and activation of neuronal reflexes. The EAR is characterized by bronchoconstriction that generally responds to β-2 adrenergic drugs.
Late asthma reaction (LAR): the release of inflammatory mediators during the EAR primes adhesion molecules in the airway epithelium and capillary endothelium that allows eosinophils and other inflammatory cells to attach to the epithelium and endothelium. Additional inflammatory mediators are released which induce desquamation of the airway epithelium. The LAR is characterized by airway edema, increased mucous production, capillary leak and eventually, a hyperresponsive airway. This phase is more responsive to anti-inflammatory agents such as corticosteroids.

(A)

Signs and Symptoms	Mild	Moderate	Severe
Peak expiratory flow rate (PEFR)	>70% of predicted or baseline	50-70% of predicted or baseline	< 50% of predicted or baseline
Respiratory rate	30% above mean	30-50% above mean	>50% above mean
Alertness	Normal	Normal	Decreased
Dyspnea	Mild, speaking in full sentences	Moderate, speaking in partial sentences	Severe, single word speech
Accessory muscle use	Mild retractions	Moderate retractions, chest hyperinflation	Severe retractions and hyperinflation, nasal flaring
Color	Good	Pale	Cyanotic
Auscultation	End expiratory wheeze	Expiratory and inspiratory wheeze	↓ wheeze and ↓ breath sounds
Oxygen saturation	>95%	90-95%	<90%
$PaCO_2$	<35 mmHg	<40 mmHg	>40 mmHg

(B) Pulsus paradoxus – one of the most objective ways to assess severity of asthma (See p.298)
Chest radiographs should be considered to rule out pneumothorax or pneumomediastinum.

(C)

Blood gases in status asthmaticus:

	pH	$PaCO_2$	PaO_2
Mild	↑ or normal	↓ or normal	↓
Moderate	↔	↔	↓↓
Severe	↓	↑↑	↓↓↓

(D) Risk factors for severe status asthmaticus:
- child diagnosed with asthma before 1 y of age
- history of previous ICU admission with or without mechanical ventilation
- frequent ED visits/hospitalization
- less than 10% improvement in PEFR despite treatment
- poor understanding of their disease
- recent or current treatment with corticosteroids
- SpO_2 <90% despite supplemental oxygen

(E) **Albuterol** can cause tachycardia, but is generally well tolerated in children. Prolonged and especially continued use can result in tachyphylaxis. Like other β-adrenergic agents, albuterol results in kaliuresis; therefore, serum electrolytes should be monitored with continued use. **Continuous albuterol nebulization** should be considered if patient fails to improve on frequent intermittent nebulization. Basis for use is that the delivery of lower doses of drug at a continuous rate is more beneficial than repeated high intermittent doses. Has been shown to result in enough improvement in moderate to severe status asthmaticus to avoid intubation.

✳ Continued on p.236

Clinical Manifestations

(A) **HISTORY** presence of high risk factors, home medications (time of last dose) (B)
CVS tachycardia, hypertension, hypotension, **pulsus paradoxus**
RESP retractions, dyspnea, ability to speak full sentences, wheezing, air entry, cyanosis, **oxygen saturation (SpO₂)**
CNS lethargy, agitation, obtundation, syncope, seizures

Diagnostics

(C) **Blood** ABG/CBG, CBC, differential, theophylline levels if indicated, electrolytes
Imaging chest radiograph
Other peak expiratory flow rate (PEFR)

Status Asthmaticus
ED and In-patient Management

Ensure ABCs
Supplemental O₂ to maintain SpO₂ >95%
Pulse oximetry
IV access, assess hydration
Monitor BP

(D) Assess for risk factors

(E) **Bronchodilator by Nebulization**
albuterol 0.15 mg/kg/dose
MIN dose 2.5 mg
MAX dose 5 mg
May administer q 10-20 min. x 3

Begin supplemental oxygen

plus

Bronchodilator by Nebulization (F)
ipratropium bromide
< 40 kg 250 mcg/dose
> 40 kg 500 mcg/dose
or 2.5 mL (500 mcg) of 0.02% soln
Consider **levalbuterol** (G)

Reassess

Respiratory Failure
- < 10% improvement in PEFR after treatment
- SpO₂ < 92% despite supplemental oxygen
- Pulsus paradoxus > 15 mmHg
- Severe dyspnea, accessory muscle use, inability to speak more than 1 or 2 words at a time
- Inaudible wheezing with ↓ air entry
- Agitation, obtundation
- ☎ Notify ICU, obtain ABG (H)

Continue **supplemental O₂** (nonrebreather mask)

consider **epinephrine** (1:1000) 0.01 mL/kg SC (I)

methylprednisolone
2 mg/kg IV LD, then 1 mg/kg/dose q 6 h
MAX 60 mg/dose after LD

continuous albuterol nebulization (E)
0.3 – 0.45 mg/kg/h, MAX 15 mg/h

consider
continuous theophylline infusion IV (J) (K)
plus
terbutaline 2-10 mcg/kg loading dose, then begin continuous infusion 0.1-0.4 mcg/kg/min. ↑ by 0.1-0.2 mcg/kg/min q 30 min depending on clinical response
or
isoproterenol 0.05-0.5 mcg/kg/min.
↑ by 0.05 mcg/kg/min q 5-10 min if necessary

Respiratory Failure
Other Therapies to Consider

HeliOx by face mask (50:50, 60:40 or 70:30 mixture if patient's O₂ requirements allow) (L) (M)

MgSO₄ 25-50 mg/kg IV over 15-20 min. MAX ? g

(N) **Intubation and Mechanical Ventilation**
Suggested drugs for sedation and neuromuscular blockade:
ketamine 1 mg/kg/dose IV x 1
plus
midazolam 0.1 mg/kg/dose IV (O)
with or without
cisatracurium 0.1 mg/kg/dose IV

Consider **0.9 NS** 20 mL/kg IV bolus
Consider **THAM** 1 mEq/kg/dose IV for respiratory or metabolic acidosis
Use NaHCO₃ with caution (P)

- Monitor ABG, electrolytes
- Consider chest radiograph to rule out pneumothorax/ pneumomediastinum
- Maintain adequate oxygenation
- Once positive pressure ventilation is initiated, pulsus paradoxus is no longer reliable.

► ✱ Continued on p.237

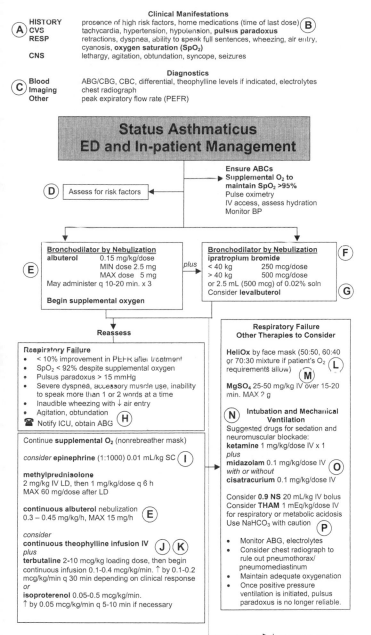

✳ Continued from p.234

Continuous albuterol: 0.3-0.45 mg/kg/h (MAX 15 mg/h). Switch to intermittent dosing when patient improves.

(F) **Ipratropium bromide** is an anticholinergic agent similar to atropine, but an additional ammonium group prevents systemic absorption. It may provide additional bronchodilation, and decreased mucous production as well, when used in combination with a β-2 agonist. It is **not** recommended for use as first-line therapy or as the sole agent for treatment of status asthmaticus.

(G) **Levalbuterol** is the pure R-isomer of racemic albuterol. 0.63 mg of levalbuterol is equal to 2.5 mg of albuterol. There have been few studies on the safety and efficacy of the use of levalbuterol in children.

(H) Indications for ICU admission:
- altered sensorium
- exhaustion
- markedly decreased air entry
- rising PCO_2 and hypoxemia despite aggressive treatment
- ICU admission is warranted for a patient with several high risk factors

Some children with severe status asthmaticus who do not respond to inhaled agents appear to benefit from **epinephrine** as a subcutaneus injection.

(J) When using intravenous β-adrenergic agents such as **terbutaline** or **isoproterenol**, it may be necessary to monitor CPK-MB levels and/or EKG tracings. These drugs increase the metabolic demands of the heart as a result of their chronotropicity. Continuous **terbutaline** IV infusion should be decreased if patient is also receiving theophylline.

(K) **Theophylline bolus**
- if previously on theophylline, **aminophylline** 3 mg/kg/dose IVB
- if **not** previously on theophylline, **aminophylline** 6 mg/kg/dose IVB
  1 mg/kg IV aminophylline ↑ serum level by 2 mcg/mL

Theophylline infusion		Adjust dose of theophylline in the presence of:
2-6 mos	0.4 mg/kg/h	• CHF
6-11 mos	0.7	• RSV infection
1-9 y	0.9	• liver dysfunction
9-12 y	0.7	• use of erythromycin, cimetidine or propranolol
> 12 y	0.5	• theophylline toxicity (See p.138)

(L) **HeliOx** has been shown to be of benefit in children with moderate to severe airway obstruction from status asthmaticus. Helium has a much lower density compared to nitrogen. Use of a helium/oxygen mixture (50:50, 60:40, 70:30) converts turbulent airflow to laminar airflow in a narrowed airway. It also increases deposition of nebulized drugs into the airway. The limitations to its use are the need for high O_2 requirements, and unavailability.

(M) **MgSO4** inhibits the slow inward calcium current through plasma membranes and competes with calcium for binding sites. It may provide some benefit in children with severe status asthmaticus. Dose 25-50 mg/kg/dose IV.

(N) Oxygen, intubation and mechanical ventilation:
- When SpO2 is persistently <90% despite aggressive therapy and supplemental oxygen, ABG should be obtained to better assess oxygenation/ventilation status.
- The MOST COMMON cause of death in asthma is HYPOXEMIA.
- Persistent hypoxemia with or without respiratory acidosis, along with altered mental status (agitation, exhaustion, lethargy or obtundation) are indications for intubation and mechanical ventilatory support.
- Goals of mechanical ventilation
  - correct hypoxemia
  - controlled hypoventilation – accept levels of PCO_2 up to 90 mmHg and pH >7.1 in attempt to minimize delivered tidal volume and peak inspiratory pressures. Ventilator rate should be maintained at no more than 12/minute, with a longer exhalation time (I:E ratio 1:3 or 1:4) to allow complete emptying of the lungs before the next breath is delivered.

(O) In selecting drugs to use for sedation and paralysis of a patient with asthma, it is preferable to avoid those which lead to further histamine release (morphine, pancuronium). Ketamine has beneficial direct smooth muscle relaxation effects, but can lead to increased secretions and arrhythmias. Addition of midazolam or other benzodiazepine is known to blunt the dissociative effects of ketamine.

(P) Intravascular volume status and metabolic acidosis: because of poor intake, vomiting, and diuresis (induced by medications), patients with severe status asthmaticus may develop inadequate volume status, metabolic acidosis, and even hypotension. Consider isotonic fluid bolus to improve intravascular volume status.
Correct acidosis with **THAM** 1 mEq/kg/dose IV or **NaHCO3** 1-2 mEq/kg/dose IVB

(Q) In children with mild to moderate asthma, **prednisone** 2 mg/kg/d PO div q 12 h is as efficacious as **methylprednisolone** 1 mg/kg/dose IV q 6 h. If IV access has not been established, and the patient is unable to tolerate PO medications, **dexamethasone** 1.5 mg/kg/dose by nebulizer may benefit children with mild to moderate asthma.

✻ Continued from p.235

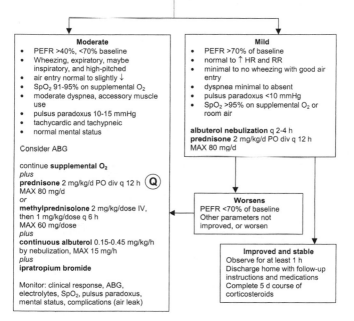

Moderate
- PEFR >40%, <70% baseline
- Wheezing, expiratory, maybe inspiratory, and high-pitched
- air entry normal to slightly ↓
- SpO_2 91-95% on supplemental O_2
- moderate dyspnea, accessory muscle use
- pulsus paradoxus 10-15 mmHg
- tachycardic and tachypneic
- normal mental status

Consider ABG

continue **supplemental O_2**
plus
prednisone 2 mg/kg/d PO div q 12 h $\textcircled{Q}$
MAX 80 mg/d
or
methylprednisolone 2 mg/kg/dose IV, then 1 mg/kg/dose q 6 h
MAX 60 mg/dose
plus
continuous albuterol 0.15-0.45 mg/kg/h by nebulization, MAX 15 mg/h
plus
ipratropium bromide

Monitor: clinical response, ABG, electrolytes, SpO_2, pulsus paradoxus, mental status, complications (air leak)

Mild
- PEFR >70% of baseline
- normal to ↑ HR and RR
- minimal to no wheezing with good air entry
- dyspnea minimal to absent
- pulsus paradoxus <10 mmHg
- SpO_2 >95% on supplemental O_2 or room air

albuterol nebulization q 2-4 h
prednisone 2 mg/kg/d PO div q 12 h
MAX 80 mg/d

Worsens
PEFR <70% of baseline
Other parameters not improved, or worsen

Improved and stable
Observe for at least 1 h
Discharge home with follow-up instructions and medications
Complete 5 d course of corticosteroids

NOTES

Dislodged Tracheostomy Tube

Mary Lieh-Lai

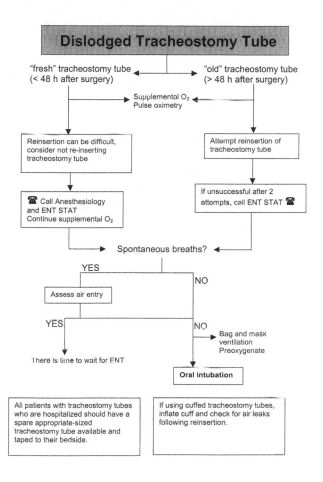

All patients with tracheostomy tubes who are hospitalized should have a spare appropriate-sized tracheostomy tube available and taped to their bedside.

If using cuffed tracheostomy tubes, inflate cuff and check for air leaks following reinsertion.

Croup/Laryngotracheobronchitis (LTB)

Mary Lieh-Lai

Croup or laryngotracheobronchitis (LTB) is a viral infection that affects the subglottic trachea and leads to extrathoracic airway obstruction. It is generally a mild disease, commonly seen during the winter months. Occasionally, a child with severe croup may require hospitalization and rarely, endotracheal intubation.

(A) Age: commonly 6 month – 3 years
Etiology: parainfluenza, influenza, RSV
Prodrome: URI symptoms and low-grade fever
Differential diagnoses: epiglottitis, bacterial tracheitis, retropharyngeal abscess, congenital or acquired subglottic stenosis, laryngeal web, or subglottic hemangioma.
In children with recurrent episodes of croup, history of BPD, prolonged intubation or subglottic stenosis, notify ENT for evaluation ☎

(B) Radiographic finding: "steeple sign", narrowing of the trachea at the level of the pyriform sinus which results from intraluminal edema. Consider magnified airway radiographs.

(A) Clinical Manifestations

barky cough, retractions can be severe, low-grade fever, URI prodrome, loud inspiratory stridor

Diagnostics
(B) ABG/CBG, CBC, differential, AP/lateral neck radiographs

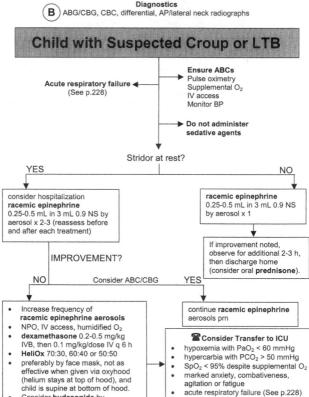

Child with Suspected Croup or LTB

Ensure ABCs
Pulse oximetry
Supplemental O₂
IV access
Monitor BP

Acute respiratory failure ◄
(See p.228)

▶ **Do not administer sedative agents**

Stridor at rest?

YES | **NO**

consider hospitalization
racemic epinephrine
0.25-0.5 mL in 3 mL 0.9 NS by aerosol x 2-3 (reassess before and after each treatment)

racemic epinephrine
0.25-0.5 mL in 3 mL 0.9 NS by aerosol x 1

If improvement noted, observe for additional 2-3 h, then discharge home (consider oral **prednisone**).

IMPROVEMENT?

NO — Consider ABC/CBG — **YES**

- Increase frequency of **racemic epinephrine** aerosols
- NPO, IV access, humidified O₂
- **dexamethasone** 0.2-0.5 mg/kg IVB, then 0.1 mg/kg/dose IV q 6 h
- **HeliOx** 70:30, 60:40 or 50:50
- preferably by face mask, not as effective when given via oxyhood (helium stays at top of hood), and child is supine at bottom of hood.
- Consider **budesonide** by nebulization

continue **racemic epinephrine** aerosols prn

☎ **Consider Transfer to ICU**
- hypoxemia with PaO₂ < 60 mmHg
- hypercarbia with PCO₂ > 50 mmHg
- SpO₂ < 95% despite supplemental O₂
- marked anxiety, combativeness, agitation or fatigue
- acute respiratory failure (See p.228)

Acute Epiglottitis

Thomas Brousseau

Acute epiglottitis is an emergency that if untreated, can progress rapidly to complete airway obstruction and death. Historically, acute epiglottitis was commonly due to *Haemophilus influenzae* type B. Incidence has decreased dramatically since the introduction of the *H. influenza* type B vaccine. Other organisms have recently been implicated (group A β-hemolytic streptococci, *S. pneumococcus*) as causative agents.

Clinical Manifestations

GEN	"toxic looking", anxious appearance, characteristic pose of sitting up, leaning forward with mouth open, drooling, fever
RESP	**abrupt onset** of dyspnea, nasal flaring, soft stridor

Diagnostics

CBC, differential, blood and throat culture (only after airway has been established)

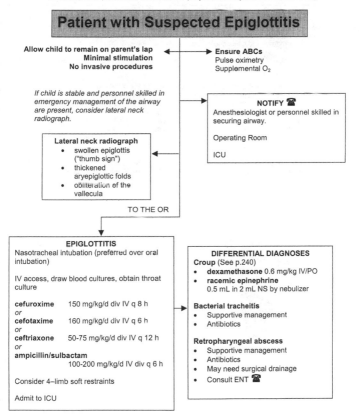

Patient with Suspected Epiglottitis

Allow child to remain on parent's lap
Minimal stimulation
No invasive procedures

Ensure ABCs
Pulse oximetry
Supplemental O$_2$

If child is stable and personnel skilled in emergency management of the airway are present, consider lateral neck radiograph.

NOTIFY ☎
Anesthesiologist or personnel skilled in securing airway.

Operating Room

ICU

Lateral neck radiograph
- swollen epiglottis ("thumb sign")
- thickened aryepiglottic folds
- obliteration of the vallecula

TO THE OR

EPIGLOTTITIS
Nasotracheal intubation (preferred over oral intubation)

IV access, draw blood cultures, obtain throat culture

cefuroxime	150 mg/kg/d div IV q 8 h
or	
cefotaxime	160 mg/kg/d div IV q 6 h
or	
ceftriaxone	50-75 mg/kg/d div IV q 12 h
or	
ampicillin/sulbactam	
	100-200 mg/kg/d IV div q 6 h

Consider 4–limb soft restraints

Admit to ICU

DIFFERENTIAL DIAGNOSES
Croup (See p.240)
- **dexamethasone** 0.6 mg/kg IV/PO
- **racemic epinephrine** 0.5 mL in 2 mL NS by nebulizer

Bacterial tracheitis
- Supportive management
- Antibiotics

Retropharyngeal abscess
- Supportive management
- Antibiotics
- May need surgical drainage
- Consult ENT ☎

Foreign Body Aspiration

Laila Tutunji

Foreign body aspiration is one of the most important, preventable causes of unintentional deaths in children under 5 years of age. It accounts for 10% of deaths in children < 1 y of age. Less than 30% of children who aspirate foreign bodies come to medical attention within the first 24 hours of the event. Unless the foreign body is causing complete airway obstruction, the initial symptoms may subside.

A

Organic	Inorganic
peanuts (most common)	toy parts
hot dogs and bread (most dangerous)	crayons
vegetables (most irritating)	coins
popcorn kernels	pins
seeds	needles
bones	bullets

B Signs and symptoms depend on the location of the foreign body. Unlike adults, aspirated objects do not always tend to lodge in the right main stem bronchus. Children can present immediately with coughing, gagging, choking or in respiratory arrest, but may also present days to months after the event with fever and signs and symptoms of pneumonia.

C ABG/CBG may show hypoxemia, hypercarbia or both depending on the degree and site of obstruction.

D Radiopaque foreign bodies will be visible on chest or lateral neck radiographs. With a radiolucent foreign body, effects of the object on the airway and lungs may still allow localization. Aspirated objects may cause partial obstruction, leading to a ball valve effect, causing differential expansion secondary to air trapping on the obstructed side and tracheal shift to the contralateral side. Inspiratory and expiratory films best detect this. If the child is unable to cooperate for inspiratory and expiratory films, left and right lateral decubitus radiographs can be obtained. The side with the foreign body will not deflate when placed on the dependent position. Complete obstruction leads to atelectasis and collapse with tracheal shift to the affected side.

E If antibiotics are indicated, provide coverage for anaerobic organisms. Occasionally, children with intense inflammatory reaction to organic material aspiration may benefit from a course of corticosteroids.

Clinical Manifestations

(A) History
history of possible foreign body aspiration, toys at home with small detachable parts, work-up should be pursued in all patients with clinical signs and symptoms of foreign body aspiration despite the lack of a witnessed event

(B) Initial presentation
choking, stridor, gagging, coughing, wheezing, with or without cyanosis, inability to vocalize, respiratory arrest may occur with complete airway obstruction.

Late presentation
persistent and localized wheezing and coughing, recurrent pneumonia with or without fever, hyperresonance on percussion

Diagnostics

(C) Blood
ABG/CBG, CBC, differential

(D) Imaging
PA and lateral chest radiograph, inspiratory and expiratory chest radiographs, lateral decubitus chest radiographs if indicated, occasionally, chest CT may be needed for localization of foreign body

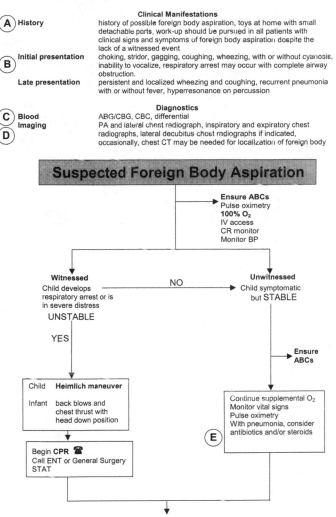

Suspected Foreign Body Aspiration

Ensure ABCs
Pulse oximetry
100% O$_2$
IV access
CR monitor
Monitor BP

Witnessed — NO → **Unwitnessed**
Child develops respiratory arrest or is in severe distress — Child symptomatic but STABLE

UNSTABLE

YES

Ensure ABCs

Child **Heimlich maneuver**

Infant back blows and chest thrust with head down position

Begin **CPR**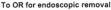
Call ENT or General Surgery STAT

Continue supplemental O$_2$
Monitor vital signs
Pulse oximetry
With pneumonia, consider
(E) antibiotics and/or steroids

To OR for endoscopic removal

Wheezing Other Than Asthma

Jyoti Panicker

> Wheezing is a high-pitched musical sound generally heard during the phase of exhalation. Not all that wheezes is asthma. Any obstruction in the intrathoracic extrapulmonary or intrapulmonary airway can lead to wheezing.

Common Causes of Wheezing in Infants and Children

Inflammatory	Mechanical Obstruction	Cardiac	Metabolic/Others
• bronchiolitis • cystic fibrosis • immotile cilia syndrome • aspiration • GERD • smoke inhalation • anaphylaxis • pneumonitis • immunodeficiency	• enlarged lymph nodes (tumors, TB) • vascular rings and slings • congenital anomalies of the airway • bronchial or pulmonary cysts • bronchopulmonary sequestration • lobar emphysema	• congestive heart failure • pulmonary venous obstruction	• hypocalcemic tetany • psychogenic

Differential Diagnosis of Wheezing

(A)

Clinical Manifestations	Diagnostics	Diagnosis/Initial Management
Abrupt onset, coughing, choking	chest radiograph, may need inspiratory/expiratory films	**foreign body aspiration** (See p.242) ENT or Pediatric Surgery consult ☎ Rigid bronchoscopy for removal
Fever, URI symptoms <6-12 mos of age, first episode	RSV nasal wash (See p.226)	**Bronchiolitis** (See p.226)
Respiratory distress observed after feeding, history of vomiting, spitting up or choking	pH probe, scintiscan or barium swallow	**GERD** may need therapy with propulsive agents or in severe cases, fundoplication
History of prematurity with mechanical ventilation	chest radiograph	bronchopulmonary dysplasia **(CHF)** may need diuretics
Recurrent pneumonia, failure to thrive, sinusitis	sweat chloride test immune function studies ciliary function studies	**cystic fibrosis immunodeficiency state immotile cilia**
Heart murmur, tachycardia, may have cardiomegaly or hepatomegaly	cardiac ECHO, EKG	**congestive heart failure, myocarditis, cardiomyopathy,** congenital heart disease **(CHD),** arrhythmias
Persistent wheezing despite bronchodilator therapy	barium swallow, chest CT or MRI, cardiac ECHO may be necessary	**vascular ring** consult CV surgery
Signs of tetany	serum Ca^{++}	**Hypocalcemic tetany** calcium supplementation
Adolescent with recurrent wheezing and no obvious cause	psychological evaluation	**Psychogenic**

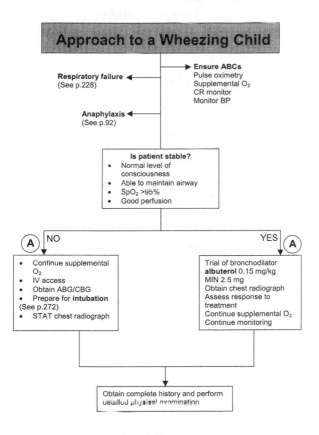

Approach to a Wheezing Child

Respiratory failure ◄──── ➤ **Ensure ABCs**
(See p.228)   Pulse oximetry
                                   Supplemental O₂
                                   CR monitor
                                   Monitor BP

Anaphylaxis ◄────
(See p.92)

Is patient stable?
- Normal level of consciousness
- Able to maintain airway
- SpO₂ >95%
- Good perfusion

(A) NO   YES (A)

- Continue supplemental O₂
- IV access
- Obtain ABG/CBG
- Prepare for **intubation** (See p.272)
- STAT chest radiograph

Trial of bronchodilator
albuterol 0.15 mg/kg
MIN 2.5 mg
Obtain chest radiograph
Assess response to treatment
Continue supplemental O₂
Continue monitoring

Obtain complete history and perform detailed physical examination

Chapter 14 ♣ Smoke Inhalation and Surface Burns

Burns: Thermal, Chemical and Electrical

Michelle Rubinstein

> Burn - an injury to tissue resulting from direct thermal insult, exposure to caustic chemicals or radiation, or contact with an electrical current.

(A) Degree of burns

First degree: superficial burns

 Epidermis only, painful, minimal edema, skin function remains intact

Second degree: partial thickness burns

- Superficial partial thickness

 Epidermal destruction plus < ½ of the dermis, pain, edema with blisters, superficial dermal capillary network still intact. Heals within 7-14 d with minimal scarring.

- Deep partial thickness

 Epidermal destruction plus > ½ of the dermis, white leathery, marble-like appearance to the skin. Dry speckled pattern seen secondary to thrombosed vessels, +/- pain. Heals slowly. Dense scarring occurs if skin heals by primary intention.

Third degree: full thickness burns

 Epidermis, dermis, and subcutaneous tissues destroyed. Skin pale or charred, +/- blisters. Skin grafting usually required.

Percentage of Surface Area of Head and Legs at Various Ages

Area in Diagram	Age in Years				
	0	1	5	10	15
A=1/2 of head	9 ½	8 ½	6 ½	5 ½	4 ½
B=1/2 of 1 thigh	2 ¾	3 ¼	4	4 ¼	4 ½
C=1/2 of 1 lower leg	2 ½	2 ½	2 ¾	3	3 ¼

From Solomon JR, Pediatric burns. Crit Care Clin, 1:161, 1985. With permission.

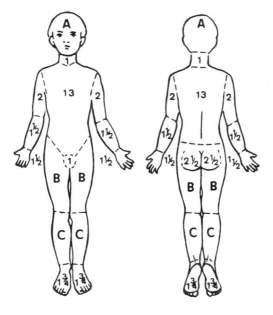

✳ Continued on p.248

Clinical Manifestations

Determine   degree of burn

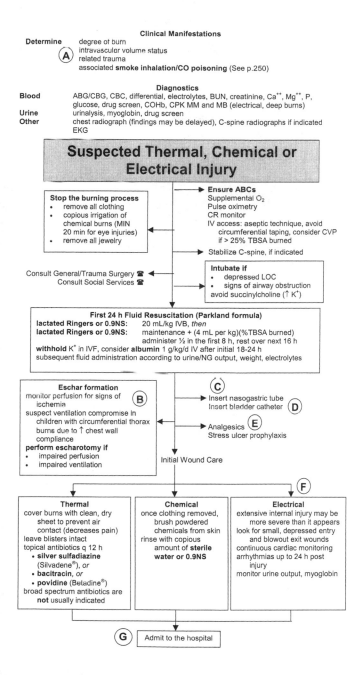

(A)   intravascular volume status

     related trauma

     associated **smoke inhalation/CO poisoning** (See p.250)

Diagnostics

Blood   ABG/CBG, CBC, differential, electrolytes, BUN, creatinine, Ca^{++}, Mg^{++}, P, glucose, drug screen, COHb, CPK MM and MB (electrical, deep burns)

Urine   urinalysis, myoglobin, drug screen

Other   chest radiograph (findings may be delayed), C-spine radiographs if indicated EKG

Suspected Thermal, Chemical or Electrical Injury

Ensure ABCs
Supplemental O_2
Pulse oximetry
CR monitor
IV access: aseptic technique, avoid circumferential taping, consider CVP if > 25% TBSA burned

Stop the burning process
- remove all clothing
- copious irrigation of chemical burns (MIN 20 min for eye injuries)
- remove all jewelry

Stabilize C-spine, if indicated

Consult General/Trauma Surgery ☎
Consult Social Services ☎

Intubate if
- depressed LOC
- signs of airway obstruction
avoid succinylcholine (↑ K^+)

First 24 h Fluid Resuscitation (Parkland formula)
lactated Ringers or 0.9NS: 20 mL/kg IVB, *then*
lactated Ringers or 0.9NS: maintenance + (4 mL per kg)(%TBSA burned)
     administer ½ in the first 8 h, rest over next 16 h
withhold K^+ in IVF, consider **albumin** 1 g/kg/d IV after initial 18-24 h
subsequent fluid administration according to urine/NG output, weight, electrolytes

Eschar formation
monitor perfusion for signs of ischemia (B)
suspect ventilation compromise in children with circumferential thorax burns due to ↑ chest wall compliance
perform escharotomy if
- impaired perfusion
- impaired ventilation

(C)
Insert nasogastric tube
Insert bladder catheter (D)

Analgesics (E)
Stress ulcer prophylaxis

Initial Wound Care

(F)

Thermal
cover burns with clean, dry sheet to prevent air contact (decreases pain)
leave blisters intact
topical antibiotics q 12 h
- **silver sulfadiazine** (Silvadene®), *or*
- **bacitracin**, *or*
- **povidine** (Betadine®)
broad spectrum antibiotics are **not** usually indicated

Chemical
once clothing removed, brush powdered chemicals from skin
rinse with copious amount of **sterile water or 0.9NS**

Electrical
extensive internal injury may be more severe than it appears
look for small, depressed entry and blowout exit wounds
continuous cardiac monitoring
arrhythmias up to 24 h post injury
monitor urine output, myoglobin

(G) → Admit to the hospital

✳ Continued from p.246

Obtain the following history:
　　Did the injury occur in a closed space? Assume **CO poisoning** (See p.250)
　　Were hazardous chemicals involved?
　　Was the patient intoxicated?
　　Check tetanus status.
　　A history of pre-existing cardiac or renal disease is significant in patients with electrical burns
　　　or myoglobinuria.

(B) Edema under the eschar impairs venous return, causing decreased arterial blood flow, ischemia, and gangrene. Observe for numbness, pain, cyanosis, and weak or absent peripheral pulses.

(C) TBSA burns ≥15% are associated with paralytic ileus, which may cause gastric distension.

(D) Monitor urine output. The most common cause of oliguria is inadequate fluid administration. Increased fluid requirements in patients with burns are associated with inhalation and electrical injuries, fractures, edema formation, delayed resuscitative efforts, and concomitant alcohol intoxication. See p.200 for management of **acute renal failure** and myoglobinuria.

(E) **Morphine sulfate** 0.1-0.15 mg/kg IV (**not** IM/SC) may be administered **only after** adequate circulation has been established and significant associated injuries have been ruled out, particularly due to its histamine-related vasodilatory effects and blunting of sensorium. Rule out other causes of agitation such as occult trauma, early shock, and hypoxia.

(F) Most electrical injuries are associated with low voltage 120V/AC. Newer data recommends a less aggressive approach. Patients with low voltage (< 1000V) electrical injuries who are asymptomatic and have only minor injuries/burns may be discharged home, after a thorough history and physical exam; extensive diagnostic and cardiac evaluation is not usually indicated. Children sustain oral injuries by mouthing electrical plugs, possibly requiring follow-up by Plastic Surgery.

(G)

Admission criteria

partial thickness burn ≥10% TBSA	
full thickness burns ≥2%TBSA	
burn areas with high risk for disability or poor cosmetic outcome	• 1% burn to the face, perineum, hands, feet • circumferential burns • burns overlying joints
chemical and electrical burns	• loss of consciousness • water contact • sustained tetany • entry and exit wounds on different extremities • current path crosses the heart • oral commissural burns
evidence of smoke inhalation or CO poisoning (See p.250)	
children with burns + associated trauma	
suspected child abuse	• burn pattern does not match history provided • submersion injuries are well-demarcated, symmetrical or circumferential burns of the buttocks, hands or feet • cigarette burns are deep, small and circular • contact burns with deep, geometric patterns or sharply demarcated borders

NOTES

Smoke Inhalation Injury and Carbon Monoxide (CO) Poisoning

Michelle Rubinstein

> Smoke inhalation becomes evident in the airway and lungs within the first 5 days following the inhalation of thermal and chemical products of combustion.
> - Chemical injury can occur at any level of the respiratory tract, because chemicals and their metabolites cause cellular damage. Typically causes lower airway (subglottic) injury.
> - Thermal injury is usually limited to the upper airway (supraglottic).

(A) Cherry-red color of the lips and skin classically associated with CO poisoning, is clinically infrequent and may be due to thermal injury instead. Victims may also exhibit pallor secondary to vasoconstriction.

(B) Chest radiograph may show diffuse interstitial infiltration or local areas of atelectasis and edema.

(C) Upper airway lesions
Usually due to thermal inhalation that actually causes burns and severe edema of the naso/oropharynx and laryngeal structures. In severely hypovolemic patients, supraglottic edema may not manifest until after fluid resuscitation is initiated.

(D) Lower airway lesions
Usually due to chemical inhalation.
The immediate effects of smoke inhalation include loss of ciliary action, mucosal edema, bronchiolitis, alveolar epithelial damage, and impaired gas exchange. Areas of atelectasis worsen V/Q mismatch. Later effects include sloughing of the tracheobronchial mucosa and mucopurulent membrane formation, with increased risk of infection. After 24 h, pathology resembles that of acute respiratory distress syndrome.

(E) CO poisoning
Is also seen with the use of improperly vented stoves, faulty or rear-vented exhaust systems in open trucks, faulty or non-vented fireplaces, etc.

COHb level	Manifestations
0.3-1% (endogenous)	none
1-10% (asymptomatic)	↑ threshold to visual stimuli, ↓ angina threshold
10-20% (mild toxicity)	mild headache and/or confusion
20-40% (moderate toxicity)	worsening headache, nausea, vomiting, irritability, weakness, dizziness, mental status changes, shortness of breath, shock
40-60% (severe toxicity)	as above, plus ↑ HR, ↑RR, seizures, syncope, death
> 60%	coma, usually death

Use of **Hyperbaric Oxygen (HBO)**
The t ½ of COHb in room air is 4-6 h. Half-life is reduced to 45-60 min when 100% oxygen is administered and to 20-30 min when using HBO.

Considerations for HBO treatment
- symptomatic patients with persistent neurologic and cardiovascular symptoms
- COHb levels ≥25-40%
- recurrent (up to 3 weeks) and/or persistent (> 6 h) symptoms after initial treatment with 100% O_2
- pregnant women with COHb levels > 15-20% or if fetal monitoring indicates distress, regardless of the mother's COHb level

(F) Cyanide has a t ½ of approximately 1 h, so levels are difficult to detect. Cyanide antidote kit should only be used if poisoning is highly suspect. The first step consists of administering nitrite that may result in methemoglobinemia; may skip to step 2. The second step consists of administering thiosulfate. This treatment enhances detoxification and elimination of cyanide.

(G) Consider admission for the following:
- history of stupor or loss of consciousness at the scene
- abnormal vital signs at the scene or vital signs remain abnormal
- elevated COHb due to a house fire
- persistent mental status changes or confusion
- COHb ≥15-20%

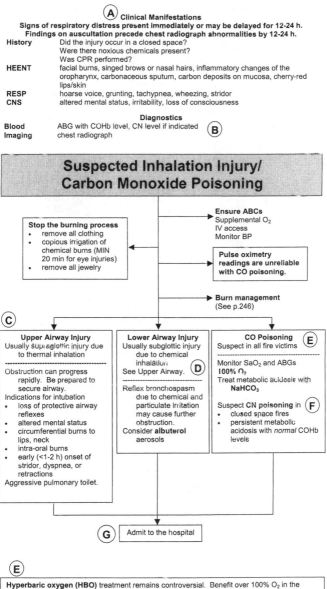

(A) Clinical Manifestations

Signs of respiratory distress present immediately or may be delayed for 12-24 h.
Findings on auscultation precede chest radiograph abnormalities by 12-24 h.

History	Did the injury occur in a closed space? Were there noxious chemicals present? Was CPR performed?
HEENT	facial burns, singed brows or nasal hairs, inflammatory changes of the oropharynx, carbonaceous sputum, carbon deposits on mucosa, cherry-red lips/skin
RESP	hoarse voice, grunting, tachypnea, wheezing, stridor
CNS	altered mental status, irritability, loss of consciousness

Diagnostics

Blood	ABG with COHb level, CN level if indicated (B)
Imaging	chest radiograph

Suspected Inhalation Injury/ Carbon Monoxide Poisoning

Ensure ABCs
Supplemental O₂
IV access
Monitor BP

Stop the burning process
- remove all clothing
- copious irrigation of chemical burns (MIN 20 min for eye injuries)
- remove all jewelry

Pulse oximetry readings are unreliable with CO poisoning.

► Burn management
(See p.246)

(C)

Upper Airway Injury
Usually supraglottic injury due to thermal inhalation

Obstruction can progress rapidly. Be prepared to secure airway.
Indications for intubation
- loss of protective airway reflexes
- altered mental status
- circumferential burns to lips, neck
- intra-oral burns
- early (<1-2 h) onset of stridor, dyspnea, or retractions
Aggressive pulmonary toilet.

Lower Airway Injury
Usually subglottic injury due to chemical inhalation
See Upper Airway. (D)

Reflex bronchospasm due to chemical and particulate irritation may cause further obstruction.
Consider **albuterol** aerosols

CO Poisoning (E)
Suspect in all fire victims

Monitor SaO₂ and ABGs
100% O₂
Treat metabolic acidosis with **NaHCO₃**

Suspect **CN poisoning** in (F)
- closed space fires
- persistent metabolic acidosis with *normal* COHb levels

(G) Admit to the hospital

(E)

Hyperbaric oxygen (HBO) treatment remains controversial. Benefit over 100% O₂ in the immediate care setting has not been shown.
Treatment with 100% O₂ should not be delayed, while awaiting transport to a facility with HBO. Patients must be stable for transport.
An HBO chamber and qualified staff must be available to perform the procedure safely.

Chapter 15 ♣ Trauma

Stabilization of the Trauma Patient

Michelle Rubinstein

Trauma is defined in terms of extent (local vs multiple), mechanism (blunt vs penetrating), and severity. It is the **number one** cause of death in children > 1 y of age in the US. 80% of all pediatric trauma is secondary to blunt injury. The most common causes of traumatic deaths in decreasing order are motor vehicular accidents (approximately 50%), homicide, suicide, drowning, pedestrian/motor vehicular accidents, and burns.

Always begin with the **primary survey/ABCDE** of trauma resuscitation:

(A)
- **A – Airway** and C-spine stabilization
- **B – Breathing** and ventilation
- **C – Circulation** and hemorrhage control
- **D – Disability** (neurologic status)
- **E – Exposure** and environment control

(B) The Pediatric GCS: 14-15 is normal and ≤ 8 represents severe neurologic deficit/injury. Patients with GCS ≤ 8 require intubation. CT scan of the head is recommended **only after stabilization** of the airway and circulation.

Eye Opening		Motor response	
4	Spontaneous	6	Spontaneous (obeys verbal commands)
3	To speech	5	Localizes pain
2	To pain	4	Withdraws to pain
1	No response	3	Decorticate posture
		2	Decerebrate posture
		1	No response

Best verbal response (pediatric adaptation)

5	Oriented	Social smile, orients to sound, follows objects, coos, converses, interacts appropriately with environment
4	Confused/disoriented	Consolable crying, aware of environment, uncooperative interactions
3	Inappropriate words	Inappropriate persistent crying, moaning, inconsistently aware of environment/inconsistently consolable
2	Incomprehensible words	Agitated, restless, inconsolable crying, unaware of environment
1	No response	No response

From Rubinstein JS, Hageman HR. Monitoring of critically ill children. *Critical Care Clinics* 4:621,1988 with permission

Vital Signs by Age

(C)

Age	Weight (kg)	Heart Rate (bpm)	Systolic BP (mmHg)	Respiratory Rate
Preterm	2	120-180	40-60	55-65
Term Newborn	3	90-170	52-92	40-60
1 month	4	110-180	60-104	30-50
6 months	7	110-180	65-125	25-35
1 y	10	80-160	70-118	20-30
2 y	12	80-130	73-117	20-30
4 y	16	80-120	65-117	20-30
6 y	20	75-115	76-116	18-24
8 y	25	70-110	79-119	18-22
10 y	30	70-110	82-122	16-20
12 y	40	60-110	84-128	16-20
14 y	50	60-105	84-136	16-20

From Iliff A, Lee VA, Pulse rate, respiratory rate, and body temperature of children between two months and eighteen years of age. *Child Dev* 23:237, 1952. With permission.

The Pediatric Trauma Score

(D)

PTS	+ 2	+ 1	- 1
Airway	Normal	Oral/nasal airway required	Intubated, tracheostomy, invasive
Level of consciousness	Completely awake	Obtunded or any LOC	Comatose
Weight	> 20 kg	10-20 kg	< 20 kg
BP (systolic)	> 90 mmHg	50-90 mmHg	< 50 mmHg
Open wound	None	Minor	Major or penetrating
Fractures	None	Minor	Open or multiple fractures, gunshot wounds

The pediatric trauma score is used to assess injury severity, and is based on factors known to increase mortality and morbidity. A score of ≤ 8 indicates significant trauma and these patients should be transferred to the nearest pediatric trauma center.

Adapted from the Committee on Trauma of the American College of Surgeons. *Advanced Trauma Life Support Course for Physicians* 1993, p.394. American College of Surgeons, with permission.

✱ Continued on p.254

"Assume every injury until proven otherwise"

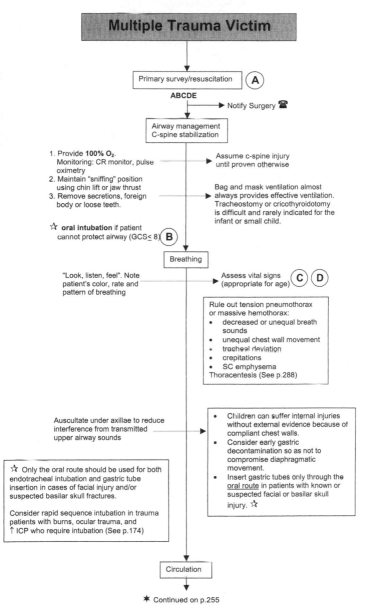

Multiple Trauma Victim

Primary survey/resuscitation (A)

ABCDE

→ Notify Surgery ☎

Airway management
C-spine stabilization

1. Provide **100% O₂**.
   Monitoring: CR monitor, pulse oximetry
2. Maintain "sniffing" position using chin lift or jaw thrust
3. Remove secretions, foreign body or loose teeth.

→ Assume c-spine injury until proven otherwise

→ Bag and mask ventilation almost always provides effective ventilation. Tracheostomy or cricothyroidotomy is difficult and rarely indicated for the infant or small child.

☆ **oral intubation** if patient cannot protect airway (GCS ≤ 8) (B)

Breathing

"Look, listen, feel". Note patient's color, rate and pattern of breathing

→ Assess vital signs (C) (D)
(appropriate for age)

Rule out tension pneumothorax or massive hemothorax:
- decreased or unequal breath sounds
- unequal chest wall movement
- tracheal deviation
- crepitations
- SC emphysema
Thoracentesis (See p.288)

Auscultate under axillae to reduce interference from transmitted upper airway sounds

- Children can suffer internal injuries without external evidence because of compliant chest walls.
- Consider early gastric decontamination so as not to compromise diaphragmatic movement.
- Insert gastric tubes only through the <u>oral route</u> in patients with known or suspected facial or basilar skull injury. ☆

☆ Only the oral route should be used for both endotracheal intubation and gastric tube insertion in cases of facial injury and/or suspected basilar skull fractures.

Consider rapid sequence intubation in trauma patients with burns, ocular trauma, and ↑ ICP who require intubation (See p.174)

Circulation

✱ Continued on p.255

✳ Continued from p.252

(E) Fractures and musculoskeletal injuries occur frequently in children but are rarely life threatening, except in the following situations (obtain STAT surgical consult ☎):
1. Pelvic fractures that can result in significant blood loss
2. Arterial hemorrhage from either blunt or penetrating injury
   - cool, pale, pulseless extremity
   - rapidly expanding hematoma
3. Crush injuries that lead to rhabdomyolysis and renal failure

(F) Limb-threatening injuries
1. Open fractures
   - immobilization, systemic antibiotics, cover area with sterile dressing
   - consult Orthopedics service ☎ following stabilization of patient
2. Vascular injuries and amputations
3. Compartment syndrome: vascular insufficiency and compromise due to increased pressure within a fascial compartment usually resulting from edema or hemorrhage. Irreversible muscle necrosis can occur within 6-8 hours of onset. If suspected, consult **Orthopedics** STAT ☎.
   - most common in lower leg, forearm, feet and hands
   - signs and symptoms: pain, paresthesias, pallor, pulselessness, paralysis
4. Nerve injuries
   - usually associated with fracture and/or dislocation
   - reduction of fracture/dislocation should only be attempted by skilled personnel

✱ Continued from p.253

Circulation

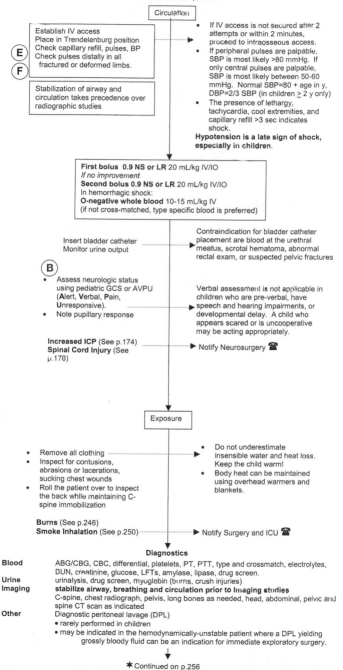

Ⓔ
Ⓕ
Establish IV access
Place in Trendelenburg position
Check capillary refill, pulses, BP
Check pulses distally in all
fractured or deformed limbs.

Stabilization of airway and
circulation takes precedence over
radiographic studies

- If IV access is not secured after 2
  attempts or within 2 minutes,
  proceed to intraosseous access.
- If peripheral pulses are palpable,
  SBP is most likely >80 mmHg. If
  only central pulses are palpable,
  SBP is most likely between 50-60
  mmHg. Normal SBP=80 + age in y,
  DBP=2/3 SBP (in children ≥ 2 y only)
- The presence of lethargy,
  tachycardia, cool extremities, and
  capillary refill >3 sec indicates
  shock.
  **Hypotension is a late sign of shock,
  especially in children.**

First bolus 0.9 NS or LR 20 mL/kg IV/IO
If no improvement
Second bolus 0.9 NS or LR 20 mL/kg IV/IO
In hemorrhagic shock:
O-negative whole blood 10-15 mL/kg IV
(if not cross-matched, type specific blood is preferred)

Insert bladder catheter
Monitor urine output

Contraindication for bladder catheter
placement are blood at the urethral
meatus, scrotal hematoma, abnormal
rectal exam, or suspected pelvic fractures

Ⓑ
- Assess neurologic status
  using pediatric GCS or AVPU
  (**A**lert, **V**erbal, **P**ain,
  Unresponsive).
- Note pupillary response

Verbal assessment is not applicable in
children who are pre-verbal, have
speech and hearing impairments, or
developmental delay. A child who
appears scared or is uncooperative
may be acting appropriately.

Increased ICP (See p.174)
Spinal Cord Injury (See
p.170)

Notify Neurosurgery ☎

Exposure

- Remove all clothing
- Inspect for contusions,
  abrasions or lacerations,
  sucking chest wounds
- Roll the patient over to inspect
  the back while maintaining C-
  spine immobilization

- Do not underestimate
  insensible water and heat loss.
  Keep the child warm!
- Body heat can be maintained
  using overhead warmers and
  blankets.

Burns (See p.246)
Smoke Inhalation (See p.250)

Notify Surgery and ICU ☎

Diagnostics

Blood	ABG/CBG, CBC, differential, platelets, PT, PTT, type and crossmatch, electrolytes, BUN, creatinine, glucose, LFTs, amylase, lipase, drug screen.
Urine	urinalysis, drug screen, myoglobin (burns, crush injuries)
Imaging	**stabilize airway, breathing and circulation prior to imaging studies**
	C-spine, chest radiograph, pelvis, long bones as needed, head, abdominal, pelvic and spine CT scan as indicated
Other	Diagnostic peritoneal lavage (DPL)
	• rarely performed in children
	• may be indicated in the hemodynamically-unstable patient where a DPL yielding grossly bloody fluid can be an indication for immediate exploratory surgery.

✱ Continued on p.256

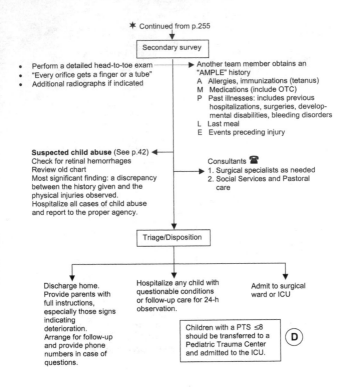

✳ Continued from p.255

Secondary survey

- Perform a detailed head-to-toe exam
- "Every orifice gets a finger or a tube"
- Additional radiographs if indicated

Another team member obtains an "AMPLE" history
A Allergies, immunizations (tetanus)
M Medications (include OTC)
P Past illnesses: includes previous hospitalizations, surgeries, developmental disabilities, bleeding disorders
L Last meal
E Events preceding injury

Suspected child abuse (See p.42)
Check for retinal hemorrhages
Review old chart
Most significant finding: a discrepancy between the history given and the physical injuries observed.
Hospitalize all cases of child abuse and report to the proper agency.

Consultants ☎
1. Surgical specialists as needed
2. Social Services and Pastoral care

Triage/Disposition

Discharge home. Provide parents with full instructions, especially those signs indicating deterioration. Arrange for follow-up and provide phone numbers in case of questions.

Hospitalize any child with questionable conditions or follow-up care for 24-h observation.

Admit to surgical ward or ICU

Children with a PTS ≤8 should be transferred to a Pediatric Trauma Center and admitted to the ICU. **D**

NOTES

Near Drowning

Michael Fiore

Drowning is the 2nd most common cause of injury-related deaths in children 1-14 years of age.
Drowning: death from asphyxia within 24 hours of a submersion injury.
Near drowning: survival beyond 24 hours after a submersion episode. May also be fatal.
Wet drowning: aspiration of fluid into the lungs (90% of drowning)
Dry drowning: drowning without fluid aspiration, presumably from laryngospasm and hypoxemia
Warm water $\geq 20°$ C, cold water $< 20°$ C, very cold water $\leq 5°$ C

(A)

Risk Factors
Age: Bimodal distribution
Children < 4 years old
swimming pools, bathtubs, and buckets
must consider child abuse in drowning in children < 1 year of age
Adolescents 15 – 19 years old
natural bodies of water (ponds, lakes, rivers, oceans)
frequently associated with boating, alcohol, and high risk behavior
• Gender: male to female ratio 4:1
• Warm weather months
• Lack of adult supervision
• Improper safety barriers enclosing residential swimming pools
• Substance use
• Predisposing factors: seizures, mental retardation, arrhythmias, neuromuscular disease, head or spine injury, syncope, apnea, hyperventilation, hypoglycemia, suicide
Infant/toddler swimming lesson programs do not prevent drowning.

The pathophysiology of near drowning is related to the multi-organ effects of hypoxemia which is the most important factor in morbidity and mortality.

The type of water aspirated (fresh or salt water) has little clinical significance. End result is interruption of the alveolar/capillary unit, pneumonitis, atelectasis, pulmonary edema, and hypoxemia.

The success or failure of initial basic life support provided at the scene of the immersion is the most important determinant of outcome. Patients without cardiac activity upon arrival to the Emergency Department have a very poor prognosis. **(B)**

Points to consider in rescue of a near drowning victim
- Rescue breathing should be initiated ASAP, even while still in the water.
- Chest compressions are not effective when performed in water.
- The Heimlich maneuver is not effective in removing aspirated water.
- Any debris visualized in the oropharynx should be removed.
- Anticipate vomiting, attempt to prevent aspiration.

Intravascular volume depletion is common, due to pulmonary edema and intracompartmental fluid shifts, regardless of the type of fluid aspirated.

Patients with severe hypothermia after very cold water immersions should be fully warmed before cessation of resuscitation efforts.

(C)

Conn-Barker Classification of Severity
Most applicable within 10 minutes of initial resuscitation efforts
Category A (awake)
Conscious with normal neurologic function
GCS 15
Asymptomatic or minimal respiratory symptoms
May have mild alterations in chest radiograph, blood gas analysis
Category B (blunted)
Impaired cortical function (obtunded or stuporous)
Normal brainstem function (normal respiratory pattern and purposeful movements to pain)
Respiratory distress with abnormalities in blood gas and chest radiograph
Category C (comatose)
Cortical dysfunction and brainstem dysfunction (abnormal respiratory pattern, abnormal response to painful stimuli)
• C1 (decorticate) – Cheyne-Stokes respirations
• C2 (decerebrate) – central hyperventilation
• C3 (flaccid) – apneic or terminal respiratory effort, GCS 3
• C4 (death) – cardiopulmonary arrest
* Categories C3 and C4 have a poor prognosis for intact neurologic survival

Clinical Manifestations

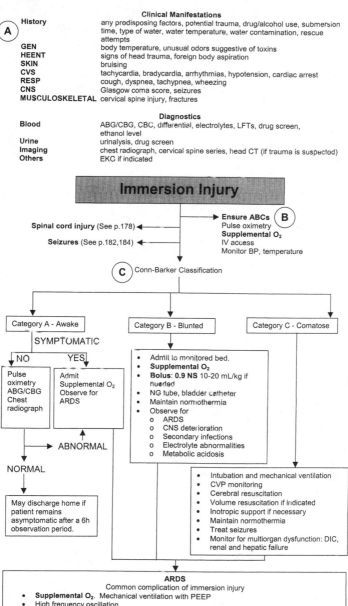

History	any predisposing factors, potential trauma, drug/alcohol use, submersion time, type of water, water temperature, water contamination, rescue attempts
GEN	body temperature, unusual odors suggestive of toxins
HEENT	signs of head trauma, foreign body aspiration
SKIN	bruising
CVS	tachycardia, bradycardia, arrhythmias, hypotension, cardiac arrest
RESP	cough, dyspnea, tachypnea, wheezing
CNS	Glasgow coma score, seizures
MUSCULOSKELETAL	cervical spine injury, fractures

Diagnostics

Blood	ABG/CBG, CBC, differential, electrolytes, LFTs, drug screen, ethanol level
Urine	urinalysis, drug screen
Imaging	chest radiograph, cervical spine series, head CT (if trauma is suspected)
Others	EKG if indicated

Immersion Injury

Ensure ABCs (B)
Pulse oximetry
Supplemental O₂
IV access
Monitor BP, temperature

Spinal cord injury (See p.178) ◄

Seizures (See p.182,184) ◄

(C) Conn-Barker Classification

Category A - Awake

SYMPTOMATIC

NO / YES

NO →
Pulse oximetry
ABG/CBG
Chest radiograph

YES →
Admit
Supplemental O₂
Observe for ARDS

→ ABNORMAL

NORMAL

May discharge home if patient remains asymptomatic after a 6h observation period.

Category B - Blunted

- Admit to monitored bed.
- **Supplemental O₂**
- **Bolus: 0.9 NS** 10-20 mL/kg if needed
- NG tube, bladder catheter
- Maintain normothermia
- Observe for
  - ARDS
  - CNS deterioration
  - Secondary infections
  - Electrolyte abnormalities
  - Metabolic acidosis

Category C - Comatose

- Intubation and mechanical ventilation
- CVP monitoring
- Cerebral resuscitation
- Volume resuscitation if indicated
- Inotropic support if necessary
- Maintain normothermia
- Treat seizures
- Monitor for multiorgan dysfunction: DIC, renal and hepatic failure

ARDS
Common complication of immersion injury

- **Supplemental O₂.** Mechanical ventilation with PEEP
- High frequency oscillation
- ECMO and surfactant therapy of unproven benefit.
- Aggressive management for ARDS in near drowning should be tempered by the severity of hypoxic-ischemic CNS injury

NOTES

Section III ♣ Procedures

- Abdominal Paracentesis
- Radial Arterial Puncture
- Double Volume Exchange Transfusion
- Femoral Vein Cannulation
- Intraosseous Needle Placement
- Endotracheal Intubation
- Partial Exchange Transfusion
- Percutaneous Pericardiocentesis
- Rapid Sequence Intubation (RSI)
- Subclavian Catheter Placement
- Subdural Tap
- Suprapubic Bladder Aspiration
- Thoracentesis: Needle Aspiration of Pneumothorax
- Umbilical Vein/Artery Cannulation (UVC/UAC)
- Tapping a Ventriculoperitoneal Shunt (VPS)
- Conscious Sedation
- Non-Invasive Monitoring
- Temporary Cardiac Pacing
- Measurement of Pulsus Paradoxus

Abdominal Paracentesis

Russell Clark

Indications
- Diagnostic: ascites associated with unexplained fever, leukocytosis, suspicion of spontaneous bacterial peritonitis, abdominal pain.
- Therapeutic: massive ascites and respiratory compromise, or risk of rupture of umbilical or abdominal hernia

Contraindications: coagulopathy, immunocompromised state, pregnancy, suspected intraabdominal adhesions or obstruction

Complications: bleeding, infection, perforation of internal organ, ascitic leak, hypotension

Equipment and supplies

- bladder catheter
- sterile gloves, gown, hat, mask and drapes x 4
- several sterile 4x4 gauze
- povidone-iodine solution
- 5 mL 1% lidocaine with epinephrine
- 5 mL syringe, 10 mL syringe, 50 mL syringe
- 25-gauge x 1 inch needle, 14 to 18-gauge x 2 inch angiocatheter
- 1 liter evacuated collection bottles as required
- IV tubing
- 3 way stopcock
- aerobic and anaerobic culture bottles
- 4 red top tubes for chemistry studies, one purple top tube for cell count and differential
- assistant
- bag and mask, O_2, CR monitor, pulse oximeter, automated blood pressure machine

Procedure

1. Empty urinary bladder, electively or via bladder catheter.
2. Position patient supine or with head and chest up at 30° as desired.
3. Confirm presence of ascitic fluid (physical examination or abdominal ultrasound).
4. Select site on abdomen for tap A or B (See figure on p.263)
5. A is 1-2 cm caudad to the umbilicus in the midline
6. B is 2-4 cm cephalad to the anterior superior iliac spine, just lateral to the rectus abdominis sheath.
7. Prepare and drape skin in sterile fashion.
8. Anesthetize location on skin with 1% lidocaine with epinephrine, and using Z track technique anesthetize the parietal peritoneum and subcutaneous fatty tissue 1 cm below the skin site.
9. Assemble 10 mL syringe - 3 way stopcock and 18 gauge angiocatheter in series with the IV tubing on the "T" port of the stopcock, and lever off to IV tubing.
10. Apply gentle suction while entering the peritoneal cavity, along the same Z track anesthetized above. When ascitic fluid returns, advance the angiocatheter over the needle and remove the needle. Withdraw 10 mL peritoneal fluid for studies.
11. Attach 50 mL syringe in place of 10 mL on stopcock and withdraw 50-100 mL fluid for further diagnostic studies. Introduce opposite end of IV tubing into a 1 liter evacuated collection bottle and turn stopcock for therapeutic paracentesis, repeat as desired to withdraw preselected volume.
12. Apply dressing
13. Procedure note.

Studies: specific gravity, protein, albumin, glucose, LDH, amylase (If suspecting pancreatitis, also send serum amylase), cell count and differential, Gram stain, culture, acid fast bacillus stain & culture, fungal stain & culture, cytology (suspected neoplasm), triglyceride, bilirubin.

NOTE: Notify pathology for cellblock studies.

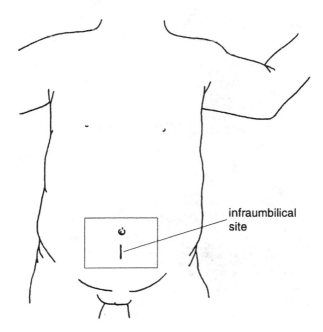

infraumbilical
site

Abdominal paracentesis

Radial Arterial Puncture

Thomas Brousseau

Indications: to obtain blood for blood gas analysis, blood chemistries

---

Equipment/supplies

- 22 gauge Butterfly® needle
- alcohol and povidone-iodine wipes
- tuberculin syringe with a minute amount of heparin
  (too much heparin can result in a falsely low pH)
- 2 x 2 or 4 x 4 gauze
- gloves

Procedure

1. Refer to diagram for landmarks of radial artery.
2. Perform the Allen test to confirm good ulnar collateral circulation.
3. Palpate radial pulse to ascertain location of the vessel.
4. Clean area with povidone-iodine and alcohol.
5. Attach tuberculin syringe to Butterfly® needle, unless using arterial blood sampler
   (e.g., Smooth-E®).
6. Using the non-dominant hand, relocate the site of maximal pulsation. Insert and direct needle
   (at 20° to 30° angle) towards the pulsation. Allow the plunger to rise with the arterial pressure.
   If there is no blood return, gradually withdraw the needle. If both walls were punctured, a
   sample may be obtained during withdrawal. If unable to obtain sample, retract the needle
   until it is just deep in the dermis and redirect the needle.
7. After collecting sample, remove needle.
8. Apply pressure on area for at least 5 minutes.
9. Apply sterile gauze.
10. Remove air bubbles from the sample. If blood gas analysis cannot be done immediately, the
    sample may be stored in ice for up to 1 hour with minimum deterioration.
11. Procedure note.

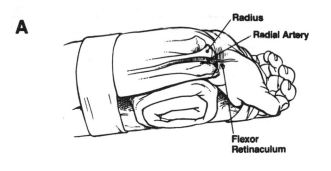

Arterial puncture. (From L Chameides, *Textbook of Pediatric Advanced Life Support.* Dallas: American Heart Association, 1994, p.45. With permission.)

NOTES

Double Volume Exchange Transfusion

Adiaha Spinks

Indications
- Hyperbilirubinemia
- Sepsis/DIC, e.g., meningococcemia
- Acute leukemia with WBC > 250,000/mm^3

Equipment/supplies

- One central venous and one arterial line are preferred. If unavailable, 2 large-bore venous lines can be used, but this may make the procedure difficult, especially in larger patients.
- 4-way or 6-way stopcock
- Tubing: one line connected to a container for discarded blood; one line connected to a filter and transfusion bag
- 10-mL, 20-mL, or 60-mL syringes depending on the aliquots planned
- Sterile drapes, gowns, gloves
- Type and crossmatched PRBC reconstituted with FFP (total volume 160 mL/kg)
- If a large volume of blood is going to be used, it may be necessary to administer Ca^{++} and glucose IV to the patient halfway through the procedure.
- Bag and mask, oxygen, pulse oximeter, CR monitor, automated blood pressure machine
- Progress note or exchange transfusion sheet, and an assistant to record ins and outs

Procedure

1. Obtain pre-exchange blood work: CBC with differential, total and direct bilirubin, PT, PTT, TT, Coomb's, serum electrolytes, glucose, Ca^{++}, P.
2. Blood should be at room or near body temperature.
3. Have equipment ready. This procedure is preferably done with two individuals—one removing blood from the arterial catheter, and the other administering fresh blood into the venous line. Aliquots can be 5-mL, 10-mL, 20-mL, or 60-mL removed or administered depending on the patient size.
4. Remember to administer Ca^{++} and glucose as needed during the procedure.
5. Monitor vital signs, O$_2$ saturation.
6. Obtain post-exchange labs: same as pre-exchange labs.
7. Procedure note.

Femoral Vein Cannulation

Adiaha Spinks

Indications: CVP monitoring, central venous access, and hyperalimentation

Complications: bleeding, infection, inadvertent arterial puncture

Equipment/supplies

- 1% lidocaine
- vascular access tray
- 3-mL, 5-mL, 10-mL, syringes
- sterile drape, gloves, mask
- 4 x 4 gauze
- povidone-iodine solution
- suture kit
- If patient requires sedation, bag and mask, O_2, pulse oximeter, automated blood pressure machine, CR monitor

Procedure

1. Place patient on back with leg externally rotated at 45° angle (frog leg position).
2. Palpate the femoral pulse. The femoral vein lies medial to the femoral artery.
   (Remember: **NAVEL**—from lateral to medial—**N**erve, **A**rtery, **V**ein, **E**mpty space, **L**ymphatics)
3. Prepare and drape area using sterile technique.
4. Anesthetize the area with 1% lidocaine.
5. Insert needle medial to femoral pulse 1-2 cm below inguinal ligament.
6. Advance needle at 45° angle directed at umbilicus until free flow of blood is obtained.
7. After successful cannulation of vessel, complete procedure using the Seldinger technique (placing a guidewire through needle into vein and introducing a sheath around the guidewire).
8. Check placement of CVC by radiograph. Secure with sutures and dress in same manner as other CVC.
9. Procedure note.

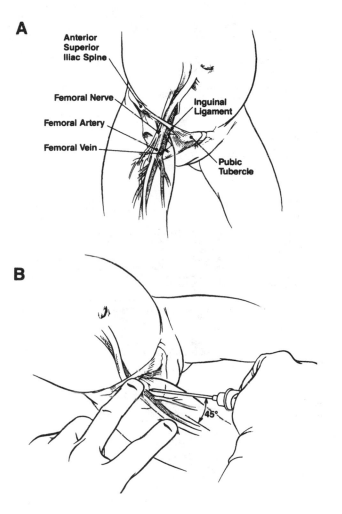

A

Anterior
Superior
Iliac Spine

Femoral Nerve

Femoral Artery

Femoral Vein

Inguinal
Ligament

Pubic
Tubercle

B

45°

Femoral vein cannulation. (From L Chameides, *Textbook of Pediatric Advanced Life Support*. Dallas: American Heart Association, Dallas, Texas, 1998. With permission.)

Intraosseous Needle Placement

Sujatha Kannan

> **Indications**: for emergency vascular access when venous route cannot be established
> **Complications**
> - extravasation of fluids/medication
> - infection, subcutaneous abscess, osteomyelitis
> - epiphyseal injury, fracture
> - fat embolism

Equipment/supplies

- intraosseous (IO) needle
- hemostat
- IV solution and set up
- povidone-iodine solution
- 4 x 4 sterile gauze
- sterile gloves

Procedure

1. Preferred site in children: proximal tibia. Distal tibia/distal femur may also be used
2. See illustration for landmarks
3. Cleanse area thoroughly with povidone-iodine solution.
4. Hold IO needle between index, middle finger and thumb. Insert the needle at a right angle to the tibia but aiming towards the foot. With slow and gentle rocking/twisting motion, enter the IO space. At this stage the resistance decreases and the needle can stand without support.
5. Unscrew "door-knob-like" attachment from needle.
6. Attach IV tubing to needle.
7. Aspiration of bone marrow confirms placement (not a consistent finding).
8. Clamp needle with hemostat at the level of the skin and secure to limb.
9. Check for soft tissue infiltration while infusing IV solution.
10. Procedure note

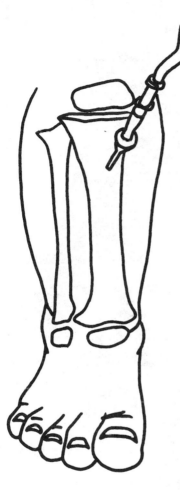

Intraosseous needle placement

Endotracheal Intubation

Sujatha Kannan

Indications: cardiopulmonary resuscitation, respiratory failure with hypoxemia or hypercarbia, absent pharyngeal reflexes as in coma/brainstem dysfunction, unstable airway from facial trauma or an airway abnormality

Complications: hypoxemia or cardiac arrest, bronchial intubation, vomiting/aspiration of gastric contents, dislodgement of teeth, laryngeal trauma, esophageal intubation

	Equipment and Supplies
Suction	wall suction, various size suction catheters, Yankauer tips, NG tube
Oxygen	self-inflating bag (preferred) with PEEP valve attachment, high flow oxygen with flow meter, non-rebreather mask
Airway	appropriate size ventilating mask, endotracheal tubes (including one size smaller and one size bigger), functioning laryngoscope, stylet, oral and pharyngeal airways of different sizes

If performing nasotracheal intubation: Magill forceps, lubricant, phenylephrine 0.25% solution
CR monitor, oxygen, pulse oximeter, automated blood pressure machine

Procedure (See p.273)

Orotracheal Intubation
1. Provide 100% oxygen via bag and mask ventilation
2. All equipment should be ready, available and in good working condition
3. Patient should be connected to pulse oximeter and EKG monitor
4. Sedate and paralyze patient using appropriate agents (See p.278,279)
5. Ascertain integrity of spinal column
6. Place patient supine in "sniffing" position. Slightly extend neck using a neck roll. (contraindicated in spinal cord injury)
7. Place laryngoscope blade in right corner of the mouth.
8. Displace tongue by directing the laryngoscope to the left of midline.
9. Hold handle at 45°.
10. Elevate the mandible by lifting the blade along the axis of the laryngoscope handle to expose the posterior pharyngeal wall. Avoid any pressure on the dentoalveolar ridge.
11. When using a straight blade, the epiglottis is lifted with the blade exposing the vocal cords.
12. Pressure on the cricoid may be necessary to permit view of the vocal cords.
13. If no laryngeal structure is seen after cricoid pressure, retract the blade gently. The most common error is to advance the blade into the esophagus.
14. Advance the endotracheal tube from the right side of the mouth to avoid blocking the view during tube passage
15. Pass it approximately 2-3 cm into the trachea
16. Attach ET tube to a bag and provide manual breaths with 100% oxygen.
17. Confirm tube position
    - Auscultation for equal breath sounds bilaterally
    - Appearance of condensation in the endotracheal tube
    - Improvement in oxygenation and heart rate
    - STAT chest radiograph to determine position
18. Secure endotracheal tube using tape and tincture of benzoin
19. An oropharyngeal airway may be used to prevent patient from biting the endotracheal tube.
20. Procedure note.

Nasotracheal Intubation (Contraindicated in coagulopathy, basilar skull fractures, and severe injuries to the hypopharynx)
1. Provide 100% oxygen by bag and mask ventilation
2. All equipment should be ready, available and in good working condition
3. Patient should be connected to pulse oximeter and EKG monitor
4. Sedate and paralyze patient using appropriate agents (See p.278,279)
5. Ascertain integrity of spinal column
6. Place patient supine in "sniffing" position. Slightly extend neck using neck roll. (Contraindicated in spinal cord injury)
7. Apply topical vasoconstrictor (phenylephrine 0.25%) to nasal mucosa
8. Guide lubricated endotracheal tube into the nasal cavity, direct endotracheal tube posteriorly so that it enters the nasopharynx
9. Visualize nasal tube tip in the nasopharynx
10. Advance endotracheal tube past the vocal cords. Magill forceps may be used to advance tube
11. Pass it approximately 2-3 cm into the trachea
12. Attach ET tube to a bag and provide manual breaths with 100% oxygen
13. Confirm tube position as above
14. Secure endotracheal tube using tape and tincture of benzoin.
15. Procedure note

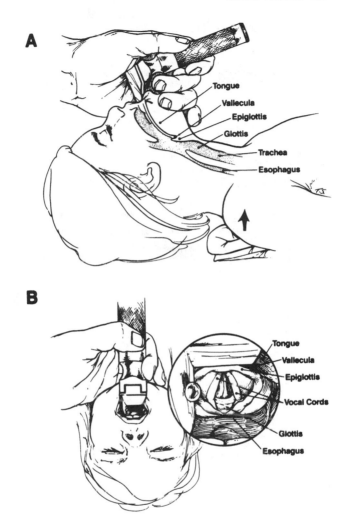

A

- Tongue
- Vallecula
- Epiglottis
- Glottis
- Trachea
- Esophagus

B

- Tongue
- Vallecula
- Epiglottis
- Vocal Cords
- Glottis
- Esophagus

Intubation technique and landmarks. (From L Chameides, *Textbook of Pediatric Advanced Life Support.* Dallas: American Heart Association, Dallas, Texas, 1998. With permission.)

Partial Exchange Transfusion

Thomas Brousseau

Indications for partial exchange transfusion in sickle cell disease: cerebrovascular accident (CVA), priapism, sepsis or acute chest syndrome. The goal of therapy is to reduce the amount of red blood cells that have undergone "sickling". This helps in further decreasing aggregation at sites of RBC accumulation.

Equipment/supplies

- IV supplies for obtaining central or peripheral IV access. Catheter should be no smaller than 20 gauge.
- type and crossmatch 12 mL/kg sickle cell negative PRBCs
- syringes for drawing off blood
- container for discarded blood
- Bag and mask, oxygen, CR monitor, pulse oximeter, automated blood pressure machine.

Procedure

1. Obtain IV access. Preferably establish two IV access sites—one for removal of blood and one for infusion of PRBCs.
2. Remove 5 mL/kg of patient's blood. Monitor vital signs closely. Obtain quantitative hemoglobin A/S levels.
3. If patient is hemodynamically unstable, proceed in a stepwise fashion. Remove 2 mL/kg and then transfuse 5 mL/kg of PRBCs. Remove an additional 3 mL/kg and then transfuse 7 mL/kg of PRBCs.
4. Procedure note.

NOTES

Percutaneous Pericardiocentesis

Russell Clark

Indications
- Therapeutic: relief of tamponade that is causing significant hemodynamic compromise
- Diagnostic: ascertain etiology of effusion

Complications
Ventricular puncture/laceration, coronary artery laceration, arrhythmias, pericardial tamponade, diaphragm perforation, infection

---

Equipment and supplies

- sterile 4 x 4 gauze
- povidone-iodine solution
- sterile gloves, gown, mask, hat
- 1% lidocaine
- 16 or 18 gauge 2-inch angiocatheter or 16 or 18 gauge 12-18 cm cardiac or spinal needle (short bevel)
- 10-mL and 50-mL syringe
- 3-way stopcock
- IV tubing
- specimen vials and culture tubes
- bag and mask, oxygen, CR monitor, pulse oximeter, automated blood pressure machine
- code cart
- volume expanders at bedside
- sterile alligator clip attached to EKG monitor (if available)
- flexible sterile guidewire

Procedure

1. Place the patient supine, or ideally, with the torso elevated 30° to 45° (this brings the heart closer to the anterior chest wall).
2. Obtain IV access. Attach patient to cardiac (EKG) monitor.
3. If patient is hemodynamically stable and respiratory status is not compromised, consider premedication/conscious sedation (See p.293). Premedication with atropine may help prevent vasovagal response.
4. Prepare and drape entire lower xiphoid and epigastric area using aseptic technique.
5. Anesthetize site with 1% lidocaine
6. Setup 3-way stopcock with lever off to middle port. Attach syringe to stopcock in-line port. Attach angiocatheter or spinal needle to stopcock, and alligator clip (if available) to the hub of the needle.
7. NOTE: after the skin has been punctured, monitor EKG by attaching the sterile cord from the pericardial needle (as above) to lead V of the EKG machine.

   Left paraxiphoid approach (preferred): applying gentle suction, slowly advance the catheter at 45° angle to the coronal plane below the left costal margin adjacent to the xiphoid toward the left midclavicular parasagittal plane. (Some operators prefer to aim for the left shoulder, the left mid scapula, or the right shoulder.) Pericardial resistance may be felt, and a "pop" may be felt upon pericardial puncture. Observe EKG monitor for changes in pattern, e.g., ST segment elevation with ventricular epicardial contact, PR segment elevation with atrial epicardial contact.

   Left parasternal approach: applying gentle suction, advance needle perpendicular to the chest wall, over top of 5th rib and adjacent to the sternal border. When the needle is deep to the costal arch, redirect towards the left shoulder. Pericardial resistance may be felt, and a "pop" felt upon pericardial puncture. Observe EKG monitor as above.

8. When fluid returns, attach a hemostat to the needle at the skin surface to prevent accidental over-penetration.
9. Withdraw desired amount of fluid and send for necessary tests: bacterial/viral/fungal cultures, cell count with differential, glucose, protein, LDH, gram stain, amylase.
10. Remove needle and apply dressing.
11. Repeat chest radiograph and echocardiogram after the procedure and in 6 hours.
12. Continue to monitor the patient closely for the next few hours.
13. Procedure note.

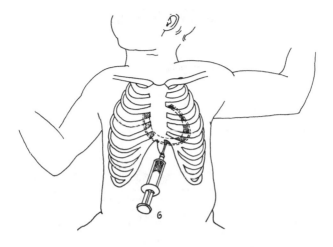

Percutaneous pericardiocentesis

Rapid Sequence Intubation (RSI)

Sujatha Kannan

> Rapid sequence intubation (RSI) is the rapid induction of general anesthesia that induces unconsciousness and muscle relaxation to facilitate intubation under optimal conditions with minimal adverse effects.
>
> Only physicians familiar with the medications, who are skilled at procedures to secure the airway and have appropriate medical assistance and monitoring equipment to carry out these procedures, should perform RSI

(A) RSI should **not** be initiated until ALL equipment is available and ready for use.

(B) Preoxygenation with 100% oxygen causes N_2 washout creating an oxygen reservoir in the FRC of the lungs. This can be achieved by using a well fitting mask (non-rebreathing mask) in a spontaneously breathing patient. When bag-valve mask ventilation is necessary, e.g., apneic patients and patients with inadequate respirations, it may be advantageous to use a paralyzing agent. Cricoid pressure (Sellick maneuver) must be applied to prevent gastric distention. Also, in spontaneously breathing patients, **do not** use a self-inflating bag to administer oxygen. No oxygen is delivered unless the bag is squeezed. This will lead to gastric distention and aspiration.

(C) Medications are given to reduce the effects of laryngoscopy and subsequent placement of the endotracheal tube.

(D)

COMMONLY USED SEDATIVES IN RAPID SEQUENCE INTUBATION

DRUG	Effect CVS	Effect ICP	Advantages	Disadvantages
Midazolam	minimal or ↓	minimal	amnestic, anticonvulsant, reversible (**flumazenil**)	respiratory depression esp. if combined with other drugs; broad dosing range because of variable sedation effects.
Etomidate	minimal	↓ ICP	Anticonvulsant (**fentanyl** 1-2 mcg/kg IV may be used to blunt sympathetic effects)	adrenocortical suppression, myoclonic movements, nausea and vomiting, no analgesic effect
Ketamine	minimal	↑ ICP	bronchodilation, amnestic, analgesia, preserves spontaneous respiration	emergence reaction, increased secretions, laryngospasm
Thiopental	↓ BP	↓ ICP	anticonvulsant, blunts sympathetic response to laryngoscopy and intubation	hypotension, histamine release (bronchospasm), dose dependent respiratory depression
Propofol	↓ BP	↓ ICP	anticonvulsant, amnestic	hypotension
Fentanyl	variable	variable	analgesic, reversible (**naloxone**)	Risk of chest wall rigidity, respiratory depression especially if given rapidly

Example of sedative combinations

No hypotension/hypovolemia	thiopental, etomidate, midazolam
Mild hypotension/hypovolemia with head injury	thiopental, etomidate
Mild hypotension/hypovolemia without head injury	ketamine, etomidate
Severe hypotension/hypovolemia	ketamine (no additional sedative)
Status asthmaticus	ketamine, midazolam, propofol
Status epilepticus	thiopental, midazolam, propofol

(E) Succinylcholine may produce muscle fasciculations as it depolarizes the cell membrane. This causes ↑ ICP, ↑ intragastric pressure, ↑ IOP, hyperkalemia, myoglobinuria, and muscle pain. It can also trigger malignant hyperthermia and cause masseter spasm. A defasciculating dose at 10% of the normal paralytic dose of any muscle relaxant may be administered 1-3 minutes prior to giving succinylcholine. Its use in the pediatric population is limited to emergent situations. Use of non-depolarizing paralytic agent is preferred for elective procedures.

(F) Cricoid pressure (Sellick maneuver) must be applied until proper placement of the endotracheal tube is ascertained.

G COMMONLY USED PARALYTIC AGENTS IN RAPID SEQUENCE INTUBATION

	SUCCINYLCHOLINE	VECURONIUM	ROCURONIUM
Mechanism	Depolarizing	Non-depolarizing	Non-depolarizing
Onset	30 to 60 seconds	90-240 seconds	30-90 seconds
Duration	4 – 6 minutes	90-120 minute	25-60 minutes
IV dose	< 10 kg 1-2 mg/kg IV > 10 kg 1-1.5 mg/kg IV	0.15-0.2 mg/kg IV	0.6-1.2 mg/kg IV
IM dose	4 mg/kg IM	not applicable	infants 1 mg/kg IM older children 1.8 mg/kg IM
Comments	Contraindications • Malignant hyperthermia • Neuromuscular disease • 48-72 hours (up to 60 days) after burns or massive tissue injury • Hyperkalemia • Cholinesterase deficiency	Slower onset than rocuronium, longer duration than succinylcholine. Has minimal hemodynamic effects.	Effects reversed by **edrophonium** (0.5-1 mg/kg IV) and **atropine** (0.01-0.02 mg/kg IV)

Cisatracurium is preferred in patients with hepatic or renal impairment as it spontaneously dissociates into inert metabolites. However, it produces histamine release when injected rapidly.

Pancuronium has few cardiovascular effects but it can cause histamine release. It has a slow onset and long duration of action.

Succinylcholine causes ↑ ICP. Ensure deep anesthesia, use IV lidocaine, and a defasciculating dose of a nondepolarizing muscle relaxant if there is a possibility of ↑ ICP, e.g., head injury.

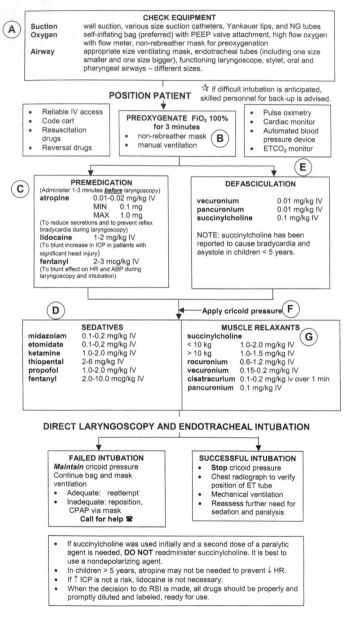

A

CHECK EQUIPMENT

Suction   wall suction, various size suction catheters, Yankauer tips, and NG tubes
Oxygen   self-inflating bag (preferred) with PEEP valve attachment, high flow oxygen
            with flow meter, non-rebreather mask for preoxygenation
Airway   appropriate size ventilating mask, endotracheal tubes (including one size
            smaller and one size bigger), functioning laryngoscope, stylet, oral and
            pharyngeal airways – different sizes.

POSITION PATIENT   ☆ if difficult intubation is anticipated,
                              skilled personnel for back-up is advised.

- Reliable IV access
- Code cart
- Resuscitation
  drugs
- Reversal drugs

**PREOXYGENATE FiO₂ 100%
for 3 minutes**
- non-rebreather mask
- manual ventilation   **B**

- Pulse oximetry
- Cardiac monitor
- Automated blood
  pressure device
- ETCO₂ monitor

E

C

PREMEDICATION
(Administer 1-3 minutes ***before*** laryngoscopy)
atropine   0.01-0.02 mg/kg IV
              MIN   0.1 mg
              MAX   1.0 mg
(To reduce secretions and to prevent reflex
bradycardia during laryngoscopy)
lidocaine   1-2 mg/kg IV
(To blunt increase in ICP in patients with
significant head injury)
fentanyl   2-3 mcg/kg IV
(To blunt effect on HR and ABP during
laryngoscopy and intubation)

DEFASCICULATION

vecuronium   0.01 mg/kg IV
pancuronium   0.01 mg/kg IV
succinylcholine   0.1 mg/kg IV

NOTE: succinylcholine has been
reported to cause bradycardia and
asystole in children < 5 years.

D

SEDATIVES
midazolam   0.1-0.2 mg/kg IV
etomidate   0.1-0.2 mg/kg IV
ketamine   1.0-2.0 mg/kg IV
thiopental   2-6 mg/kg IV
propofol   1.0-2.0 mg/kg IV
fentanyl   2.0-10.0 mcg/kg IV

Apply cricoid pressure **F**

MUSCLE RELAXANTS   **G**
succinylcholine
< 10 kg   1.0-2.0 mg/kg IV
> 10 kg   1.0-1.5 mg/kg IV
rocuronium   0.6-1.2 mg/kg IV
vecuronium   0.15-0.2 mg/kg IV
cisatracurium 0.1-0.2 mg/kg iv over 1 min
pancuronium   0.1 mg/kg IV

DIRECT LARYNGOSCOPY AND ENDOTRACHEAL INTUBATION

FAILED INTUBATION
Maintain cricoid pressure
Continue bag and mask
ventilation
- Adequate: reattempt
- Inadequate: reposition,
  CPAP via mask
  Call for help ☎

SUCCESSFUL INTUBATION
- **Stop** cricoid pressure
- Chest radiograph to verify
  position of ET tube
- Mechanical ventilation
- Reassess further need for
  sedation and paralysis

- If succinylcholine was used initially and a second dose of a paralytic
  agent is needed, **DO NOT** readminister succinylcholine. It is best to
  use a nondepolarizing agent.
- In children > 5 years, atropine may not be needed to prevent ↓ HR.
- If ↑ ICP is not a risk, lidocaine is not necessary.
- When the decision to do RSI is made, all drugs should be properly and
  promptly diluted and labeled, ready for use.

NOTES

Subclavian Catheter Placement

Thomas Brousseau

Indications: CVP monitoring, central venous access, hyperalimentation

Complications: pneumothorax, bleeding, inadvertent subclavian artery puncture

Equipment/supplies

- 1% lidocaine
- vascular access tray
- 3-mL, 5-mL, 10-mL syringe
- IV tubing
- sterile drape, gloves, gown
- suture kit
- If patient requires sedation, bag and mask, O_2, CR monitor, pulse oximeter, automated blood pressure machine

Procedure

1. Place the child in Trendelenburg position (head of bed down 20° to 30°) with the child's head turned towards the opposite side to where the line is to be inserted. Confirm that the child has good breath sounds in both lung fields before starting the procedure.
2. Locate the suprasternal notch and the junction of the middle and medial thirds of the clavicle (see illustration).
3. Prepare and drape the area using sterile technique.
4. Anesthetize skin with 1% lidocaine.
5. Fill all ports of the central line catheter with sterile saline.
6. With a syringe attached to the introducer needle, insert needle just under the clavicle at the junction of the middle and medial thirds of the clavicle. The needle should be parallel to the frontal plane and should be directed toward a fingertip placed at the suprasternal notch. While advancing the needle under the clavicle, a small amount of negative pressure should be applied to the attached syringe.
7. When free flow of blood is achieved, the bevel of the needle should be rotated downward to facilitate placement of catheter into superior vena cava.
8. Disconnect syringe and place thumb or finger over the hub of the needle to prevent air from entering the system and possibly causing air embolism.
9. Complete catheter placement using the Seldinger technique.
10. Once good flow of blood is ascertained through each port, secure the catheter with suture and apply an occlusive dressing.
11. Obtain a chest radiograph to confirm proper catheter placement. Catheter tip should be located at the junction of the SVC and right atrium. Also look for signs of pneumothorax on chest radiograph.
12. Procedure note.

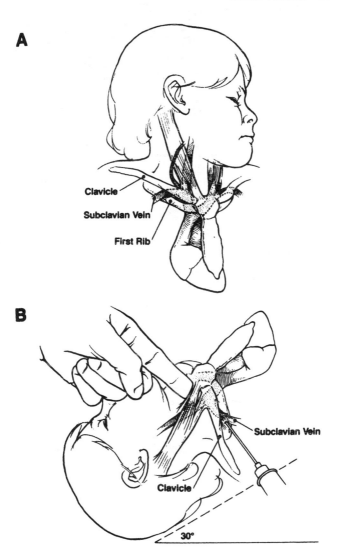

A

Clavicle

Subclavian Vein

First Rib

B

Subclavian Vein

Clavicle

30°

Subclavian vein cannulation. (From L Chameides, *Textbook of Pediatric Advanced Life Support*. Dallas: American Heart Association, Dallas, Texas 1998. With permission.)

Subdural Tap

Russell Clark

Indications: evacuation of pressurized subdural fluid collection in a child (with patent anterior fontanel) with signs and symptoms of increased ICP.

Contraindications: coagulopathy

Complications: intracranial hemorrhage, intracranial vessel rupture, cerebral contusion, subgaleal collection of fluid, air, or blood, infection, brain parenchymal puncture or laceration

---

Equipment and supplies

- 19- to 20-gauge subdural or spinal needle (check patency)
- 10 mL syringe
- razor
- povidone-iodine solution
- several sterile 4 x 4 gauze
- alcohol swabs
- sterile gloves
- bag & mask, O_2, CR monitor, pulse oximeter, automated blood pressure machine

Procedure

1. Attach CR monitor, pulse oximeter, 100% O_2
2. Restrain infant supine.
3. Shave scalp to fully expose all borders of the anterior fontanelle.
4. Prepare and drape patient in sterile fashion.
5. Palpate the coronal suture at a lateral aspect of the anterior fontanelle.
6. Firmly grasp subdural or spinal needle with the hub between the thumb and index finger of dominant hand; steady heel of this hand against infant's scalp. Steady heel of nondominant hand against scalp on opposite side of skull. With thumb of nondominant hand, displace skin laterally over anterior fontanelle for Z-track insertion technique. Advance the needle, at 90° to the skull, through skin at lateral aspect of coronal suture of anterior fontanelle. Dural resistance may be noticeable, and a "pop" indicates subdural penetration; do not advance needle more than 5-8 mm. See illustration.
7. Remove stylet to drain subdural fluid/blood. **Do not aspirate**.
8. Replace stylet, remove needle, apply dressing.
9. Send fluid for cell count, differential, gram stain, culture, protein, and glucose.
10. Repeat procedure on opposite side, as required.
11. Procedure note.

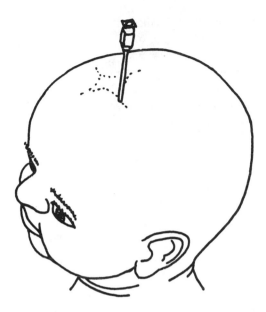

Subdural tap

Suprapubic Bladder Aspiration

Adiaha Spinks

Indications
- Used most commonly in infants < 6 months of age, but may be performed in children less than 2 years of age.
- When sterile urine culture is necessary
- When there are urethral anomalies
- When urine is unable to be obtained via less invasive procedures

Contraindications
- Patient has voided within one hour of the procedure
- Bladder is not percussed
- When patient has other genitourinary tract anomalies

Equipment/supplies

- povidone-iodine solution and 70% alcohol
- 22- or 24-gauge 1-inch needle
- 10 mL syringe
- sterile specimen container

Procedure

1. Ascertain that the infant has not voided in the past 60 minutes before the procedure. **Do not** perform this procedure if the patient has voided within the last hour.
2. Restrain the infant in a frog-leg position.
3. The bladder should be palpated above the pubic symphysis; percuss the borders of the bladder.
4. Clean the region between the pubic symphysis and umbilicus with povidone-iodine and alcohol.
5. The urethral meatus should be occluded to prevent the loss of urine during the procedure. Occlude the urethral meatus by applying mild pressure to the urethral meatus of the female or by squeezing the penile urethra of the male.
6. With the needle attached to the syringe, enter the bladder 2 cm above the pubic symphysis in the midline. Introduce the needle at a 20° angle to the skin, aiming cranially. Apply gentle suction to the syringe until urine is obtained. Do not advance the needle more than 2.5 cm.
7. Remove needle. Transfer sample to appropriate container.
8. Procedure note.

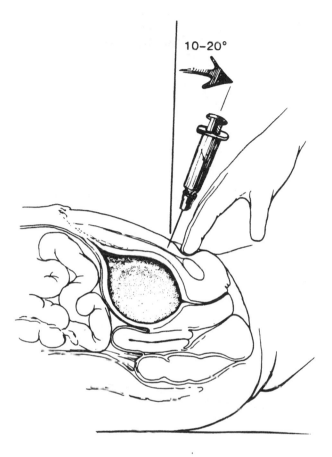

10–20°

Suprapubic Bladder Aspiration. (From Fleisher GR, Ludwig S, Henretig FM, Ruddy RM, and Silverman BK (eds), *Textbook of Pediatric Emergency Medicine, 4e*. Philadelphia: Lippincott Williams & Wilkins, 2000. With permission.)

Thoracentesis:
Needle Aspiration of Pneumothorax

Adiaha Spinks

Indication: pneumothorax with cardiovascular compromise

Equipment/supplies

- 20-gauge or 18-gauge angiocatheter
- 3-way stopcock
- 60 mL syringe
- povidone-iodine solution
- 4 x 4 gauze
- sterile drapes, sterile gloves, masks
- bag and mask, oxygen, pulse oximeter, CR monitor, automated blood pressure monitor
- petrolatum-impregnated gauze

Procedure

1. Cleanse area with povidone-iodine solution.
2. Prepare and drape area, using sterile technique.
3. With patient supine, locate the 2nd intercostal space at the midclavicular line on the side of the pneumothorax.
4. Make sure the 3-way stopcock lever is turned such that it is off to the middle port. Attach syringe to the stopcock.
5. With a syringe attached to the angiocatheter, approach the area at about a 45° angle. Enter the pleural cavity between the ribs, staying close to the superior border of the rib to avoid hitting blood vessels and nerves. Continue aspirating while advancing the needle. A popping sensation is usually felt when the intrapleural space is entered.
6. Remove needle; attach the stopcock with syringe attached to the angiocatheter and aspirate. To "discard" aspirated air turn stopcock lever off to patient and discard through middle port. Continue to aspirate intrapleural air in this fashion, until you can no longer get air without meeting resistance.
7. Apply petrolatum occlusive dressing to area after catheter removal.
8. Obtain post-thoracentesis radiograph.
9. Procedure note.

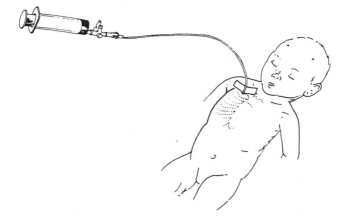

Thoracentesis: needle aspiration of pneumothorax. (From Halliday HL, McCluire G, and Reid H (eds), *Handbook of Neonatal Intensive Care*. Philadelphia: WB Saunders Co., 1989, p. 93. With permission.)

Umbilical Vein/Artery Cannulation (UVC/UAC)

Russell Clark

Indications: venous or arterial pressure monitoring, blood sampling or infusion (UVC) of medications and fluids in newborns.

Equipment and supplies:
- 3.5 or 5.0 F single lumen catheter
- sterile measuring tape, umbilical tape
- sterile hemostat
- sterile drapes, gloves, gown
- 3-way stopcock
- syringe with saline flush, povidone-iodine solution
- 4 x 4 gauze
- scalpel, blade, needle holder, sutures
- dilator

Procedure

1. Secure infant in supine position
2. Determine length of catheter to be inserted for either high (T6-T9) or low (L3-L4) placement (See chart on p.291).
3. Flush catheter with sterile saline solution before insertion.
4. Cleanse umbilical stump using sterile technique.
5. Place sterile drapes.
6. Tie umbilical string around base of umbilical stump.
7. Hold umbilical stump with hemostat and cut cord with a scalpel 2 cm above the skin line.
8. Identify the vessels. Normally, the umbilical vein is the thin-walled, single vessel that is larger than the two thicker-walled arteries.
9. Gently dilate the vein if necessary.
10. Insert umbilical catheter into umbilical vein or artery to desired length. Check for adequacy of blood return.
11. Secure catheter with suture and tape bridge (See p.291)
12. Confirm placement of catheter by abdominal radiograph.

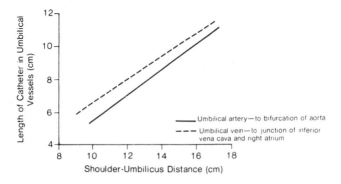

Graph for determination of length of umbilical catheter to be inserted. (From Fletcher MA and Macdonald MG (eds), *Atlas of Procedures in Neonatology*. Philadelphia: JB Lippincott Co., p.156. With permission.)

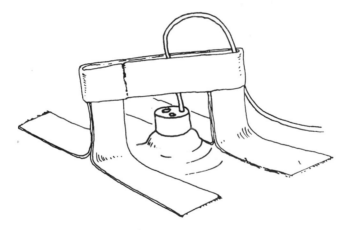

Tape bridge to secure umbilical catheter. From Halliday HL, McCluire G, and Reid H (eds), *Handbook of Neonatal Intensive Care*. Philadelphia: WB Saunders Co., 1989, p99. With permission.)

Tapping a Ventriculoperitoneal Shunt (VPS)

Thomas Brousseau

Background
A ventriculoperitoneal shunt is used to divert cerebrospinal fluid from the ventricles to the peritoneal cavity.
Indications for VP shunt tap
- In cases of suspected shunt malfunction and/or infection.
- To decrease ICP prior to surgery.

Equipment/supplies

- razor
- povidone-iodine solution
- sterile drape, gown, gloves, mask
- CSF collection tubes X 4
- 23 gauge Butterfly® needle and syringe (larger gauge needles can damage reservoir and predispose to persistent leaks)
- sterile transparent occlusive patch
- sterile dressing
- bag and mask, O_2, CR monitor, pulse oximeter, automated blood pressure machine

Procedure

1. Determine area of shunt reservoir by palpation or radiograph.
2. Shave hair over reservoir if applicable.
3. Prepare and drape area of reservoir in a sterile manner.
4. Place sterile transparent occlusive patch over area.
5. Enter reservoir at an oblique angle using a 23 gauge Butterfly® needle.
6. Estimate opening pressure by holding open end of Butterfly® tubing up and measuring column of CSF in cm.
7. Obtain CSF and send for cell count, Gram stain, culture, protein, and glucose.
8. Remove needle.
9. Cover puncture site with sterile gauze dressing.
10. Procedure note

Conscious Sedation

Sujatha Kannan

Conscious sedation is defined by the American Society of Anesthesiologists (ASA) is a medically controlled state of depressed consciousness that 1) allows protective reflexes to be maintained; 2) retains the patient's ability to maintain a patent airway independently and continuously; and 3) permits appropriate response by the patient to physical stimulation or verbal command. That loss of consciousness is unlikely is an important aspect of this definition. Therefore, drugs used for conscious sedation should have enough of a safety margin such that loss of consciousness is highly unlikely.

Deep sedation: medically controlled state of depressed consciousness or unconsciousness from which the patient is not easily aroused. It may be accompanied by partial or complete loss of protective reflexes, and includes the inability to maintain a patent airway independently and respond purposefully to physical stimulation or verbal command.

General anesthesia: a medically controlled state of unconsciousness accompanied by loss of protective reflexes, including the inability to maintain a patent airway independently and respond purposefully to physical stimulation or verbal command.

ASA Physical Status Classification

Class I   A normally healthy patient
Class II   A patient with mild systemic disease
Class III   A patient with severe systemic disease
Class IV   A patient with severe systemic disease that is a constant threat to life
Class V   A moribund patient who is not expected to survive without the operation

Appropriate candidates for conscious or deep sedation: Class I and II.

Possible complications
- vomiting
- seizures
- anaphylaxis
- anaphylactoid reactions
- respiratory depression
- hypotension
- cardiorespiratory arrest

Information regarding current and past illnesses should be obtained:
- airway problems
- pulmonary disease
- congestive heart failure
- rhythm disturbances
- need for prophylaxis for endocarditis
- seizures
- neuropathies and myopathies
- pregnancy
- sickle cell disease
- diabetes
- congenital adrenal hyperplasia
- allergies
- past experience with anesthesia
- medications

Personnel:
1. Practitioner: the individual administering conscious sedation must be skilled in these techniques, and should have the ability to provide the necessary level of monitoring. The practitioner should have training in basic life support at the very least. Training in pediatric advanced life support is strongly encouraged.
2. Support staff: a person other than the practitioner, who can assist in monitoring, as well as resuscitative measures if necessary. Training in basic pediatric life support is recommended. This individual should be very familiar with the emergency cart and resuscitation equipment.
3. Monitoring:
Baseline (before the procedure): obtain informed consent from the parent or legal guardian. Full set of vital signs.
During the procedure: document name, route, site, time and dosage of all drugs administered. Continuous quantitative monitoring of oxygen saturation (pulse oximetry) and heart rate. Intermittent recording of respiratory rate and blood pressure. Airway patency should be ensured throughout the procedure. A functioning suction apparatus should be available at all times.
After the procedure: continuous monitoring in a properly equipped facility until patient is suitable for discharge (see p.294)

Equipment:
Drugs
- oxygen
- 50% glucose for IV
- atropine
- epinephrine (1:1000, 1:10,000)
- phenylephrine
- dopamine
- albuterol for nebulization
- diazepam
- isoproterenol
- calcium chloride or gluconate
- sodium bicarbonate
- lidocaine
- naloxone
- flumazenil
- diphenhydramine HCl
- hydrocortisone
- methylprednisolone
- aminophylline
- racemic epinephrine

✳ Continued on p.294

✳ Continued from p.293

Intravenous equipment
- 24-, 22-, 20-, 18-, 16-
  gauge angiocath
- tourniquets
- alcohol wipes

- adhesive tapes
- assorted syringes
- IV tubing
- IV fluid: 0.9 NS and LR

- IV boards
- IO needle
- sterile gauze pads

Equipment for managing the airway
- face masks (infant, child, small adult,
  medium adult, large adult)
- breathing valve and bag set
- oral airways (infant, child, small,
  medium and large adult)
- nasal airways (small, medium, large)
- laryngoscope blades (straight 1, 2, 3
  and curved 2, 3)

- laryngoscope handles
- endotracheal tubes (from 2.5 to 8.0 mm)
- stylettes
- surgical lubricant
- suction catheters
- nebulizer
- gloves

Monitoring and resuscitation equipment
- pulse oximetry
- EKG monitor

- automated blood
  pressure monitor
- defibrillator

- external pacemaker
- suction machine

Dietary precautions
1. Infants 0-5 months: no milk or solids for 4 h prior to procedure
2. Infants 6-36 months: no milk or solids for 6 h prior to procedure
3. Children > 36 months: no milk or solids for 8 h prior to procedure
4. All patients may have clear liquids until 2-3 hours before the procedure

Patients at risk for aspiration
1. History of GE reflux
2. Extreme obesity
3. Pregnancy
4. History of previous esophageal dysfunction

Drugs Used for Conscious Sedation

Drug	Dose	Route	Onset (min)	Duration (h)
diazepam	0.1-0.2 mg/kg/dose	IV, PO, PR	1.5-3	1
lorazepam	0.05 mg/kg/dose MAX single dose: 2 mg	IV, IM, PO, PR	IV 1-5	3-4
midazolam	0.05 mg/kg/dose MAX single dose 0.2 mg/kg	IV, IM, PR	IV 1-3	1-2
pentobarbital	0.5-1 mg/kg/dose	IV	1-10	1-4
chloral hydrate	25-100 mg/kg MAX 2 g	PO, PR	30-60	
morphine	0.1 mg/kg/dose MAX dose 15 mg	IV, IM	IV 1-2 IM 10-25	IV .25-1 IM 1-4
fentanyl	1-2 mcg/kg/dose MAX 5 mcg/kg	IV, IM,	IV/IM 1-2	0.5-1
ketamine	IV 0.5-1 mg/kg/dose IM 2-4 mg/kg/dose MAX 13 mg/kg	IV, IM	IV 30 sec IM 12-25	12-25 min

Discharge criteria
1. Patients should be alert and oriented, infants and patients with abnormal neurologic or mental status should have returned to their baseline function.
2. Vital signs should be stable and within acceptable limits.
3. Patients who need pharmacologic antagonists to reverse oversedation must be monitored for at least 1 hour to detect and treat recurrence and any adverse effects.
4. Outpatients must be discharged to a responsible adult who is capable of reporting any complications resulting from the procedure or sedation.
5. Outpatients must be provided with oral and written instructions regarding post-procedure diet, medications and activity level; what complications to look for, and the appropriate action in case of emergency.

Non-Invasive Monitoring

Mary Lieh-Lai

Pulse oximetry

Pulse oximetry represents a continuous, non-invasive modality of measuring oxygen saturation. Oximetry utilizes the principles of spectrophotometry to determine hemoglobin oxygen saturation. Spectrophotometry is based on the Beer-Lambert law that states the relationship of concentration of solute to the intensity of light transmitted through a solution. The oximeter probes contain light emitting diodes (LEDs) which emit lights of 2 wavelengths, infrared (940 nm), and red (660 nm). Oxyhemoglobin absorbs less red light than deoxyhemoglobin, while the opposite is true with infrared light. This difference in light absorption is used to calculate oxygen saturation. Based on the oxygen-hemoglobin dissociation curve, the oxygen saturation (SaO_2) can be related to PaO_2.

Benefits of pulse oximetry:
1. Non-invasive
2. Continuous monitoring
3. Readily available

Pitfalls of pulse oximetry:
1. Inaccurate with decreased perfusion or with increased motion
2. Does not distinguish between oxy-, carboxy-, or methemoglobin
3. Reading is inaccurate in the presence of nail polish or with high levels of ambient light
4. Influenced by the shape of the oxygen-hemoglobin dissociation curve. Since this curve is sigmoidal, the pulse oximeter does not detect a significant drop in SaO_2 at higher levels of oxygenation. In cases where patients are receiving oxygen supplementation, PaO_2 may drop to detrimental levels before detection.

Transcutaneous oxygen/carbon dioxide monitoring

Transcutaneous oxygen ($tcPO_2$) and carbon dioxide ($tcPCO_2$) measurements can be obtained via a polarographic electrode (Clark electrode). The transcutaneous method of oxygen and carbon dioxide measurement is very accurate. When the polarograph is exposed to PO_2 in the gaseous phase, correlation is linear from 0 to 100% O_2, and even in hyperbaric conditions. This method was highly popular in the 70's to 80's, but fell to disuse with the advent of pulse oximetry and improved capnometry.

Benefits of transcutaneous monitoring:
1. Non-invasive
2. Ease of use
3. Accuracy

Disadvantages of transcutaneous monitoring:
1. Need for frequent calibration
2. Heating the electrode to 45°C causes burns

Capnometry

Carbon dioxide is produced from aerobic metabolism, transported via the circulation, and eliminated by ventilation. Capnometry is the measurement of end-tidal carbon dioxide ($ETCO_2$) at the proximal airway during breathing.

The most common method used for measurement is infrared absorption, which is based on the fact that infrared light energy absorption is directly related to carbon dioxide concentration.

Two methods of infrared capnometry:
1. Mainstream: sensor is placed directly at the end of the endotracheal tube (in intubated patients), and CO_2 is measured as the gas stream passes directly through the beam of light.
Advantage: higher accuracy
Disadvantage: bulky sensor can result in significant drag on the endotracheal tube and occasionally cause accidental extubation.
2. Sidestream: may be used in non-intubated patients, but requires constant aspiration of the gas by a pump. The gas is then transported to the sensor for measurement.
Advantage: can be used in non-intubated patients and is not bulky
Disadvantage: the constant aspiration frequently draws in moisture which renders the tubing susceptible to clogging

A rough estimate of CO_2 levels can also be obtained using colorimetric CO_2 detectors, a form of litmus paper which changes color according to the pH present in the gas.

$\uparrow ETCO_2$:
1. $\uparrow$ muscle activity
2. Malignant hyperthermia
3. $\downarrow$ minute ventilation
4. Bicarbonate infusion

$\downarrow ETCO_2$
1. Hypothermia
2. Pulmonary embolism
3. Bronchospasm
4. $\uparrow$ minute ventilation

Toe or Peripheral Temperature

A complex capillary network in the epidermis-dermis allows the skin to perform one of its most important functions, which is thermoregulation. Under normal conditions, up to 70% of these capillaries are perfused. Measurement of toe temperature provides an estimation of the adequacy of peripheral perfusion.

In an individual with normal cardiac output and perfusion, the toe (peripheral) temperature should closely approximate that of core temperature (37°C). When the toe temperature approximates that of room temperature (22° – 24°C), this can be an indication that peripheral perfusion (and perhaps cardiac output) is not adequate to maintain normal capillary perfusion. Along with heart rate, blood pressure and urine output, toe temperatures may be used for non-invasive and objective assessment of cardiac output and the potential need for appropriate therapy.

Temporary Cardiac Pacing

Adiaha Spinks

Indications
- Bradycardia refractory to medications
- Patients with Sick Sinus Syndrome
- Patients with complete heart block or AV asynchrony

Contraindications
- Severe hypothermia (physiologic bradycardia)
- Asystole > 20 minutes

Equipment/supplies

- Transcutaneous external pacemaker
- 2 patch electrodes with adhesive backs (large size for patients >15 kg; small or medium for patients < 15 kg)
- EKG electrodes
- Bag and mask, oxygen, pulse oximeter, CR monitor, automated blood pressure monitor
- Code cart at the bedside

Procedure

1. Attach EKG electrodes to patient as indicated (right arm, left arm, left leg)
2. Attach patch electrodes to patient: (pacing patches should not touch EKG electrodes)
   - Negative electrode is to be placed on the anterior chest over the heart or on the left fourth intercostal space in the midaxillary line (near the cardiac apex)
   - Positive electrode is to be placed on the back behind the heart or on the anterior chest on the right side beneath the right clavicle
3. Connect electrodes to output cable
4. Set output to 0 mA.
5. Set pacing rate to 10% above the normal average heart rate for child's age (e.g., 120-160 bpm for neonate)
6. Increase output mA until capture is achieved, i.e., when there is a pacing spike before each QRS wave on the EKG.
7. Procedure note.

Measurement of Pulsus Paradoxus

Thomas Brousseau

Definition: exaggeration of the normal drop in blood pressure during inspiration.

In cardiac tamponade, increased blood return to the right ventricle during inspiration causes the intraventricular septum to bulge into the left ventricle. This causes compression of the left ventricle with decreased stroke volume and consequently, cardiac output.

In the presence of airway obstruction, there is an increase in negative pleural pressure during inspiration. This results in increased afterload and decreased arterial pressure.

Pulsus paradoxus can be seen in cardiac tamponade, constrictive pericarditis, restrictive cardiomyopathy, severe obstructive lung disease (including severe asthma), mitral stenosis with right heart failure, pulmonary embolism, and RV infarction.

Equipment/supplies

- sphygmomanometer
- stethoscope

Procedure

1. With the patient in the supine position with head and chest at 30° to 45° angle, attach blood pressure cuff.
2. Inflate blood pressure cuff above systolic blood pressure.
3. Deflate cuff slowly.
4. Listen for point at which first Korotkoff sounds are heard during expiration.
5. Continue to deflate cuff slowly.
6. Note point at which Korotkoff sounds are heard throughout all phases of the respiratory cycle.
7. Pulsus paradoxus is significant if the difference between the two pressures is greater than 10 mmHg.

Section IV ♣ Appendix

- Antimicrobial Formulary Agents
- Samples of Continuous Infusion Calculation
- Formulae
- Table of Forced Vital Capacity Normalized for Height and Weight Values
- ICU Card
- Insulin Coverage
- Laboratory Findings in Patients with Abnormal Serum Sodium
- Toxicology Panels
- Pharmacokinetic Calculations
- Hyperalimentation for ICU Patients
- Antihypertensive Agents

Antimicrobial Formulary Agents

Recommended Pediatric Doses

Agent	Route	Dosage (mg/kg/d)	Interval (in h)	Maximum (g/d)	Comments
Acyclovir	IV	30	8		infuse over 1 hr
Acyclovir	PO	80	6	3.2	
Amikacin	IV	15-22.5	8	1.5	obtain serum levels
Amoxicillin	PO	25-80	8-12	2-3	
Amoxicillin/ Clavulanate	PO	25-40	8-12	1.5	dosed on amoxicillin component
Amphotericin B (conventional)	IV	1	24		• needs test dose • causes hypokalemia
Amphotericin B, lipoid (Abelcet®)	IV	5	24		systemic fungal infection with renal impairment
Ampicillin	IV	< 7 d: 75-150	8		
		> 7 d: 100-200	6		
		100-200	4-6	12	• non-meningitic dose
		400	4-6	12	• meningitic dose
Ampicillin/ sulbactam (Unasyn®)	IV	100-200	4-6	8	dosed on ampicillin component
Azithromycin	PO	5-12	24	1 (1 dose)	non-gonococcal urethritis/ cervicitis
	PO	10 (day 1) then 5 x 4d	24	250-500 mg	otitis media/pneumonia
	PO	12	24 x 5d	500 mg	pharyngitis
Cefazolin	IV	50-100	8	6	
Cefepime	IV	100	12	4	
	IV	150	8	6	febrile neutropenia only
Cefotaxime	IV	0-1 wk: 100	12	12	• for serious bacterial
	IV	1-4 wk: 150	8	12	infections, in neonates,
	IV	> 4 wk: 160	6	12	patients with HIV & hematologic malignancies
	IV	100-200	6	12	• non-meningitic dose
	IV	200-300	6	12	• meningitic dose
Cefoxitin	IV	80-160	6	12	
Ceftazidime	IV	150	8	6	
Ceftriaxone	IV/IM	50-75	12-24	2	• non-meningitic
		100	12-24	4	• meningitic
Cefuroxime	IV	150	8	4.5	
Cefuroxime	PO	30	12	1	
Cephalexin	PO	25-50	6	4	
Clindamycin	IV	25-50	6-8	4.8	
Clindamycin	PO	20-30	6-8	1.8	
Cloxacillin	PO	50-100	6	4	
Dicloxacillin	PO	25-50	6	2	
Doxycycline	IV, PO	2-4	12	200 mg	for patients > 8 yrs of age
Erythromycin ethylsuccinate	PO	40-50	6	3.2	
Erythromycin lactobionate	IV	20-40	6	4	infuse over 1-2 hours
Fluconazole	PO, IV	3-6	24	200	PO route is recommended
Foscarnet	IV	180	8		• treatment of CMV, HSV
		90-120	24		• prophylaxis of CMV, HSV
Ganciclovir	IV	10	12		• treatment of CMV
	IV	5	24		• prophylaxis of CMV
Gentamicin	IV	5-7.5	8-12	300 mg	obtain serum levels
Isoniazid	PO	10-20	24	300 mg	
Ketoconazole	PO	5-10	12-24	800 mg	
Metronidazole	IV	30	6	4	
	PO	15-35	8	4	
Nystatin	topical	100,000 U	6		suspension for oral candidiasis

Oxacillin	IV	100-200	4-6	12	
Penicillin					
G benzathine	IM	50,000 U	1 dose	2.4 MU	
G potassium	IV	0.2-0.4 MU	4	24 MU	1.7 mEq K⁺ per 1 MU
G procaine	IM	50,000 U	24	4.8 MU	
G sodium	IV	0.2-0.4 MU	4	24 MU	2 mEq Na⁺ per 1 MU
Penicillin VK	PO	25-50	6-8	3 g	
Piperacillin	IV	300	4-6	24	
Piperacillin-tazobactam	IV	300	6-8		dosed based on piperacillin component
Pyrazinamide	PO	30	24	2	
Rifampin	PO	10-20	24	600	• tuberculosis
	PO	20	24 x 4d	600	• *H. influenzae* prophylaxis
	PO	20	12 x 2d	600	• meningococcal prophylaxis
Tobramycin	IV	5-7.5	8-12	300	obtain serum levels
Trimethoprim-sulfamethoxazole (TMP/SMZ)	IV, PO	8/40	8-12	320 mg TMP	• for general infections
	IV, PO	20/100	6		• for Pneumocystis only
Vancomycin	IV	40	6	2	• for most infections; infuse over 1 hour
	IV	60	6	2	• for meningitis
	PO	25-50	6	2	• for *C. difficile* only

Samples of Continuous Infusion Calculation

1. Dopamine
   weight   5 kg
   desired dose 10 mcg/kg/minute

a. concentration of solution is 200 mg of dopamine in 250 mL of D_5Water

$$\frac{200 \text{ mg}}{250 \text{ mL}} = \frac{0.8 \text{ mg}}{\text{mL}} \times \frac{1000 \text{ mcg}}{\text{mg}} = \frac{800 \text{ mcg}}{\text{mL}}$$

$$\frac{800 \text{ mcg/mL}}{5 \text{ kg}} \times \frac{10 \text{ mcg/kg/minute}}{x \text{ mL}}$$

$$800 \text{ x} = 50$$

$$x = \frac{50}{800} = 0.6 \text{ mL/minute} \times 60 = 3.75 \text{ mL/hour (infusion rate)}$$

b. concentration of solution is 400 mg of dopamine in 250 mL D_5Water

$$\frac{400 \text{ mg}}{250 \text{ mL}} = \frac{1.6 \text{ mg}}{\text{mL}} \times \frac{1000 \text{ mcg}}{\text{mg}} = \frac{1600 \text{ mcg}}{\text{mL}}$$

$$\frac{1600 \text{ mcg/mL}}{5 \text{ kg}} \times \frac{10 \text{ mcg/kg/minute}}{x \text{ mL}}$$

$$1600 \text{ x} = 50$$

$$x = \frac{50}{1600} = 0.03 \text{ mL/minute} \times 60 = 1.8 \text{ mL/hour (infusion rate)}$$

Note: inotropic solutions are generally packaged as standard solutions with specific concentrations. It is for this reason that the above calculations are more practical than the often recommended formula:

$$6 \times \frac{\text{desired dose (mcg/kg/minute)}}{\text{desired rate (mL/hour)}} \times \text{weight in kg} = \frac{\text{mg drug}}{100 \text{ mL of fluid}}$$

With this formula, varying concentrations will be needed, which may not always be available.

Formulae

Sujatha Kannan

Plasma osmolality	Plasma Osmolality = $2(Na) + \dfrac{glucose}{18} + \dfrac{BUN}{2.8}$
Osmolar gap	Osmolar gap = measured osmolality - calculated osmolality
Anion gap	Anion gap = (Serum Na + K) - (Cl$^-$+HCO$_3^-$)
Alveolar O_2 tension	PAO$_2$ = [FiO$_2$ x (P$_B$ -47)] - $\dfrac{PaCO_2}{R}$
A-a gradient	AaDO$_2$ = PAO$_2$ - PaO$_2$
Shunt fraction	$\dfrac{Qs}{Qt} = \dfrac{CcO_2 - CaO_2}{CcO_2 - CvO_2}$
Arterial O_2 content	CaO$_2$ = [Hgb x 1.34 x SaO$_2$] + [PaO$_2$ x 0.003]
Mixed venous O_2 content	CvO$_2$ = [Hgb x 1.34 x SvO$_2$] + [PvO$_2$ x 0.003]
End capillary O_2 content	CcO$_2$ = [Hgb x 1.34 x SaO$_2$] + [PAO$_2$ x 0.003]
O_2 consumption	VO$_2$ = Q$_T$ x C(a - v)O$_2$
AV O_2 difference	A-vDO$_2$ = CaO$_2$ - CvO$_2$
Cardiac index	CI = $\dfrac{Cardiac\ output}{BSA}$
Mean arterial pressure	MAP = $\dfrac{systolic + 2\ (diastolic)}{3}$
Systemic vascular resistance	SVR = (MAP – CVP or mean RAP) x $\dfrac{80}{CO}$
Pulmonary vascular resistance	PVR = (mean PA – PCWP) x $\dfrac{80}{CO}$
QT duration	QTc = QT(sec) / $\sqrt{}$R-R interval (sec)
Creatinine clearance	C$_{cr}$ = $\dfrac{k\ x\ Ht\ (cm)}{serum\ Cr}$ or $\dfrac{(140\text{-}age)\ (Wt\ in\ kg)}{72\ x\ serum\ Cr}$ k = 0.45 in babies<1; 0.55 if > 1 year and in adult females; 0.7 in adolescent and adult males
Renal failure index	RFI = $\dfrac{Urine\ Na\ x\ Plasma\ Cr}{Urine\ Cr}$ x 100
Winter's formula for determining the adequacy of respiratory compensation for metabolic acidosis	pCO$_2$ = 1.5 [HCO$_3$] + 8 $\pm$ 2 or Δ10 mm Hg PCO$_2$ = Δ 0.08 pH
Fractional excretion of sodium	FE$_{Na}$ = $\dfrac{Urine\ Na\ x\ Plasma\ Cr}{Urine\ Cr\ x\ Plasma\ Na}$ x 100 < 1% pre-renal > 1% renal failure
Body surface area (m^2)	BSA = $\dfrac{4\ x\ Wt\ (kg) + 7}{Wt + 90}$ or $\{[Ht\ (cm)\ x\ Wt\ (kg) \div 3600\}^{1/2}$
Insensible water loss	IWL = 400 mL/m^2/d
Correction for sodium in hyperglycemia	Na + [(glucose - 100) x 0.016]
Corrected calcium	[0.8 x (normal albumin - patient albumin)] + total Ca^{++}
Centigrade	°C = (°F - 32) x 5/9
Fahrenheit	°F = (°C x 9/5) + 32
Size of ETT	$\dfrac{[16 + age\ (y)]}{4}$

Table of Forced Vital Capacity Normalized for Weight and Height Values

Summary of Normal Values and SD* for Lung Volumes in Children

HEIGHT (cm.)	VC(ml.) Male		VC(ml.) Female		FEV$_{1.0}$(ml.) Male + Female		FRC(ml.) Male		FRC(ml.) Female		RV(ml.) Male		RV(ml.) Female		TLC(ml.) Male		TLC(ml.) Female	
	Mean	±2SD	Mean	±2SD	Mean	±2SD	Mean	±2SD	Mean	±2SD	Mean	±2SD	Mean	±2SD	Mean	±2SD	Mean	±2SD
110	1252	216	1223	294	1053	258	662	356	693	244	369	130	369	130	1539	504	1513	496
120	1592	214	1554	260	1403	252	873	300	893	210	453	134	453	134	1980	374	1953	368
130	1979	230	1916	268	1457	228	1110	266	1118	204	545	130	545	130	2470	282	2437	242
140	2411	288	2323	300	2146	304	1375	270	1367	224	653	122	653	122	3016	270	2974	242
150	2883	400	2770	366	2586	412	1673	284	1643	266	773	118	773	118	3633	304	3576	326
160	3421	546	3270	502	3080	568	2003	318	1942	322	907	134	907	134	4308	444	4242	520
170	4038	802	3856	782	3629	724	2372	424	2323	452	1056	182	1056	182	5070	732	5039	822

*SD calculated for mean values by different authors around the overall mean.

ICU Card

A. Sarnaik, M. Lieh-Lai, K. Meert, S. Heidemann, C. Reid
Division of Critical Care Medicine, Children's Hospital of Michigan

Average Dimensions of Endotracheal Tubes

Age	Internal diameter (mm)	Oral: mouth to mid-trachea (cm)	Nasal: nares to mid-trachea (cm)
Premature	2.5-3.0	9	10
Full-term	3.0-3.5	10	11
6 mos	4.0	11	13
12-24 mos	4.5	13-14	16-17
4 y	5.0	15	17-18
6 y	5.5	17	19-20
8 y	6.0	19	21-22
10 y	6.5	20	22-23
12 y	7.0	21	23-24
14 y	7.5	22	24-25
Adults	8-9.5	23-25	25-28

Glasgow Coma Scale

Eyes		
Open	Spontaneously	4
	To verbal command	3
	To pain	2
	No response	1
Best Verbal		
	Oriented/conversant	5
	Disoriented/conversant	4
	Inappropriate words	3
	Incomprehensible sounds	2
	No response	1
Best Motor		
To verbal command	Obeys	6
To painful stimulus	Localizes	5
	Flexion/withdrawal	4
	Flexion/abnormal	3
	Extension	2
	No response	1
TOTAL		3-15

Therapeutic/Normal Levels

Carbamazepine		4-12 mcg/mL
Calcium, ionized		1.18-1.32 mmol/L
Clonazepam		15-20 mcg/mL
Cyclosporine trough (whole blood) early post-treatment		250-800 ng/mL (RIA) 100-450 ng/mL (HPLC)
Digoxin		0.8-2.0 ng/mL
Gentamicin/ tobramycin	peak trough	6-10 mcg/mL < 2 mcg/mL
Lidocaine		2-6 mcg/mL
Phenytoin, total free		10-20 mcg/mL 1-2 mcg/mL
Phenobarbital		10-20 mcg/mL
Theophylline (for bronchospasm)		10-15 mcg/mL
Thiocyanate		< 10 mg/dL
Valproic acid		50-150 mcg/mL
Vancomycin	peak trough	30-40 mcg/mL < 7.5 mcg/mL

INFUSIONS

DRUG	DILUTION	CONC	USUAL DOSE RANGE
Dobutamine	200 mg in 250 mL 400 mg in 250 mL 800 mg in 250 mL 1600 mg in 250 mL	800 mcg/mL 1600 mcg/mL 3200 mcg/mL 6400 mcg/mL	2-20 mcg/kg/min
Dopamine	200 mg in 250 mL 400 mg in 250 mL 800 mg in 250 mL 1600 mg in 250 mL 3200 mg in 250 mL	800 mcg/mL 1600 mcg/mL 3200 mcg/mL 6400 mcg/mL 12800 mcg/mL	2-25 mcg/kg/min
Esmolol	2500 mg in 250 mL	10 mg/mL	loading: 500 mcg/kg infusion: 50-500 mcg/kg/min
Epinephrine	1-10 mg in 100 mL	10-100 mcg/mL	0.02-1 mcg/kg/min
Fentanyl	1 mg in 50 mL 2 mg in 100 mL	20 mcg/mL 40 mcg/mL	2-10 mcg/kg/h
Heparin	12,500 U in 250 mL 25,000 U in 250 mL 50,000 U in 250 mL	50 U/mL 100 U/mL 200 U/mL	loading: 50 U/kg Infusion: 10-25 U/kg/**h**
Isoproterenol	1 mg in 100 mL 1 mg in 50 mL	10 mcg/mL 20 mcg/mL	0.05-1 mcg/kg/min
Labetalol		1 mg/mL	0.4-1 mg/kg/h MAX 3 mg/kg/h
Lidocaine	500 mg in 250 mL 1 g in 250 mL 2 g in 250 mL	2000 mcg/mL 4000 mcg/mL 8000 mcg/mL	20-50 mcg/kg/min
Midazolam	undiluted	1 mg/mL	0.4-6 mcg/kg/min

		5 mg/mL	MAX 8 mcg/kg/min
Milrinone	undiluted	1 mg/mL	loading: 50 mcg/kg infusion: 0.375-0.75 mcg/kg/min
Nitroglycerine	50 mg in 250 mL 100 mg in 250 mL 150 mg in 250 mL 200 mg in 250 mL 250 mg in 250 mL	200 mcg/mL 400 mcg/mL 600 mcg/mL 800 mcg/mL 1000 mcg/mL	0.25-5 mcg/kg/min
Nitroprusside	50 mg in 250 mL 100 mg in 250 mL 150 mg in 250 mL 200 mg in 250 mL 250 mg in 250 mL	200 mcg/mL 400 mcg/mL 600 mcg/mL 800 mcg/mL 1000 mcg/mL	0.5-10 mcg/kg/min
Procainamide	500 mg in 250 mL 1 g in 250 mL	2000 mg/mL 4000 mcg/mL	loading: 2-6 mg/kg/dose over 5 min MAX 100 mg/dose
Prostaglandin E$_1$	0.25 mg in 50 mL 0.50 mg in 50 mL 0.50 mg in 25 mL	5 mcg/mL 10 mcg/mL 20 mcg/mL	0.05-0.2 mcg/kg/min
Vasopressin	10 U in 1000 mL	10 milliunits/mL	esophageal varices: 0.3 U/kg IVB infusion: 70 milliunits/kg/h DI: 3 milliunits/kg/h, ↑ as needed

Commonly Used Emergency Drugs

DRUG	ROUTE	DOSE	FREQUENCY
Adenosine	IV	0.05-0.25 mg/kg IV rapid push, followed by rapid 0.9NS flush	↑ by 0.05 mg/kg q 2 min up to 0.25 mg/kg
Amiodarone	IV	5 mg/kg over 30 min followed by continuous infusion 5-10 mcg/kg/min	
Atropine	IV	0.02 mg/kg MIN 0.1 mg MAX 2 mg	repeat in 20 min
Bumetanide	IV or PO	0.015-0.1 mg/kg/d	
Calcium chloride 10%	IV	10-30 mg/kg MAX 1 g	q 15-30 min
Calcium gluconate 10%	IV	100 mg/kg MAX 1 g	q 15-30 min
Captopril	PO	0.15-0.5 mg/kg/dose MAX 6 mg/kg/24 h	qd-qid
Cisatracurium	IV	0.1 mg/kg	q 1 h
Diazoxide	Rapid IV	1-3 mg/kg MAX 150 mg/dose	q 5-15 min
Electric countershock		cardioversion 0.5 J/kg defibrillation 2 J/kg	double and repeat if unsuccessful
Enoxaparin (low mol. weight heparin)	SC	DVT treatment 1.5 mg/kg DVT prophylaxis 1 mg/kg	q 12 h q 12 h
Epinephrine (1:10,000) Epinephrine (1:1000)	IV ET	0.1 mL/kg 0.1 mL/kg	q 5-15 min
Fentanyl	IV	3-10 mcg/kg	q 1-2 h
Flumazenil	IV	initial dose 0.01 mg/kg MAX 0.2 mg, then 0.005-0.01 mg/kg MAX 3 mg in 1 h	q 1 min initial q 20 min subsequent
Glucagon	IV	0.025-0.1 mg/kg	q 20-30 min
Hydralazine	IV	0.15 mg/kg	q 4-6 h
Kayexalate	PR	1 g/kg	q 6 h
Ketamine	IV	0.5-3 mg/kg	single dose
Lidocaine	IV	1 mg/kg	q 5-10 min
Lorazepam	IV	0.03-0.1 mg/kg MAX 4 mg	q 15 min
Mannitol	IV	0.25-1 g/kg	q2-8 h
Midazolam	IV	0.05-0.2 mg/kg	q 1-2 h
Morphine	IV	0.1 mg/kg	q 1-2 h
Naloxone	IV	0.1 mg/kg	q 15-30 min
Nifedipine	SL/NG	0.25-0.5 mg/kg	q 6-8 h
Pancuronium	IV	0.1 mg/kg	q 1 h
Pentobarbital	IV	1-2 mg/kg	q 2-3 h
Phenobarbital	IV	20 mg/kg loading dose	x 1
Phenytoin	IV	20 mg/kg loading dose MAX infusion rate ≤ 1 mo: 0.5 mg/kg/min, > 1 mo: 1 mg/kg/min	x 1
Ranitidine	IV	2 mg/kg/day	div q 6-8 h
Sodium chloride, 3%	IV	5 mL/kg (to ↑ serum Na$^+$ by 4 mEq/L)	x 1, check serum Na$^+$
THAM (tris-hydroxy-amino-methane) – buffer (0.3 mEq/mL)	IV	according to base deficit: 0.3 x body wgt in kg x base deficit	x 1, check ABG/CBG
Vecuronium	IV	0.1 mg/kg	q 30-60 min

NOTES

Insulin Coverage

Sujatha Kannan

Scales for supplemental coverage at 0600, 1130, 1600, 2000, 2400 and 0300 (Coverage for urine ketones and/or increased blood sugars using regular insulin)		
Urine Ketones	**If blood sugar > 180 mg/dL (supplement)**	**If blood sugar < 180 mg/dL (supplement)**
Small	10% total daily dose (N + R)	5% total daily dose (N + R)
Moderate	15% total daily dose	7.5% total daily dose
Large	20% total daily dose	10% total daily dose

- Coverage for ketones always overrides coverage for increased blood sugar
- If a patient has ketones in a 6 am void and has not had any ketones in the last 12 hours or the midnight or 3 am blood glucose test was < 80, **do not cover for ketones** but use the coverage based on blood sugar. This elevated sugar and urinary ketones may be a Somogyi phenomenon.

Coverage for blood sugar

Chemstrip	10-20 kg	20-40 kg	40-60 kg	60-80 kg	>80 kg
At 6am, 11:30 am, 4:00 pm, 8:00 pm					
180-240	1 u R	1 u R	2 u R	2 u R	3 u R
240-320	1 u R	2 u R	3 u R	4 u R	6 u R
320-400	2 u R	3 u R	4 u R	6 u R	9 u R
For 12:00 midnight and 3:00 am					
180-240	-----	-----	2 u R	2 u R	3 u R
240-320	1 u R	2 u R	2 u R	3 u R	4 u R
320-400	2 u R	2 u R	3 u R	4 u R	5 u R

Note: 1 unit can be added to the basal dose; do not give 1u as a single separate dose

from: the diabetic protocol, Division of Endocrinology, Department of Pediatrics, Children's Hospital of Michigan

Laboratory Findings in Patients with Abnormal Serum Sodium

	Serum			Urine						
	Na$^+$ (mEq/L)	K$^+$ (mEq/L)	osm (mOsm/L)	Na$^+$ (mEq/L)	K$^+$ (mEq/L)	osm (mOsm/L)	sp. gr.	BUN UUN	FE$_{Na}$ (%)	Urine volume
Hypernatremic dehydration	↑	↔	↑	<40	↔	>500	>1.030	>1:10	<1	↓
ATN		variable		>40	↔	≈ serum	≈1.010	<1:10	>3	↑ or ↓
SIADH	↓	↔	↓	>40	↑	>300	>1.020	>1:20	>1, <3	↓
Central DI	↑	↔	↑	<10	↓	<100	<1.005	<1:5	<1	↑
Salt poisoning	↑	↔	↑	>50	↔	>300	↔ or ↑	variable	>3	↔
Factitious hyponatremia* (e.g., hyperglycemia)	↓	↑ or ↓	↑	variable	↑	>250	↔ or ↑	variable	>1	↑ or ↔
Pseudohyponatremia (hyperlipidemia)	↓	↔	↔	↔	↔	↔	↔	variable	<1	↔
Adrenal insufficiency	↓	↑	↓	>40	↓	↔	↔	↔	>1	variable

* an increase in blood sugar by 100 mg/dL reduces serum sodium by 1.6 mEq/L because of ECF dilution
Source: Ashok P. Sarnaik MD, Chief of Critical Care Medicine, Children's Hospital of Michigan

Toxicology Panels

Randy Prescilla

Toxicology panels vary between institutions
(The panels listed below are available at the Detroit Medical Center Laboratories)

Serum drug screen, individual[a]

acetaminophen	ethanol	ethylene glycol
salicylates	acetone	propylene glycol
benzodiazepines	methanol	
barbiturates	isopropanol	

[a]Send a minimum of 1 mL whole blood in lavender-top tube

Serum drug screen (SDS)[a]

acetaminophen salicylates benzodiazepines barbiturates	cyclic antidepressants ethanol

[a]Send a minimum of 2 mL whole blood in lavender-top tube

Serum drug screen (SDS)[a]

acetone ethanol methanol isopropanol

[a]Send a minimum of 1 mL whole blood in lavender-top tube

Urine drugs of abuse (DA2)[a]

amphetamines barbiturates benzodiazepines cocaine (benzoylecgonine) cannabinoids	opiates phencyclidine propoxyphene methadone methaqualone

[a] Send minimum of 5 mL urine

Urine drugs of abuse (DA2)[a]

acetaminophen salicylates cyclic antidepressants HPLC (REMEDi)[b]

[a] Send minimum of 10 mL of urine
[b] HPLC (REMEDi) screens for approximately 916 drugs and metabolites, and should be used when the substance is unknown, but ingestion is strongly suspected.

Pharmacokinetic Calculations

Randy Prescilla

Steady state concentration (Css):

$$Css = \frac{Rinf}{Cl} \text{ where Rinf = rate of infusion and Cl = clearance}$$

example: if the infusion rate of drug x is 2 mg/min, and its clearance is 60 L/h, what steady state concentration can be expected?

$$Css = \frac{Rinf}{Cl} = \frac{120 \text{ mg/h}}{60 \text{ mg/h}} = 2 \text{ mg/L}$$

New concentration (C_2):

$$C_2 = C_1 (e^{-kt}) \quad \text{where } k = 0.693/t_{1/2}$$

example: a patient with digoxin toxicity has a level of 5.6 ng/mL. The physician wants to hold the digoxin dose until the digoxin level has dropped to about 0.5 ng/mL. How long should the drug be held assuming a half-life ($t_{1/2}$) of 36 h and an apparent distribution of 5 L/kg?

$$C_2 = C_1 (e^{-kt}) \text{ and } k = 0.693/36 = 0.019$$
$$0.5 = 5.6 (e^{-0.019t})$$
$$t = 140 \text{ h}$$

Rate of infusion (Rinf):

$$Rinf = \text{target Css} \times \frac{Cl}{F} \qquad \text{where F = frequency of dosing = 1 in IV dosing}$$

example: if a steady state concentration of 15 mcg/mL of theophylline is desired in a 68-kg nonsmoker who is otherwise normal, what should be the infusion rate of a drug? Cl of theophylline = 0.65 mL/kg/min

$$Rinf = \text{target Css} \times \frac{Cl}{F} = 15 \text{ mcg/mL} \times 0.65 \text{ mL/kg}$$
$$= 9.75 \text{ mcg/kg/min}$$
$$= 40 \text{ mg/h of theophylline}$$

Loading dose (LD):

$$LD = (Vd)(Cp) \qquad \text{where Cp is desired plasma concentration}$$

example: calculate the loading dose for an ethanol solution given the following:
0.7 L/kg = Vd = volume of distribution in child
100-150 mg/dL = desired serum concentration
0.79 = specific gravity of 100% ethanol = 0.79
79 mg/mL = 10% ethanol (10 mL 100% ethanol + 90 mL 5% dextrose)

$$LD = \frac{(0.7 \text{ L})}{kg} \times \frac{(10 \text{ dL})}{L} \times \frac{(100 \text{ mg})}{dL} = \frac{(700 \text{ mg})}{kg} \times \frac{(1 \text{ mL})}{79 \text{ mg}} = 8.86 \text{ or } 9 \text{ mL/kg}$$

Hyperalimentation for ICU Patients

Varsha Gharpure

FLUID VOLUME: total amount should be individualized based on disease state

General Guidelines

Body Weight	Estimated Fluid Requirement per Day
1-10 kg	100 mL/kg
11-20 kg	1000 mL + 50 mL/kg for each kg > 10 kg
> 20 kg	1500 mL + 20 mL/kg for each kg >20 kg

Post-operative Cardiovascular Patients

Day	Open Heart Surgery	Closed Heart Surgery
Operative day	750 mL/m^2	1000 mL/m^2
Post-op day 1	1000 mL/m^2	1200 mL/m^2
Post-op day 2	1200 mL/m^2	1500 mL/m^2
Post-op day 3	1500 mL/m^2	

To optimize total caloric intake in fluid-restricted or in patients on multiple drug infusions
- mix infusions in dextrose 10% in infants (except for arterial lines, use 0.9 NS only)
- consider concentrating inotropic solutions (discuss with pharmacy and nursing staff)

CARBOHYDRATES: 3.4 kcal/g of dextrose

Age	Initial day	Subsequent days
Neonates	5 g/kg/d	2 g/kg/d
Infants > 1 month of age	10 g/kg/d	5 g/kg/d
Older children/adolescents	dextrose 10%	↑ by 2.5-5% daily

LIPIDS: 9 kcal/g, 20% (2 g/100 mL) lipid solution in glycerol provides 2 kcal/mL

Age	Initial day	Subsequent days
Premature/LBW infants	0.5 g/kg/d	↑ by 0.5 g/kg/d MAX 3 g/kg/d
Infants, children, adolescents	1 g/kg/d	↑ by 0.5-1 g/kg/d MAX 3 g/kg/d

CALORIC INTAKE: desired goal for non-protein caloric intake for normal children

Age	Energy Requirement (kcal/kg/d)
Premature infants	70-90
full term to 1 year	80-95
2-9 years	60-70
10-13 years	50-60
Adolescents	40

- Caloric goal generally cannot be met on day 1. Both carbohydrate and lipid intake should be increased as tolerated until caloric goal is reached.
- Maintain blood glucose < 200 mg/dL without causing glucosuria
- If increasing amount of lipids, obtain serum triglycerides immediately before starting infusion each day. Maintain serum triglyceride level < 200 mg/dL
- Sepsis and surgery may increase caloric needs by almost 25%
- Patients who are receiving sedation and neuromuscular blockade may have less caloric needs

DISTRIBUTION OF NON-PROTEIN CALORIES
- 30-50% should be derived from lipids and 70% from carbohydrates
- In patients with chronic respiratory failure, up to 60% of non-protein calories may be derived from lipids in order to ↓ CO_2 production

PROTEINS: 6.25 g of protein = 1 g of nitrogen. Begin at 1-1.5 g/kg/d, advance as tolerated

Age	Protein Requirement (g/kg/d)
Premature infants	2.0-3.5
Birth-1year	2.0-2.5
2-9 years	1.5-2.0
10-13 years	1.5-2.0
Adolescents	1.0-1.5

- For children ≥ 3 kg: use Travasol® - contains both essential and non-essential amino acids
- For neonates < 5 kg: use TrophAmine® - contains cysteine, taurine, tyrosine (considered essential amino acids for neonates) and higher concentrations of branch chain amino acids and less amounts of glycine, methionine, and phenylalanine.
- Reduce protein intake in patients with hepatic encephalopathy or acute renal failure who are not on dialysis. Use HepatAmine® and NephrAmine® should be reserved for those with severe hepatic or renal failure respectively.
- Amino acid solution is usually available as a 10% solution (10 g/100 mL).

NON-PROTEIN CALORIE TO NITROGEN RATIO: to enhance efficient use of proteins for anabolism, calories and protein must be provided in proportion (ratio = 150-250:1). Patients on restricted protein intake should be provided with a ratio of 300-350:1.

$$\text{Ratio} = \frac{\text{non-protein calories (CHO calories + lipid calories)}}{\text{g of nitrogen}}$$

ELECTROLYTES, TRACE ELEMENTS AND MULTIVITAMINS

Sodium	2-4 mEq/kg/d	available as NaCl, Na acetate or Na phosphate (1 mM PO_4 = 1.33 mEq Na^+)
Potassium	2-3 mEq/kg/d	available as KCl, K acetate, K phosphate (1 mM of PO_4 = 1.47 mEq K^+)
Chloride	2-3 mEq/kg/d	as NaCl or KCl
Acetate	1-4 mEq/kg/d	as Na or K acetate
Magnesium	0.25-0.5 mEq/kg/d	as $MgSO_4$, 1 mEq of $MgSO_4$ = 12.5 mg of elemental Mg^{++}
Calcium	neonate 300-500 mg/kg infant 100-200 mg/kg adolescent 50-100 mg/kg	1 g Ca gluconate contains 4.65 mEq = 96 mg of elemental Ca^{++}
Phosphate	neonate 1-1.5 mM/kg/d infant 1 mM/kg/d adolescent 0.5-1 mM/kg/d	1 mM of PO_4 = 31 mg elemental P

- Concentration of electrolytes may have to be altered depending on patient needs
- Amounts of Ca^{++} and P are limited by precipitation. Avoid precipitation by maintaining Ca^{++}(mEq) + P (mM) $\leq$ 30/L when using Travasol® solutions and $\leq$ 40/L when using TrophAmine® solutions.
- Trace elements must include zinc, copper, manganese, chromium and selenium
  - children $\leq$ 11 y, use PTE-5 (0.2 mL/kg/d, MAX 5 mL/day)
  - older children, use MTE-5 (2.5 mL/d)
  - for children < 5 kg, provide additional 100 mcg/kg/d zinc supplement
  - additional zinc supplementation may be needed for ↑ loss
  - avoid chromium and copper in patients with cholestasis
  - omit molybdenum in patients with renal failure
- Supply both lipid and water soluble vitamins
  - children $\leq$ 11 y, MVI-Pediatric (2 mL/kg, MAX 5 mL)
  - older children, MVI-12 (10 mL/day) + Vit K every week
  - for patients with renal failure, ↓ amount of fat-soluble vitamins
  - **failure to provide thiamine can lead to thiamine deficiency, with shock (cardiac beri beri), tissue anoxia and severe metabolic acidosis (lactic acidosis)**

MONITORING FOR PATIENTS ON TPN

Monitoring Parameter	Frequency
weight, intake/output, blood glucose	daily
urine glucose	q shift
triglycerides	daily until MAX reached, then once weekly
electrolytes	3-4 times/week
CBC, differential, BUN, creatinine, Ca^{++}, Mg^{++}, P	2 times/week
albumin	as needed
LFT's	weekly
length, head circumference	weekly

- Sicker patients may require more frequent monitoring
- If available determine resting energy expenditure (REE) and respiratory quotient (RQ)

Additional points:
1. Watch the units and decimal points to avoid iatrogenic complications
2. If only peripheral venous access is available:
     dextrose concentration < 12.5%
     amino acids $\leq$ 20 g/L
     calcium $\leq$ 8 mEq/L
     potassium $\leq$ 40 mEq/L
     total osmolality $\leq$ 900 mOsm/L

Antihypertensive Agents

K. Jane Lee

Drug	Dose	Onset	Duration	Comment
sodium nitroprusside arterial and venous vasodilator	0.5–8.0 mcg/kg/min IV	30 sec	very short	requires continuous blood pressure monitoring, if not contraindicated, ideal agent for use in hypertensive crisis/encephalopathy because dose can be titrated with rapid response, monitor cyanide, thiocyanate levels, USE with CAUTION in patients with renal failure
nitroglycerin venous vasodilator	1–5 mcg/kg/min IV	immediate	very short	adjust dose according to renal function
nifedipine calcium channel blocker	0.25–0.5 mg/kg PO/SL/NG q 15 min, then q 3–4 h	10–30 min	4–6 h	5 mg cap ≈ 0.175 mL 10 mg cap ≈ 0.35 mL
labetalol alpha and beta blocker	0.25 mg/kg IV over 1–2 min q 10–15 min or 0.015–0.05 mg/kg/min MAX 3.25 mg/kg/total dose	immediate	10 h	use with caution in patients with bradycardia, CHF or asthma
propranolol beta blocker	0.01–0.1 mg/kg/dose IV MAX dose (infants) 1 mg/dose MAX dose (children) 3 mg/dose	15–30 min	4–6 h	contraindicated in asthma, Raynaud's syndrome, CHF and heart block
esmolol selective beta-1 blocker	500 mcg/kg IV loading dose 50–500 mcg/kg/min continuous IV	10–15 min	9 min	administer only in monitored setting; avoid in children with asthma or CHF
diazoxide	1–3 mg/kg rapid IV push	5 min	3–12 h	may cause hyperglycemia and hyponatremia

Subject Index